AHA Hospital Statistics™

2024 Edition

AHA Catalog NUMBER 082024
Telephone ORDERS 1-800-AHA-2626

ISSN 0090-6662
ISBN-13: 978-1-55648-503-9

Copyright © 1999 by Health Forum an American Hospital Association company
Copyright © 2000-2024 by Health Forum LLC, an affiliate of the American Hospital Association

All rights reserved. No portion of Hospital Statistics may be duplicated or reproduced
without prior written consent of Health Forum, LLC.
Printed in the U.S.A.

Contents

Table	Page	
	v	Acknowledgments & Advisements
	vii	How to Use this Book
	xv	Hospital Requirements
	xvii	Data Comparability
	xviii	Notes on the Survey
1	2	Historical Trends in Utilization and Personnel for Selected Years from 1946 through 2022
2	9	2022 U.S. Hospitals: Utilization and Personnel
3	12	Total United States
4	14	Bed Size Categories
5	32	U.S. Census Divisions
6	50	States
7	153	2022 Facilities and Services in the U.S. Census Divisions and States
8	171	Community Hospitals by Metropolitan Area: Utilization and Personnel
	203	Statistics for Multihospital Health Care Systems
	205	Glossary
	217	2022 AHA Annual Survey of Hospitals

AHA Hospital Statistics © 2024 Health Forum LLC, an affiliate of the American Hospital Association **iii**

Acknowledgments & Advisements

Acknowledgments

The 2024 edition of *AHA Hospital Statistics* is published by Health Forum, an affiliate of the American Hospital Association, Rick Pollack, President and CEO.

Advisements

The data published here should be used with the following advisements: The data are based on replies to an annual survey that seeks a variety of information, not all of which is published in this book. The information gathered by the survey includes specific services, but not all of each hospital's services. Therefore, the data do not reflect an exhaustive list of all services offered by all hospitals. For information on the availability of additional data, please contact Health Forum, ahadatainfo@aha.org.

Health Forum does not assume responsibility for the accuracy of information voluntarily reported by the individual institutions surveyed. The purpose of this publication is to provide basic data reflecting the delivery of health care in the United States and associated areas, and is not to serve an official and all-inclusive list of services offered by individual hospitals.

How to Use this Book

For more than seven decades, *AHA Hospital Statistics*™ has reported aggregate hospital data derived from the AHA Annual Survey and is the definitive source when doing trend analysis with data by bed size category, U.S. Census Divisions, States, and Metropolitan Areas. As the health care delivery system changes, so have the data tracked by the survey and presented in this report. Recent additions include:

- **Community health indicators** that offer readers a connection to the community for their analysis and planning: the data are broken down into beds, admissions, inpatient days, ER outpatient visits, and other indicators per 1000 population, as well as expense per capita.

- **Utilization and personnel** by all CBSAs in the United States.

- **Five-year trend data** on insurance products, and managed care contracts enable you to identify changes in relationships between hospitals and other health care systems and providers.

- **Tables 3 through 6 have been organized** to show breakdowns between inpatient and outpatient care to better reflect market shifts toward outpatient-centered care. Additional clarity is gained by the breakdown between total facility data (which includes nursing home type units under the control of the hospital) and hospital units (which exclude the nursing home data).

TABLE 6	ALABAMA				
	U.S. Community Hospitals (Nonfederal, short-term general and other special hospitals)				
	Utilization, Personnel, Community Health Indicators 2018–2022				
	2022	**2021**	**2020**	**2019**	**2018**
TOTAL FACILITY (Includes Hospital and Nursing Home Units)					
Utilization - Inpatient					
Beds	15,554	15,366	15,377	15,248	15,278
Admissions	602,107	601,414	589,081	637,490	628,561
Inpatient Days	3,842,006	3,790,463	3,524,600	3,633,143	3,614,731
Average Length of Stay	6.4	6.3	6.0	5.7	5.8
Inpatient Surgeries	176,756	176,827	202,040	206,790	184,009
Births	59,789	62,177	66,659	64,583	54,302
Utilization - Outpatient					
Emergency Outpatient Visits	2,064,969	2,073,805	1,956,700	2,488,864	2,340,055
Other Outpatient Visits	6,687,101	6,563,709	5,847,372	7,547,271	7,671,113
Total Outpatient Visits	8,752,070	8,637,514	7,804,072	10,036,135	10,011,168
Outpatient Surgeries	513,797	441,932	432,214	485,735	416,529
Personnel					
Full Time RNs	24,180	24,036	24,472	24,821	24,371
Full Time LPNs	1,285	1,136	1,152	1,047	1,104
Part Time RNs	10,684	11,670	8,679	8,374	7,433
Part Time LPNs	736	721	491	411	332
Total Full Time	76,519	75,583	75,332	75,955	73,116
Total Part Time	30,559	33,889	25,988	24,837	21,425

Example of five-year trend data

- **Facilities and Services information** on more than 100 categories of hospital facilities and services in Table 7. At a glance, you can determine the number and percentage of hospitals offering a specific service such as Oncology, Palliative Care Program, Complementary Medicine, Women's Health Services and Tobacco Cessation.

- **Plus, System and Group Purchasing Organizations** that demonstrate ways in which organizations are linked.

AHA Hospital Statistics © 2024 Health Forum LLC, an affiliate of the American Hospital Association

The survey instrument and the glossary

A good place to begin your analysis is the AHA Annual Survey instrument. Found on page 219, it includes the instructions, questions, and terms that were used to gather the data for fiscal year 2022. This can be extremely valuable for a clearer understanding of the data we collect and the tables presented in *AHA Hospital Statistics*.

Please also review the glossary in the back of the book. The glossary contains complete definitions for specific terms used in the tables and text of *AHA Hospital Statistics*. These definitions will clarify how terminology is being used.

As mentioned above, it is important to note that the primary focus of the most detailed data contained in *AHA Hospital Statistics* is community hospitals. As defined, community hospitals are all non-federal, short-term general and special hospitals whose facilities and services are available to the public. If the majority of a hospital's patients are admitted to units where the average length of stay is 30 days or less, a hospital may still be classified as short-term even if it includes a nursing-home-type unit. (For a more complete definition of community hospitals, please see the glossary definition, located on page 205.)

Getting the most out of *AHA Hospital Statistics*
This section of the book provides an introduction for getting the most out of your *AHA Hospital Statistics* 2024 edition. Here, you'll find a guide to the book, with insights into each table.

> **Beds:** The number of beds regularly maintained (set up and staffed for use) for inpatients as of the close of the reporting period. Excludes newborn bassinets.
>
> **Extracorporeal shock wave lithotripter (ESWL):** A medical device used for treating stones in the kidney or urethra. The device disintegrates kidney stones noninvasively through the transmission of acoustic shock waves directed at the stones.
>
> **Fitness center:** Provides exercise, testing, or evaluation programs and fitness activities to the community and hospital employees.
>
> **Stroke care:** Stroke telemedicine is a consultative modality that facilitates the care of patients with acute stroke by specialists at stroke centers.

Example of Glossary definitions.

CLASSIFICATION	YEAR	HOSPITALS	BEDS (in thousands)	ADMISSIONS (in thousands)	AVERAGE DAILY CENSUS (in thousands)	ADJUSTED AVERAGE DAILY CENSUS (in thousands)
Table 1						
Historical Trends in Utilization and Personnel for Selected Years from 1946 through 2022						
Total United States	1946	6,125	1,436	15,675	1,142	—
	1950	6,788	1,456	18,483	1,253	—
	1955	6,956	1,604	21,073	1,363	—
	1960	6,876	1,658	25,027	1,402	—
	1965	7,123	1,704	28,812	1,403	—
	1970	7,123	1,616	31,759	1,298	—
	1971	7,097	1,556	32,664	1,237	—
	1972	7,061	1,550	33,265	1,209	—
	1973	7,123	1,535	34,352	1,189	—
	1974	7,174	1,513	35,506	1,167	—
	1975	7,156	1,466	36,157	1,125	—
	1976	7,082	1,434	36,776	1,090	—
	1977	7,099	1,407	37,060	1,066	—
	1978	7,015	1,381	37,243	1,042	—
	1979	6,988	1,372	37,802	1,043	—
	1980	6,965	1,365	38,892	1,060	—
	1981	6,933	1,362	39,169	1,061	—
	1982	6,915	1,360	39,095	1,053	—
	1983	6,888	1,350	38,887	1,028	—
	1984	6,872	1,339	37,938	970	—
	1985	6,872	1,318	36,304	910	—
	1986	6,841	1,290	35,219	883	—
	1987	6,821	1,267	34,439	873	—
	1988	6,780	1,248	34,107	863	—
	1989	6,720	1,226	33,742	853	—
	1990	6,649	1,213	33,774	844	—
	1991	6,634	1,202	33,567	827	—
	1992	6,539	1,178	33,536	807	—
	1993	6,467	1,163	33,201	783	—
	1994	6,374	1,128	33,125	745	—
	1995	6,291	1,081	33,282	710	—
	1996	6,201	1,062	33,307	685	—
	1997	6,097	1,035	33,624	673	—
	1998	6,021	1,013	33,766	662	—
	1999	5,890	994	34,181	657	—
	2000	5,810	984	34,891	650	—
	2001	5,801	987	35,644	658	—
	2002	5,794	976	36,326	662	—

Example of Table 1

Table 1 — Historical Trends in Utilization and Personnel for Selected Years from 1946 through 2022

Table 1 at a Glance

This table is used to evaluate historical data and allows you to examine long-term trends in health care with data dating back more than sixty years. Table 1 reports on all hospitals in the United States. One important note: Hospitals included in this table include AHA-member and non-member hospitals. A hospital does not need to be an AHA member to be included.

This table segments the data into various organizational structure categories. Here's a brief look at these different classifications:

- Total United States Hospitals
- Total Non-Federal Short-term and other special hospitals
- Community hospitals
- Non-government not-for-profit community hospitals
- Investor-owned (for-profit) community hospitals
- State and local government community hospitals

Table 1 also provides input on nationwide utilization and personnel trends. You'll find answers to questions such as: *Over the past 25 years, what trends do I see comparing the average length of stay at government and non-government not-for-profit community hospitals and investor-owned for-profit community hospitals? or What has been the trend in outpatient visits?*

Table 2 — 2022 U.S. Hospitals: Utilization and Personnel

Table 2 at a Glance

This table takes a closer look at U.S. Hospitals for 2022. It offers a snapshot of utilization and personnel statistics, and breaks down this information for specialty hospitals. In addition, this is the only table that outlines data on federal hospitals. You'll be able to use this table to better understand the number of beds set-up and staffed and how many personnel and trainees are on the payroll.

Note: The 2021 performance data do not reflect the full impact of the COVID-19 pandemic.

AHA Hospital Statistics © 2024 Health Forum LLC, an affiliate of the American Hospital Association **ix**

TABLE 3

TOTAL UNITED STATES

U.S. Community Hospitals
(Nonfederal, short-term general and other special hospitals)

Utilization, Personnel, Community Health Indicators 2018–2022

	2022	2021	2020	2019	2018
TOTAL FACILITY (Includes Hospital and Nursing Home Units)					
Utilization - Inpatient					
Beds	784,112	787,967	789,354	787,995	792,417
Admissions	31,555,807	31,967,073	31,393,318	34,078,100	34,251,159
Inpatient Days	188,912,326	187,599,105	177,341,078	185,149,928	185,307,228
Average Length of Stay	5.9	5.8	5.6	5.4	5.4
Inpatient Surgeries	7,641,635	7,788,190	8,003,571	8,950,559	8,999,976
Births	3,510,787	3,485,508	3,505,115	3,567,799	3,637,593
Utilization - Outpatient					
Emergency Outpatient Visits	136,969,033	126,957,429	123,267,216	143,432,284	143,454,611
Other Outpatient Visits	662,698,100	658,639,366	593,892,101	641,802,972	622,937,901
Total Outpatient Visits	799,667,133	785,596,795	717,159,317	785,235,256	766,392,512
Outpatient Surgeries	19,773,775	19,126,174	16,975,312	19,418,138	19,168,038
Personnel					
Full Time RNs	1,292,453	1,309,064	1,342,589	1,322,217	1,306,941
Full Time LPNs	68,318	62,753	62,756	63,352	63,951
Part Time RNs	606,727	580,312	573,485	575,878	559,832
Part Time LPNs	25,584	22,785	22,180	22,403	22,170
Total Full Time	4,651,219	4,615,569	4,610,279	4,600,213	4,549,056
Total Part Time	1,769,245	1,702,146	1,676,632	1,678,799	1,632,575
HOSPITAL UNIT (Excludes Separate Nursing Home Units)					
Utilization - Inpatient					
Beds	756,787	759,533	759,530	755,167	757,609
Admissions	31,485,823	31,893,717	31,306,074	33,965,386	34,130,471
Inpatient Days	181,508,006	179,742,748	168,497,152	174,701,046	174,295,886
Average Length of Stay	5.7	5.6	5.3	5.1	5.1

Total U.S.

Example of Table 3. Helps contrast acute and long-term care

Table 3 — Total United States

Table 3 at a Glance

This table provides a look at all U.S. Community Hospitals, in terms of general overview with utilization by inpatient and outpatient, personnel and community health indicators. It provides a snapshot of the past five years, allowing you to track emerging trends.

This national information can be compared to local or regional trends, for benchmarking:

- Both inpatient and outpatient information is included, for better evaluation of data.

- Reporting by total facility *Includes hospital and Nursing Home Units* and hospital unit only *Excludes Separate Nursing Home Units* helps contrast acute and long-term care.

- Community health indicators can help uncover trends and help determine future facility needs.

Note: The 2021 performance data do not reflect the full impact of the COVID-19 pandemic.

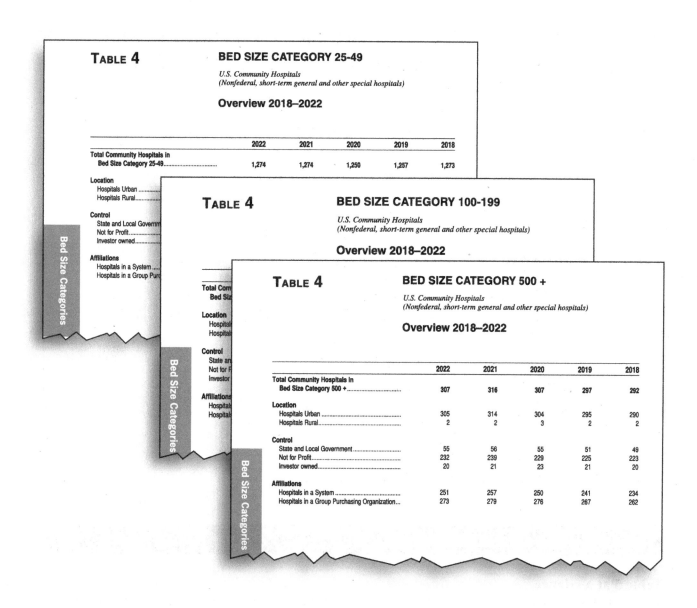

Example of Table 4. Compares facilities with peers.

Table 4 — Bed Size Categories

Table 4 at a Glance

This table provides a look at all U.S. Community Hospitals, broken down by bed size. The table includes general overview, utilization, and personnel information. These categories of bed sizes were developed by the AHA, and have become an industry standard. By categorizing each facility into a peer group, this table provides a snapshot of the past five years allowing you to compare facilities with their peers.

Note: The 2021 performance data do not reflect the full impact of the COVID-19 pandemic.

		2022	2021	2020	2019	2018
TABLE 5						

U.S. CENSUS DIVISION 2: MIDDLE ATLANTIC

U.S. Community Hospitals
(Nonfederal, short-term general and other special hospitals)

**Utilization, Personnel, Community
Health Indicators 2018–2022**

	2022	2021	2020	2019	2018
TOTAL FACILITY (Includes Hospital and Nursing Home Units)					
Utilization - Inpatient					
Beds	106,265	106,808	108,046	108,395	109,558
Admissions	4,314,139	4,513,245	4,344,122	4,847,024	4,919,808
Inpatient Days	27,976,453	27,658,029	26,282,445	28,091,060	28,429,768
Average Length of Stay	6.5	6.1	6.1	5.8	5.8
Inpatient Surgeries	1,052,716	1,086,678	1,083,481	1,210,079	1,240,226
Births	425,696	429,428	426,512	437,062	449,748
Utilization - Outpatient					
Emergency Outpatient Visits	17,442,118	16,461,972	15,516,505	18,582,130	18,746,561
Other Outpatient Visits	102,147,671	104,889,407	89,091,153	97,478,356	95,944,515
Total Outpatient Visits	119,589,789	121,351,379	104,607,658	116,060,486	114,691,076
Outpatient Surgeries	2,732,466	2,670,791	2,379,609	2,753,593	2,651,080
Personnel					
Full Time RNs	195,190	196,554	200,526	196,433	191,768
Full Time LPNs	8,038	7,824	8,134	7,996	8,418
Part Time RNs	66,230	62,118	63,475	63,586	64,203
Part Time LPNs	2,189	2,029	2,070	2,167	2,387
Total Full Time	755,472	744,665	732,489	731,633	715,362
Total Part Time	210,002	202,795	203,798	204,982	211,260

Example of Table 5. Uncovers trends to determine future facility needs.

Table 5 — U.S. Census Divisions

Table 5 at a Glance

This table provides a look at all U.S. Community Hospitals, broken down by Census Division. The table includes general overview, utilization, personnel, and community health indicator information. It provides a snapshot of the past five years, allowing you to track trends on a regional level. In addition, this allows you to compare this data to other population based health indicators, offering a more comprehensive look than the survey data alone. Community health indicators can help uncover trends and help determine future facility needs.

Table 6 — States

Table 6 at a Glance

This table provides a look at all U.S. Community Hospitals, broken down by State. The table includes general overview, utilization, personnel, and community health indicator information. It provides a snapshot of the past five years, allowing you to track trends on a state level.

Note:

You can use the information in tables 3, 4, 5 and 6 to make accurate comparisons across Total U.S., Bed Size Category, Census Division and State.

Note: The 2021 performance data do not reflect the full impact of the COVID-19 pandemic.

AHA Hospital Statistics © 2024 Health Forum LLC, an affiliate of the American Hospital Association

Table 7 — 2022 Facilities and Services in the U.S. Census Divisions and States

Table 7 at a Glance

This table examines facilities and services by both Census Division and State. A comprehensive alphabetical guide helps make each facility or service easy to find. This table will allow you to better understand what service lines are emerging and how many facilities offer a particular service in a discrete state or region.

This collection of facilities and services information data is unique to *AHA Hospital Statistics* and the list is continually growing. Recent additions include:

- Biocontainment patient care unit
- Basic interventional radiology
- Medication-assisted treatment for Opioid Use Disorder
- Prenatal and postpartum psychiatric services
- Forensic psychiatry services

Table 7 (Continued)

CLASSIFICATION	HOSPITALS REPORTING	GENETIC TESTING/ COUNSELING		GERIATRIC SERVICES		HEALTH FAIR		COMMUN EDU
		Number	Percent	Number	Percent	Number	Percent	Number
UNITED STATES	4,097	889	21.7	1,632	39.8	2,613	63.8	3,135
COMMUNITY HOSPITALS	3,682	875	23.8	1,539	41.8	2,535	68.8	3,025
CENSUS DIVISION 1, NEW ENGLAND	148	56	37.8	82	55.4	100	67.6	130
Connecticut	24	13	54.2	17	70.8	21	87.5	22
Maine	29	7	24.1	17	58.6	15	51.7	28
Massachusetts	50	18	36	23	46	32	64	39
New Hampshire	26	11	42.3	15	57.7	20	76.9	24
Rhode Island	9	4	44.4	7	77.8	7	77.8	7
Vermont	10	3	30	3	30	5	50	10
CENSUS DIVISION 2, MIDDLE ATLANTIC	357	149	41.7	187	52.4	255	71.4	279
New Jersey	71	40	56.3	44	62	51	71.8	58
New York	122	61	50	79	64.8	100	82	108
Pennsylvania	164	48	29.3	64	39	104	63.4	113
CENSUS DIVISION 3, SOUTH ATLANTIC	541	144	26.6	213	39.4	405	74.9	434
Delaware	8	3	37.5	3	37.5	5	62.5	5
District of Columbia	9	5	55.6	6	66.7	7	77.8	7
Florida	154	39	25.3	56	36.4	108	70.1	122
Georgia	88	21	23.9	28	31.8	64	72.7	72
Maryland	40	20	50	27	67.5	34	85	35
North Carolina	68	19	27.9	31	45.6	57	83.8	60
South Carolina	78	6	7.7	27	34.6	52	66.7	55
Virginia	59	23	39	23	39	49	83.1	49
West Virginia	37	8	21.6	12	32.4	29	78.4	29
CENSUS DIVISION 4, EAST NORTH CENTRAL	621	150	24.2	305	49.1	383	63.3	595
Illinois	138	37	26.8	64	46.4	108	78.3	122
Indiana	108	25	23.1	38	35.2	75	69.4	86
Michigan	120	29	24.2	63	52.5	80	66.7	104
Ohio	108	39	36.1	52	48.1	84	77.8	95
Wisconsin	147	20	13.6	88	59.9	46	31.3	128
CENSUS DIVISION 5, EAST SOUTH CENTRAL	285	44	15.4	68	23.9	178	62.5	192
Alabama	52	9	17.3	15	28.8	36	69.2	35
Kentucky	72	13	18.1	17	23.6	42	58.3	51
Mississippi	96	9	9.4	13	13.5	56	58.3	57
Tennessee	65	13	20	23	35.4	44	67.7	49
CENSUS DIVISION 6, WEST NORTH CENTRAL	556	83	14.9	235	42.3	373	67.1	451
Iowa	122	16	13.1	53	43.4	95	77.9	108
Kansas	120	19	15.8	45	37.5	68	56.7	83
Minnesota	94	12	12.8	44	46.8	67	71.3	81
Missouri	130	20	15.4	56	43.1	78	60	97
Nebraska	39	10	25.6	14	35.9	29	74.4	37
North Dakota	12	4	33.3	5	41.7	7	58.3	11
South Dakota	39	2	5.1	18	46.2	29	74.4	34
CENSUS DIVISION 7, WEST SOUTH CENTRAL	842	87	10.3	228	27.1	463	55	529
Arkansas	98	6	6.1	30	30.6	62	63.3	71
Louisiana	79	19	24.1	30	38	49	62	62
Oklahoma	99	8	8.1	25	25.3	47	47.5	62
Texas	566	54	9.5	143	25.3	305	53.9	334

Example of Table 7.

These new categories reflect the trends as hospitals expand their service lines to mirror the needs of their patients. For example, services such as acupuncture or massage therapy are now accounted for in the Complementary Medicine service item.

This table can answer questions such as: *What percentage of hospitals in the United States offer complementary medicine or wound management? or How are these new services distributed by state?*

Table 8 — Utilization and Personnel in Community Hospitals by Metropolitan Area for 2022

Table 8 at a Glance

This table provides a look at all U.S. Community Hospitals, broken down by Metropolitan Area. The table includes general overview, utilization and personnel information. It provides a snapshot of the past year.

Additional Resources

Again, in the back of the book you will find the comprehensive glossary and the 2022 annual survey questionnaire. The survey itself can be a valuable resource to understanding what was asked in order to gather the data in the book. This survey is also used to produce the *AHA Guide®* and AHA Annual Survey Database™.

Note: The 2021 performance data do not reflect the full impact of the COVID-19 pandemic.

Hospital Requirements

Hospital Requirements

An institution is considered a hospital by the American Hospital Association if it is licensed as general or specialty hospital by the appropriate state agency, and accredited as a hospital by one of the following organizations: The Joint Commission; Accreditation Commission for Health Care, Inc. (ACHC); DNV Healthcare accreditation; Center for Improvement in Healthcare Quality accreditation; or Medicare certified as a provider of acute service under Title 18 of the Social Security Act.

Types of Hospitals

Hospitals are categorized as one of four types of hospitals: general, special, rehabilitation and chronic disease, or psychiatric.

General

The primary function of the institution is to provide patient services, diagnostic and therapeutic, for a variety of medical conditions. A general hospital also shall provide:

- diagnostic x-ray services with facilities and staff for a variety of procedures
- clinical laboratory service with facilities and staff for a variety of procedures and with anatomical pathology services regularly and conveniently available
- operating room service with facilities and staff.

Special

The primary function of the institution is to provide diagnostic and treatment services for patients who have specified medical conditions, both surgical and nonsurgical. A special hospital also shall provide:

- such diagnostic and treatment services as may be determined by the Executive Committee of the Board of Trustees of the American Hospital Association to be appropriate for the specified medical conditions for which medical services are provided shall be maintained in the institution with suitable facilities and staff. If such conditions do not normally require diagnostic x-ray service, laboratory service, or operating room service, and if any such services are therefore not maintained in the institution, there shall be written arrangements to make them available to patients requiring them.
- clinical laboratory services capable of providing tissue diagnosis when offering pregnancy termination services.

Rehabilitation and Chronic Disease

The primary function of the institution is to provide diagnostic and treatment services to handicapped or disabled individuals requiring restorative and adjustive services. A rehabilitation and chronic disease hospital also shall provide:

- arrangements for diagnostic x-ray services, as required, on a regular and conveniently available basis
- arrangements for clinical laboratory service, as required on a regular and conveniently available basis
- arrangements for operating room service, as required, on a regular and conveniently available basis
- a physical therapy service with suitable facilities and staff in the institution
- an occupational therapy service with suitable facilities and staff in the institution
- arrangements for psychological and social work services on a regular and conveniently available basis

AHA Hospital Statistics © 2024 Health Forum LLC, an affiliate of the American Hospital Association **XV**

- arrangements for educational and vocational services on a regular and conveniently available basis
- written arrangements with a general hospital for the transfer of patients who require medical, obstetrical, or surgical services not available in the institution.

Psychiatric

The primary function of the institution is to provide diagnostic and treatment services for patients who have psychiatric-related illnesses. A psychiatric hospital also shall provide:

- arrangements for clinical laboratory service, as required, on a regular and conveniently available basis
- arrangements for diagnostic x-ray services, as required on a regular and conveniently available basis
- psychiatric, psychological, and social work service with facilities and staff in the institution
- arrangements for electroencephalograph services, as required, on a regular and conveniently available basis.
- written arrangements with a general hospital for the transfer of patients who require medical, obstetrical, or surgical services not available in the institution.

Data Comparability

The economic climate, demographic characteristics, personnel issues, and health care financing and payment policies differ by region, state, and city across the country. *Differences in these factors must be taken into account when using the data.* In addition, the profiles of hospitals across comparison groups vary. For example, states will differ in terms of the number and percentage of hospitals by size, ownership, services provided, types of patients treated, and so forth. *Differences in these variables also must be taken into consideration when doing a comparative analysis.*

Notes on the Survey

The 2024 edition of *AHA Hospital Statistics*[TM] draws its data from the 2022 AHA Annual Survey of Hospitals. It is the statistical complement to the 2024 edition of the *AHA Guide®*, which contains selected data about individual hospitals.

The AHA Survey was mailed to all hospitals, in the U.S. and its associated areas: American Samoa, Guam, the Marshall Islands, Puerto Rico, and the Virgin Islands. U.S. government hospitals located outside the U.S. were not included. Overall, the average response rate over the past five years has been approximately 73 percent.

Reporting Period
In completing the survey, hospitals were requested to report data for a full year, in accord with their fiscal year, ending in 2022. The statistical tables present data reported or estimated for a 12-month period, except for data on personnel, which represent situations as they existed at the end of the reporting period.

Respondents
Data for Tables 1 and 2 include 6,120 hospitals in the U.S. Data on community hospitals (nonfederal, short-term general and other special hospitals) only are presented in Tables 3-6, and Table 8.

It is important to note that the hospitals included in *AHA Hospital Statistics* are not necessarily identical to those included in *AHA Guide*. The institutions listed in the 2024 edition of *AHA Guide* include all of those institutions CMS certified, or Joint Commission accredited as of September 2023. Tables 1-6 in *AHA Hospital Statistics* present data for hospitals that were in operation during the 12-month reporting period ending 2022.

Estimates
Estimates were made of data for nonreporting hospitals and for reporting hospitals that submitted incomplete AHA Annual Survey questionnaires. Estimates were not made for beds, bassinets and facilities and services. Data for beds and bassinets of nonreporting hospitals were based on the most recent information from those hospitals. (Note that in all statistical tables, whenever bed-size categories are listed, all eight categories appear, whether or not there are hospitals in every category.)

Missing admissions, births, inpatient days, surgical operations, outpatient visits, and full-time-equivalent personnel values are estimates from regression models. For all other variables the estimates were based on ratios such as per bed averages derived from data reported by hospitals similar in size, control, major service provided, length of stay, and geographical characteristics to the hospitals that did not report this information.

Tables 1–2

Historical Trends

Table		Page
	Utilization and Personnel	
1	**Trends for Selected Years from 1946 through 2022**	2
	U.S. Hospitals	
2	**Utilization and Personnel for 2022**	9

Note: The 2021 performance data do not reflect the full impact of the COVID-19 pandemic. Please refer to the discussion in the Introduction for more information.

AHA Hospital Statistics © 2024 Health Forum LLC, an affiliate of the American Hospital Association

Note: The 2021 performance data do not reflect the full impact of the COVID-19 pandemic. Please refer to the discussion in the Introduction for more information.

Table

1

Historical Trends in Utilization and Personnel for Selected Years from 1946 through 2022

Data are for all hospitals in the United States. Data are estimated for nonreporting hospitals with the exception of newborn and outpatient data before 1972. Personnel data exclude residents, interns, and students from 1952 on; personnel data include full-time personnel and full-time equivalents for part-time personnel from 1954 on. As a result of the AHA Annual Survey validation process, the New York state data from 1976 were revised after the 1977 edition was published. The revised figures are included below. In order to provide trend data on a consistent basis, the 1970 and 1971 psychiatric and long-term data have been slightly modified. The 1982 FTE figures have updated to provide the most accurate data possible.

						ADJUSTED			NEWBORNS		FTE PERSONNEL	
				AVERAGE	AVERAGE						
				DAILY	DAILY	AVERAGE	OUTPATIENT				Per 100
		BEDS	ADMISSIONS	CENSUS	CENSUS	STAY	VISITS			Number	Adjusted
CLASSIFICATION	YEAR	HOSPITALS	(in thousands)	(in thousands)	(in thousands)	(in thousands)	(days)	(in thousands)	Bassinets	Births	(in thousands)	Census
Total United States	1946	6,125	1,436	15,675	1,142	—	—	—	85,585	2,135,327	830	—
	1950	6,788	1,456	18,483	1,253	—	—	—	90,101	2,742,780	1,058	—
	1955	6,956	1,604	21,073	1,363	—	—	—	98,823	3,476,753	1,301	—
	1960	6,876	1,658	25,027	1,402	—	—	—	102,764	3,835,735	1,598	—
	1965	7,123	1,704	28,812	1,403	—	—	125,793	101,287	3,565,344	1,952	—
	1970	7,123	1,616	31,759	1,298	—	—	181,370	97,128	3,537,000	2,537	—
	1971	7,097	1,556	32,664	1,237	—	—	199,725	94,344	3,464,513	2,589	—
	1972	7,061	1,550	33,265	1,209	—	—	219,182	92,960	3,231,875	2,671	—
	1973	7,123	1,535	34,352	1,189	—	—	233,555	90,071	3,087,210	2,769	—
	1974	7,174	1,513	35,506	1,167	—	—	250,481	88,269	3,043,386	2,919	—
	1975	7,156	1,466	36,157	1,125	—	—	254,844	86,875	3,091,629	3,023	—
	1976	7,082	1,434	36,776	1,090	—	—	270,951	85,284	3,067,063	3,108	—
	1977	7,099	1,407	37,060	1,066	—	—	263,775	83,193	3,223,699	3,213	—
	1978	7,015	1,381	37,243	1,042	—	—	263,606	80,650	3,250,373	3,280	—
	1979	6,988	1,372	37,802	1,043	—	—	262,009	79,720	3,376,467	3,382	—
	1980	6,965	1,365	38,892	1,060	—	—	262,951	79,842	3,500,043	3,492	—
	1981	6,933	1,362	39,169	1,061	—	—	265,332	78,823	3,558,274	3,661	—
	1982	6,915	1,360	39,095	1,053	—	—	313,667	77,998	3,615,751	3,746	—
	1983	6,888	1,350	38,887	1,028	—	—	273,168	77,837	3,596,146	3,707	—
	1984	6,872	1,339	37,938	970	—	—	276,566	77,845	3,563,106	3,630	—
	1985	6,872	1,318	36,304	910	—	—	282,140	77,202	3,630,961	3,625	—
	1986	6,841	1,290	35,219	883	—	—	294,634	76,002	3,680,178	3,647	—
	1987	6,821	1,267	34,439	873	—	—	310,707	74,770	3,698,294	3,742	—
	1988	6,780	1,248	34,107	863	—	—	336,208	72,568	3,794,369	3,839	—
	1989	6,720	1,226	33,742	853	—	—	352,248	71,491	3,920,384	3,937	—
	1990	6,649	1,213	33,774	844	—	—	368,184	70,539	4,046,704	4,063	—
	1991	6,634	1,202	33,567	827	—	—	387,675	69,464	4,047,504	4,165	—
	1992	6,539	1,178	33,536	807	—	—	417,874	69,052	4,007,179	4,236	—
	1993	6,467	1,163	33,201	783	—	—	435,619	67,911	3,949,788	4,289	—
	1994	6,374	1,128	33,125	745	—	—	453,584	67,311	3,886,667	4,270	—
	1995	6,291	1,081	33,282	710	—	—	483,195	66,256	3,833,132	4,273	—
	1996	6,201	1,062	33,307	685	—	—	505,455	65,138	3,790,678	4,276	—
	1997	6,097	1,035	33,624	673	—	—	520,600	64,649	3,811,522	4,333	—
	1998	6,021	1,013	33,766	662	—	—	545,481	63,485	3,795,212	4,407	—
	1999	5,890	994	34,181	657	—	—	573,461	62,714	3,829,881	4,369	—
	2000	5,810	984	34,891	650	—	—	592,673	61,915	3,940,017	4,454	—
	2001	5,801	987	35,644	658	—	—	612,276	61,527	3,929,733	4,535	—
	2002	5,794	976	36,326	662	—	—	640,515	62,151	3,934,421	4,610	—
	2003	5,764	965	36,611	657	—	—	648,560	60,699	3,976,886	4,651	—
	2004	5,759	956	36,942	658	—	—	662,131	59,660	3,965,906	4,696	—
	2005	5,756	947	37,006	656	—	—	673,689	59,073	4,048,442	4,791	—
	2006	5,747	947	37,189	653	—	—	690,425	58,670	4,126,598	4,907	—
	2007	5,708	945	37,120	645	—	—	693,510	58,429	4,128,796	5,024	—
	2008	5,815	951	37,529	649	—	—	709,960	58,133	4,109,081	5,116	—
	2009	5,795	944	37,480	641	—	—	741,551	58,078	4,001,748	5,178	—

Table 1 (Continued)

CLASSIFICATION								NEWBORNS		FTE PERSONNEL	
YEAR	HOSPITALS	BEDS (in thousands)	ADMISSIONS (in thousands)	AVERAGE DAILY CENSUS (in thousands)	ADJUSTED AVERAGE DAILY CENSUS (in thousands)	AVERAGE STAY (days)	OUTPATIENT VISITS (in thousands)	Bassinets	Births	Number (in thousands)	Per 100 Adjusted Census
2010	5,754	942	36,915	627	—	—	750,408	57,396	3,871,751	5,184	—
2011	5,724	924	36,565	615	—	—	754,454	57,022	3,767,697	5,196	—
2012	5,723	921	36,156	600	—	—	777,961	56,693	3,754,085	5,258	—
2013	6,230	940	36,095	607	—	—	795,759	57,539	3,778,696	5,456	—
2014	6,174	928	35,562	600	—	—	811,975	56,951	3,818,308	5,413	—
2015	6,180	930	35,899	608	—	—	844,487	56,606	3,826,138	5,522	—
2016	6,168	928	36,110	610	—	—	877,137	56,449	3,804,132	5,698	—
2017	6,210	931	36,510	614	—	—	880,451	55,801	3,693,124	5,841	—
2018	6,146	924	36,354	612	—	—	879,628	55,565	3,678,096	5,903	—
2019	6,090	920	36,242	611	—	—	900,689	55,085	3,608,425	5,989	—
2020	6,093	921	33,357	578	—	—	834,034	54,397	3,541,136	6,002	—
2021	6,129	920	34,011	607	—	—	903,757	54,033	3,527,429	6,001	—
2022	6,120	917	33,680	610	—	—	930,735	53,397	3,542,001	6,084	—

Note: The 2021 performance data do not reflect the full impact of the COVID-19 pandemic. Please refer to the discussion in the Introduction for more information.

Table 1 (Continued)

CLASSIFICATION	YEAR	HOSPITALS	BEDS (in thousands)	ADMISSIONS (in thousands)	AVERAGE DAILY CENSUS (in thousands)	ADJUSTED AVERAGE DAILY CENSUS (in thousands)	AVERAGE STAY (days)	OUTPATIENT VISITS (in thousands)	NEWBORNS Bassinets	NEWBORNS Births	FTE PERSONNEL Number (in thousands)	FTE PERSONNEL Per 100 Adjusted Census
Total nonfederal short-term general and other special	1946	4,444	473	13,655	341	—	9.1	—	80,987	2,087,503	505	—
	1950	5,031	505	16,663	372	—	8.1	—	86,019	2,660,982	662	—
	1955	5,237	568	19,100	407	—	7.8	—	93,868	3,304,451	826	—
	1960	5,407	639	22,970	477	—	7.6	—	98,127	3,678,051	1,080	—
	1965	5,736	741	26,463	563	620	7.8	92,631	96,782	3,413,370	1,386	224
	1970	5,859	848	29,252	662	727	8.2	133,545	93,079	3,403,064	1,929	265
	1971	5,865	867	30,142	665	736	8.0	148,423	90,444	3,337,605	1,999	272
	1972	5,843	884	30,777	664	739	7.9	166,983	89,315	3,119,446	2,056	278
	1973	5,891	903	31,761	681	768	7.8	178,939	86,851	2,987,089	2,149	280
	1974	5,977	931	32,943	701	793	7.8	194,838	85,208	2,947,342	2,289	289
	1975	5,979	947	33,519	708	806	7.7	196,311	83,834	2,998,590	2,399	298
	1976	5,956	961	34,068	715	816	7.7	207,725	82,307	2,962,305	2,483	304
	1977	5,973	974	34,353	717	820	7.6	204,238	80,228	3,117,756	2,581	315
	1978	5,935	980	34,575	720	841	7.6	204,461	78,090	3,156,570	2,662	323
	1979	5,923	988	35,160	729	841	7.6	203,873	77,277	3,287,157	2,762	328
	1980	5,904	992	36,198	748	861	7.6	206,752	77,539	3,408,699	2,879	334
	1981	5,879	1,007	36,494	764	876	7.6	206,729	76,567	3,465,683	3,039	347
	1982	5,863	1,015	36,429	763	882	7.6	250,888	75,739	3,514,761	3,110	353
	1983	5,843	1,021	36,201	750	869	7.6	213,995	75,471	3,490,629	3,102	357
	1984	5,814	1,020	35,202	703	824	7.3	216,474	75,587	3,456,467	3,023	367
	1985	5,784	1,003	33,501	650	780	7.1	222,773	74,899	3,521,296	3,003	385
	1986	5,728	982	32,410	631	774	7.1	234,270	73,688	3,584,530	3,032	392
	1987	5,659	961	31,633	624	780	7.2	247,704	72,516	3,602,416	3,120	400
	1988	5,579	949	31,480	622	795	7.2	271,436	70,361	3,706,748	3,209	404
	1989	5,497	936	31,141	619	805	7.3	287,909	69,436	3,831,051	3,307	411
	1990	5,420	929	31,203	620	820	7.3	302,691	68,443	3,958,646	3,423	417
	1991	5,370	926	31,084	612	828	7.2	323,202	67,440	3,965,489	3,539	427
	1992	5,321	923	31,053	606	832	7.1	349,397	67,095	3,925,024	3,624	436
	1993	5,289	921	30,770	593	834	7.0	368,358	66,060	3,870,392	3,681	441
	1994	5,256	904	30,739	569	814	6.8	384,880	65,728	3,809,367	3,697	454
	1995	5,220	874	30,966	549	811	6.5	415,710	64,742	3,764,756	3,718	458
	1996	5,160	864	31,116	531	800	6.2	440,845	63,646	3,723,907	3,728	466
	1997	5,082	855	31,595	529	813	6.1	450,907	63,247	3,742,240	3,794	467
	1998	5,039	842	31,830	527	821	6.0	474,366	62,162	3,726,234	3,835	467
	1999	4,977	831	32,377	527	835	5.9	495,850	61,534	3,760,295	3,840	460
	2000	4,934	825	33,102	527	850	5.8	522,970	60,845	3,880,166	3,916	461
	2001	4,927	828	33,834	534	866	5.8	539,316	60,454	3,873,395	3,990	461
	2002	4,949	823	34,501	541	887	5.7	557,336	59,974	3,870,191	4,072	459
	2003	4,918	815	34,800	540	895	5.7	563,804	59,662	3,915,842	4,112	459
	2004	4,942	810	35,098	542	910	5.6	573,126	58,710	3,931,508	4,151	456
	2005	4,956	804	35,265	542	930	5.6	587,296	58,195	3,987,766	4,260	458
	2006	4,947	805	35,403	540	940	5.6	599,597	57,832	4,075,193	4,347	462
	2007	4,915	803	35,370	535	944	5.5	603,411	57,546	4,077,962	4,468	473
	2008	5,026	810	35,776	538	963	5.5	624,185	57,301	4,073,724	4,552	473
	2009	5,023	807	35,603	529	973	5.5	643,420	57,302	3,960,432	4,594	472
	2010	4,995	806	35,160	520	974	5.4	651,617	56,610	3,818,399	4,603	473
	2011	4,983	799	34,852	514	983	5.4	657,071	56,290	3,730,342	4,654	473
	2012	5,010	802	34,438	508	992	5.4	675,223	55,987	3,715,479	4,732	477
	2013	5,372	813	34,079	509	977	5.4	684,488	56,844	3,728,411	4,874	499
	2014	5,330	804	33,545	504	1,018	5.5	700,472	56,294	3,766,328	4,829	474
	2015	5,293	802	33,861	508	1,046	5.5	731,067	55,953	3,792,223	4,948	473
	2016	5,278	801	34,052	511	1,077	5.5	757,095	55,824	3,769,965	5,088	473
	2017	5,274	800	34,351	511	1,093	5.4	766,368	55,181	3,656,809	5,217	477
	2018	5,210	794	34,268	508	1,101	5.4	766,630	54,943	3,637,593	5,239	476
	2019	5,153	789	34,094	508	1,112	5.4	785,473	54,468	3,567,799	5,316	478
	2020	5,151	791	31,410	485	1,049	5.7	717,397	53,789	3,505,115	5,318	507
	2021	5,169	789	31,982	515	1,135	5.9	785,810	53,411	3,485,508	5,332	470
	2022	5,141	785	31,571	518	1,173	6.0	799,880	52,767	3,510,787	5,394	460

Note: The 2021 performance data do not reflect the full impact of the COVID-19 pandemic. Please refer to the discussion in the Introduction for more information.

Table 1 (Continued)

CLASSIFICATION	YEAR	HOSPITALS	BEDS (in thousands)	ADMISSIONS (in thousands)	AVERAGE DAILY CENSUS (in thousands)	ADJUSTED AVERAGE DAILY CENSUS (in thousands)	AVERAGE STAY (days)	OUTPATIENT VISITS (in thousands)	NEWBORNS		FTE PERSONNEL	
									Bassinets	Births	Number (in thousands)	Per 100 Adjusted Census
Total community hospitals	1975	5,875	942	33,435	706	798	7.7	190,672	83,829	2,998,552	2,392	300
	1976	5,857	956	33,979	713	810	7.7	201,247	82,296	2,962,216	2,475	306
	1979	5,842	984	35,099	727	833	7.6	198,778	77,266	3,287,012	2,756	331
	1980	5,830	988	36,143	747	857	7.6	202,310	77,522	3,408,482	2,873	335
	1981	5,813	1,003	36,438	763	873	7.6	202,768	76,561	3,465,401	3,033	347
	1982	5,801	1,012	36,379	762	878	7.6	248,124	75,733	3,514,457	3,103	353
	1983	5,783	1,018	36,152	749	864	7.6	210,044	75,465	3,490,254	3,096	358
	1984	5,759	1,017	35,155	702	820	7.3	211,961	75,581	3,456,308	3,017	368
	1985	5,732	1,001	33,449	649	777	7.1	218,716	74,893	3,521,135	2,997	386
	1986	5,678	978	32,379	629	770	7.1	231,912	73,682	3,584,408	3,025	393
	1987	5,611	958	31,601	622	776	7.2	245,524	72,510	3,602,296	3,114	401
	1988	5,533	947	31,453	620	787	7.2	269,129	70,325	3,706,402	3,205	407
	1989	5,455	933	31,116	618	796	7.2	285,712	69,405	3,830,615	3,303	415
	1990	5,384	927	31,181	619	813	7.2	301,329	68,412	3,958,263	3,420	421
	1991	5,342	924	31,064	611	820	7.2	322,048	67,434	3,965,396	3,535	431
	1992	5,292	921	31,034	604	827	7.1	348,522	67,089	3,924,944	3,620	437
	1993	5,261	919	30,748	592	828	7.0	366,885	66,054	3,870,376	3,677	444
	1994	5,229	902	30,718	568	812	6.7	382,924	65,722	3,809,367	3,692	455
	1995	5,194	873	30,945	548	809	6.5	414,345	64,736	3,764,698	3,714	459
	1996	5,134	862	31,099	531	799	6.2	439,863	63,640	3,723,871	3,725	466
	1997	5,057	853	31,577	528	811	6.1	450,140	63,241	3,742,191	3,790	467
	1998	5,015	840	31,812	525	819	6.0	474,193	62,156	3,726,233	3,831	468
	1999	4,956	830	32,359	526	833	5.9	495,346	61,528	3,760,295	3,838	461
	2000	4,915	824	33,089	526	849	5.8	521,404	60,839	3,880,166	3,911	461
	2001	4,908	826	33,814	533	865	5.7	538,480	60,448	3,873,395	3,987	461
	2002	4,927	821	34,478	540	886	5.7	556,404	59,974	3,870,191	4,069	459
	2003	4,895	813	34,783	539	894	5.7	563,186	59,662	3,915,842	4,109	460
	2004	4,919	808	35,086	541	909	5.6	571,569	58,710	3,931,508	4,148	456
	2005	4,936	802	35,239	540	929	5.6	584,429	58,195	3,987,766	4,257	458
	2006	4,927	803	35,378	538	939	5.6	599,553	57,832	4,075,193	4,343	463
	2007	4,897	801	35,346	533	943	5.5	603,300	57,546	4,077,962	4,465	474
	2008	5,010	808	35,761	536	962	5.5	624,098	57,301	4,073,724	4,550	473
	2009	5,008	806	35,527	528	970	5.4	641,953	57,282	3,959,605	4,585	472
	2010	4,985	805	35,149	520	973	5.4	651,424	56,610	3,818,399	4,600	473
	2011	4,973	797	34,843	513	982	5.4	656,079	56,290	3,730,342	4,650	473
	2012	4,999	801	34,422	507	991	5.4	674,971	55,987	3,715,479	4,731	477
	2013	5,359	811	34,063	509	976	5.4	684,227	56,844	3,728,411	4,872	499
	2014	5,308	802	33,517	503	1,017	5.5	700,233	56,294	3,766,328	4,826	475
	2015	5,280	801	33,818	507	1,045	5.5	730,789	55,953	3,792,223	4,947	473
	2016	5,267	799	34,032	510	1,076	5.5	756,798	55,824	3,769,965	5,087	473
	2017	5,262	798	34,306	510	1,092	5.4	766,077	55,181	3,656,809	5,215	478
	2018	5,198	793	34,251	508	1,100	5.4	766,393	54,943	3,637,593	5,239	476
	2019	5,141	788	34,078	507	1,111	5.4	785,236	54,468	3,567,593	5,315	478
	2020	5,139	790	31,392	485	1,049	5.6	785,799	53,789	3,567,799	5,317	507
	2021	5,157	788	31,967	515	1,134	5.9	717,159	53,411	3,505,115	5,331	470
	2022	5,129	784	31,556	518	1,172	6.0	799,667	52,767	3,510,787	5,392	460

Note: The 2021 performance data do not reflect the full impact of the COVID-19 pandemic. Please refer to the discussion in the Introduction for more information.

Historical Trends

Table 1 (Continued)

CLASSIFICATION	YEAR	HOSPITALS	BEDS (in thousands)	ADMISSIONS (in thousands)	AVERAGE DAILY CENSUS (in thousands)	ADJUSTED AVERAGE DAILY CENSUS (in thousands)	AVERAGE STAY (days)	OUTPATIENT VISITS (in thousands)	NEWBORNS		FTE PERSONNEL	
									Bassinets	Births	Number (in thousands)	Per 100 Adjusted Census
Nongovernment not-for-profit community hospitals	1975	3,339	658	23,722	510	574	7.8	131,435	57,496	2,131,057	1,712	298
	1976	3,345	670	24,082	517	586	7.9	140,914	56,442	2,100,917	1,791	306
	1979	3,330	690	24,874	528	603	7.7	139,565	52,859	2,308,548	1,999	332
	1980	3,322	692	25,566	542	621	7.7	142,156	52,659	2,389,478	2,086	336
	1981	3,340	706	25,945	555	636	7.8	143,380	52,302	2,455,033	2,213	399
	1982	3,338	712	25,898	553	637	7.8	176,245	51,566	2,483,345	2,265	355
	1983	3,347	718	25,827	544	629	7.7	150,839	51,649	2,465,604	2,270	362
	1984	3,351	716	25,236	512	598	7.4	153,281	51,491	2,446,540	2,222	372
	1985	3,349	707	24,179	476	569	7.2	158,953	51,424	2,507,288	2,216	389
	1986	3,323	689	23,483	460	563	7.2	167,633	50,885	2,547,170	2,241	398
	1987	3,274	673	22,937	455	566	7.2	177,413	50,133	2,557,294	2,298	406
	1988	3,242	668	22,939	456	577	7.3	195,363	48,828	2,653,794	2,373	412
	1989	3,220	661	22,792	455	584	7.3	209,191	48,305	2,751,426	2,454	420
	1990	3,191	657	22,878	455	596	7.3	221,073	47,441	2,833,204	2,533	424
	1991	3,175	656	22,964	451	603	7.2	238,204	47,229	2,845,995	2,624	435
	1992	3,173	656	23,056	445	606	7.1	257,887	47,185	2,846,386	2,692	443
	1993	3,154	651	22,749	432	602	6.9	270,138	46,214	2,802,164	2,711	451
	1994	3,139	637	22,704	413	589	6.6	282,653	46,381	2,792,116	2,719	462
	1995	3,092	610	22,557	393	578	6.4	303,851	45,198	2,725,641	2,702	468
	1996	3,045	598	22,542	379	567	6.1	320,746	44,650	2,683,750	2,711	478
	1997	3,000	591	22,905	376	575	6.0	330,215	44,484	2,698,086	2,765	481
	1998	3,026	588	23,282	377	587	5.9	352,114	44,087	2,715,958	2,834	483
	1999	3,012	587	23,871	381	605	5.8	370,784	44,172	2,746,453	2,862	473
	2000	3,003	583	24,452	382	618	5.7	393,168	43,655	2,833,615	2,919	472
	2001	2,998	585	24,983	385	628	5.6	404,901	43,640	2,829,691	2,971	473
	2002	3,025	582	25,425	391	646	5.6	416,910	43,241	2,820,159	3,039	471
	2003	2,984	575	25,668	389	647	5.5	424,215	42,965	2,854,764	3,059	473
	2004	2,967	568	25,757	388	655	5.5	430,262	41,968	2,844,617	3,077	470
	2005	2,958	561	25,881	388	667	5.5	441,653	41,585	2,876,677	3,155	473
	2006	2,919	559	25,798	385	671	5.4	453,501	40,888	2,905,275	3,207	478
	2007	2,913	554	25,752	380	673	5.4	455,825	40,681	2,907,002	3,286	488
	2008	2,923	557	25,899	380	683	5.4	469,804	40,567	2,901,854	3,340	489
	2009	2,918	556	25,783	375	690	5.3	485,935	40,467	2,822,527	3,369	488
	2010	2,904	556	25,532	368	691	5.3	494,178	39,946	2,750,163	3,388	490
	2011	2,903	548	25,185	362	694	5.2	496,643	39,651	2,692,577	3,427	494
	2012	2,894	545	24,751	354	697	5.2	512,237	39,778	2,684,600	3,477	499
	2013	2,975	548	24,470	354	687	5.3	518,438	40,498	2,706,635	3,523	513
	2014	2,943	539	23,895	347	709	5.3	528,258	39,768	2,728,345	3,513	496
	2015	2,932	537	24,115	350	729	5.3	551,762	39,510	2,744,467	3,593	493
	2016	2,943	540	24,356	353	751	5.3	574,044	39,641	2,750,958	3,716	494
	2017	2,968	545	24,789	357	768	5.3	581,848	39,744	2,710,049	3,841	500
	2018	2,937	543	24,730	356	781	5.2	580,598	39,692	2,687,592	3,848	493
	2019	2,946	546	24,728	358	796	5.3	595,360	39,632	2,651,823	3,929	494
	2020	2,960	548	22,778	340	748	5.5	546,033	39,271	2,605,916	3,927	525
	2021	2,978	548	23,391	364	819	5.7	600,471	39,364	2,620,028	3,937	481
	2022	2,987	549	23,091	369	852	5.8	614,667	39,090	2,640,194	4,001	470

Note: The 2021 performance data do not reflect the full impact of the COVID-19 pandemic. Please refer to the discussion in the Introduction for more information.

Table 1 (Continued)

Investor-owned (for-profit) community hospitals

CLASSIFICATION	YEAR	HOSPITALS	BEDS (in thousands)	ADMISSIONS (in thousands)	AVERAGE DAILY CENSUS (in thousands)	ADJUSTED AVERAGE DAILY CENSUS (in thousands)	AVERAGE STAY (days)	OUTPATIENT VISITS (in thousands)	NEWBORNS		FTE PERSONNEL	
									Bassinets	Births	Number (in thousands)	Per 100 Adjusted Census
	1975	775	73	2,646	48	53	6.6	7,713	4,062	141,392	139	263
	1976	752	76	2,734	50	54	6.6	8,048	4,044	144,751	147	272
	1979	727	83	2,963	53	59	6.6	9,289	4,110	174,843	174	300
	1980	730	87	3,165	57	62	6.5	9,696	4,439	199,722	189	304
	1981	729	88	3,239	58	63	6.5	9,961	4,523	207,405	203	322
	1982	748	91	3,316	60	66	6.6	13,193	4,736	219,675	212	320
	1983	757	94	3,299	59	66	6.5	10,389	5,039	228,883	213	323
	1984	786	100	3,314	57	64	6.3	11,090	5,807	242,088	214	335
	1985	805	104	3,242	54	63	6.1	12,378	6,117	266,839	221	350
	1986	834	107	3,231	54	65	6.2	14,896	6,305	291,112	229	354
	1987	828	106	3,157	54	66	6.2	16,566	6,391	306,492	242	367
	1988	790	104	3,090	53	66	6.3	17,926	6,254	308,828	249	379
	1989	769	102	3,071	53	67	6.4	19,341	6,354	325,711	261	390
	1990	749	101	3,066	54	69	6.3	20,110	6,261	340,555	273	396
	1991	738	100	3,016	52	69	6.3	21,174	6,358	359,115	281	409
	1992	723	99	2,969	51	69	6.3	22,900	6,519	357,776	285	412
	1993	717	99	2,946	51	69	6.2	24,936	6,395	363,358	289	417
	1994	719	101	3,035	50	70	6.1	26,443	6,329	354,477	302	434
	1995	752	106	3,428	55	77	5.8	31,940	7,164	408,339	343	443
	1996	759	109	3,684	56	82	5.6	37,347	7,441	444,697	359	437
	1997	797	115	3,953	60	89	5.5	40,919	8,026	465,919	385	433
	1998	771	113	3,971	60	90	5.5	42,072	7,895	466,025	383	425
	1999	747	107	3,905	58	86	5.5	39,896	7,486	467,585	362	422
	2000	749	110	4,141	61	90	5.4	43,378	7,792	503,497	378	418
	2001	754	109	4,197	63	92	5.4	44,706	7,413	494,669	379	413
	2002	766	108	4,365	64	93	5.3	45,215	7,467	496,988	380	407
	2003	790	110	4,481	65	95	5.3	44,246	7,491	515,693	391	411
	2004	835	113	4,599	68	100	5.4	44,962	7,763	534,503	406	406
	2005	868	114	4,618	68	101	5.3	46,016	7,714	546,307	421	418
	2006	890	115	4,735	68	103	5.2	44,237	8,012	574,113	423	413
	2007	873	116	4,626	66	101	5.2	43,943	7,760	555,670	432	429
	2008	982	121	4,839	70	109	5.3	44,897	7,791	562,711	450	414
	2009	998	122	4,887	70	112	5.3	47,281	7,965	553,233	464	414
	2010	1,013	125	4,925	71	113	5.3	48,201	7,965	525,427	474	420
	2011	1,025	128	5,060	73	119	5.3	50,013	8,137	508,330	485	409
	2012	1,068	135	5,224	77	124	5.3	53,854	8,192	530,941	515	414
	2013	1,351	145	5,346	81	126	5.5	56,935	8,400	532,235	613	487
	2014	1,341	146	5,407	82	139	5.5	60,277	8,665	547,008	572	411
	2015	1,345	146	5,506	83	143	5.5	62,567	8,863	560,964	588	410
	2016	1,350	146	5,625	84	148	5.5	65,542	8,876	550,448	609	413
	2017	1,322	142	5,433	81	144	5.5	63,203	8,319	487,406	591	412
	2018	1,296	140	5,437	81	142	5.4	62,224	8,173	494,130	594	418
	2019	1,233	132	5,309	78	136	5.4	60,101	7,703	464,258	573	420
	2020	1,228	130	4,799	75	127	5.7	52,902	7,332	449,289	560	441
	2021	1,235	130	4,820	80	138	6.0	55,495	7,204	434,155	557	403
	2022	1,219	127	4,764	78	140	6.0	55,661	7,088	430,293	551	393

Note: The 2021 performance data do not reflect the full impact of the COVID-19 pandemic. Please refer to the discussion in the Introduction for more information.

Historical Trends

Table 1 (Continued)

CLASSIFICATION	YEAR	HOSPITALS	BEDS (in thousands)	ADMISSIONS (in thousands)	AVERAGE DAILY CENSUS (in thousands)	ADJUSTED AVERAGE DAILY CENSUS (in thousands)	AVERAGE STAY (days)	OUTPATIENT VISITS (in thousands)	NEWBORNS Bassinets	NEWBORNS Births	FTE PERSONNEL Number (in thousands)	FTE PERSONNEL Per 100 Adjusted Census
State and local government community hospitals	1975	1,761	210	7,067	148	171	7.6	51,525	22,271	726,103	540	316
	1976	1,760	210	7,163	146	170	7.5	52,286	21,810	716,548	537	315
	1979	1,785	211	7,262	146	171	7.4	49,924	20,297	803,621	583	341
	1980	1,778	209	7,413	149	174	7.3	50,459	20,424	819,282	598	343
	1981	1,744	210	7,255	150	174	7.6	49,427	19,736	802,963	618	354
	1982	1,715	210	7,165	149	175	7.6	58,685	19,431	811,437	627	320
	1983	1,679	207	7,025	145	170	7.6	48,816	18,777	795,767	613	360
	1984	1,622	201	6,606	133	158	7.3	47,590	18,283	767,680	581	368
	1985	1,578	189	6,028	119	145	7.2	47,386	17,352	747,008	561	387
	1986	1,521	182	5,665	114	142	7.4	49,363	16,492	746,126	555	391
	1987	1,509	180	5,507	113	144	7.5	51,544	15,986	738,510	573	399
	1988	1,501	175	5,424	112	145	7.6	55,840	15,243	743,780	583	403
	1989	1,466	170	5,253	110	145	7.7	57,179	14,746	753,478	589	406
	1990	1,444	169	5,236	111	148	7.7	60,146	14,710	784,504	614	415
	1991	1,429	168	5,084	108	148	7.8	62,670	13,847	760,286	630	424
	1992	1,396	166	5,008	108	152	7.9	67,734	13,385	720,782	643	424
	1993	1,390	169	5,054	109	157	7.8	71,811	13,445	704,854	676	430
	1994	1,371	164	4,979	104	154	7.6	73,828	13,012	662,774	672	438
	1995	1,350	157	4,961	100	154	7.4	78,554	12,374	630,718	670	435
	1996	1,330	155	4,873	96	150	7.2	81,770	11,549	595,424	654	437
	1997	1,260	148	4,720	92	148	7.1	79,007	10,731	578,186	640	433
	1998	1,218	139	4,559	87	142	7.0	80,008	10,174	544,250	614	433
	1999	1,197	136	4,583	86	143	6.9	84,667	9,870	546,257	614	430
	2000	1,163	131	4,496	83	140	6.7	84,858	9,392	543,054	614	438
	2001	1,156	132	4,634	85	145	6.7	88,873	9,395	549,035	637	438
	2002	1,136	130	4,688	84	147	6.6	94,280	9,266	553,044	651	442
	2003	1,121	129	4,634	84	152	6.6	94,725	9,206	545,385	658	434
	2004	1,117	128	4,730	85	154	6.5	96,345	8,979	552,388	666	431
	2005	1,110	128	4,740	85	161	6.5	96,760	8,896	564,782	681	424
	2006	1,119	128	4,848	86	165	6.5	101,845	8,932	595,805	713	433
	2007	1,111	131	4,967	87	169	6.4	103,532	9,105	615,290	747	443
	2008	1,105	131	5,023	86	170	6.3	109,398	8,943	609,159	760	446
	2009	1,092	127	4,857	83	168	6.2	108,738	8,850	583,845	751	447
	2010	1,068	125	4,693	80	169	6.2	109,045	8,699	542,809	738	437
	2011	1,045	121	4,598	78	170	6.2	109,423	8,502	529,435	738	434
	2012	1,037	120	4,447	77	170	6.3	108,880	8,017	499,938	739	435
	2013	1,033	118	4,247	74	163	6.3	108,854	7,946	489,541	736	451
	2014	1,024	117	4,215	74	169	6.4	111,698	7,861	490,975	741	440
	2015	1,003	118	4,197	74	173	6.4	116,460	7,580	486,792	766	442
	2016	974	113	4,051	73	177	6.5	117,212	7,307	468,559	762	431
	2017	972	111	4,084	72	180	6.4	121,026	7,118	459,354	783	434
	2018	965	110	4,084	71	177	6.4	123,571	7,078	455,871	797	450
	2019	962	110	4,041	71	179	6.5	129,775	7,133	451,718	813	454
	2020	951	112	3,815	70	174	6.7	118,224	7,186	449,910	830	478
	2021	944	110	3,756	71	177	6.9	129,631	6,843	431,325	837	472
	2022	923	108	3,701	71	180	7.0	129,339	6,589	440,300	840	466

Note: The 2021 performance data do not reflect the full impact of the COVID-19 pandemic. Please refer to the discussion in the Introduction for more information.

Table
2

2022 U.S. Hospitals: Utilization and Personnel

Excludes U.S.-Associated Areas and Puerto Rico hospitals.

CLASSIFICATION	HOSPITALS	BEDS	ADMISSIONS	INPATIENT DAYS	ADJUSTED INPATIENT DAYS	AVERAGE DAILY CENSUS	ADJUSTED AVERAGE DAILY CENSUS	AVERAGE STAY (DAYS)	SURGICAL OPERATIONS
UNITED STATES	6,120	916,752	33,679,935	222,485,102	—	609,515	—	—	28,222,203
6-24 Beds	898	14,450	352,062	1,909,290	—	5,209	—	—	897,517
25-49	1,418	46,890	1,183,711	7,926,576	—	21,706	—	—	1,833,020
50-99	1,183	84,001	2,374,276	18,234,693	—	49,957	—	—	2,262,575
100-199	1,158	165,554	5,758,739	37,801,163	—	103,559	—	—	4,611,458
200-299	581	141,853	5,479,282	34,508,915	—	94,550	—	—	4,224,712
300-399	353	121,763	4,804,061	29,813,696	—	81,681	—	—	3,474,395
400-499	194	86,028	3,490,698	21,988,335	—	60,236	—	—	2,513,233
500 or more	335	256,213	10,237,106	70,302,434	—	192,617	—	—	8,405,293
Psychiatric	668	87,582	1,247,634	23,668,281	—	64,822	—	—	2,107
Hospitals	664	86,238	1,247,548	23,245,906	—	63,665	—	—	2,107
Inst. for Intellectual Disabilities	4	1,344	86	422,375	—	1,157	—	—	0
General	4,570	773,083	31,375,620	185,310,490	—	507,697	—	—	27,065,524
Hospitals	4,555	771,968	31,359,126	185,045,928	—	506,970	—	—	27,061,775
Hospital units of institutions	15	1,115	16,494	264,562	—	727	—	—	3,749
TB and other respiratory diseases	3	168	812	34,120	—	93	—	—	0
Obstetrics and gynecology	12	1,698	75,262	346,507	—	950	—	—	66,340
Eye, ear, nose and throat	3	60	1,720	6,231	—	17	—	—	52,528
Rehabilitation	350	22,439	435,825	5,804,683	—	15,901	—	—	18,194
Orthopedic	42	1,498	59,782	173,269	—	473	—	—	201,262
Chronic Disease	3	118	389	28,368	—	77	—	—	0
Surgical	77	1,759	57,145	162,028	—	442	—	—	296,686
Cancer	16	3,138	122,137	923,516	—	2,530	—	—	153,489
Heart	15	1,016	47,244	207,887	—	569	—	—	48,984
Acute long-term care hospital	343	22,943	225,699	5,539,522	—	15,176	—	—	274,739
All other	18	1,250	30,666	280,200	—	768	—	—	42,350
Federal	207	36,886	830,278	7,527,669	—	20,633	—	—	790,515
Psychiatric	9	2,332	10,501	387,766	—	1,062	—	—	553
General and other special	198	34,554	819,777	7,139,903	—	19,571	—	—	789,962
Nonfederal	5,913	879,866	32,849,657	214,957,433	—	588,882	—	—	27,431,688
Psychiatric	659	85,250	1,237,133	23,280,515	—	63,760	—	—	1,554
Hospitals	655	83,906	1,237,047	22,858,140	—	62,603	—	—	1,554
Inst. for Intellectual Disabilities	4	1,344	86	422,375	—	1,157	—	—	0
TB and other respiratory diseases	3	168	812	34,120	34,120	93	93	42	0
Long-term general and other special	110	9,266	41,002	2,469,298	2,921,395	6,765	8,004	60.2	14,724
Short-term general and other special	5,141	785,182	31,570,710	189,173,500	428,076,927	518,264	1,172,930	6	27,415,410
Hospital units of institutions	12	1,070	14,903	261,174	261,174	717	717	17.5	0
Community Hospitals	5,129	784,112	31,555,807	188,912,326	427,815,753	517,547	1,172,213	6	27,415,410
6-24 Beds	780	12,440	297,732	1,464,202	9,723,185	4,002	26,643	4.9	868,058
25-49	1,274	41,576	1,068,234	6,629,988	26,560,246	18,151	72,871	6.2	1,821,280
50-99	900	63,469	1,885,514	13,094,514	40,335,671	35,878	110,517	6.9	2,074,217
100-199	901	130,451	5,029,382	28,789,120	73,996,383	78,873	202,738	5.7	4,460,257
200-299	483	118,181	5,163,725	28,173,136	60,302,889	77,191	165,206	5.5	3,983,762
300-399	308	106,269	4,642,693	25,800,156	52,076,626	70,684	142,680	5.6	3,424,208
400-499	176	77,736	3,394,631	20,077,453	38,908,747	54,999	106,597	5.9	2,458,513
500 or more	307	233,990	10,073,896	64,883,757	125,912,006	177,769	344,961	6.4	8,325,115
Nongovernment not-for-profit	2,987	548,752	23,091,475	134,599,636	310,819,504	368,747	851,656	5.8	20,135,388
Investor-owned (for profit)	1,219	127,027	4,763,722	28,385,960	51,151,460	77,767	140,160	6	3,757,429
State and Local Government	923	108,333	3,700,610	25,926,730	65,844,789	71,033	180,397	7	3,522,593

U.S. Hospitals

Table 2 (Continued)

CLASSIFICATION	OUTPATIENT VISITS		NEWBORNS		FULL-TIME EQUIVALENT PERSONNEL					FULL-TIME EQUIVALENT TRAINEES		
	Emergency	Total	Bassinets	Births	Physicians and Dentists	Registered Nurses	Licensed Practical Nurses	Other Salaried Personnel	Total Personnel	Medical and Dental Residents	Other Trainees	Total Trainees
UNITED STATES	141,283,079	930,734,923	53,397	3,542,001	195,994	1,737,981	110,455	4,039,195	6,083,625	139,130	23,577	162,707
6-24 Beds	3,971,545	29,678,608	619	22,394	3,812	30,567	5,107	92,090	131,576	232	250	482
25-49	9,756,977	65,685,813	3,078	113,638	9,097	76,008	11,473	231,947	328,525	575	991	1,566
50-99	12,292,949	81,169,815	4,605	208,444	12,701	122,266	13,717	321,406	470,090	2,417	1,985	4,402
100-199	27,457,834	163,779,421	10,211	554,921	27,208	256,633	21,479	649,572	954,892	9,089	1,853	10,942
200-299	23,800,482	134,610,051	9,121	609,405	24,861	252,321	17,333	584,124	878,639	10,578	4,399	14,977
300-399	18,157,321	109,007,587	7,729	539,712	20,203	222,965	10,197	461,928	715,293	12,045	2,024	14,069
400-499	13,146,504	84,430,563	4,984	383,669	16,942	170,667	8,177	367,408	563,194	14,523	1,885	16,408
500 or more	32,699,467	262,373,065	13,050	1,109,818	81,170	606,554	22,972	1,330,720	2,041,416	89,671	10,190	99,861
Psychiatric	90,545	12,110,127	9	0	3,874	33,157	6,119	163,754	206,904	477	393	870
Hospitals	90,545	12,110,127	9	0	3,863	33,002	6,077	160,205	203,147	477	393	870
Inst. for Intellectual Disabilities	0	0	0	0	11	155	42	3,549	3,757	0	0	0
General	140,113,857	893,505,517	52,748	3,482,131	183,969	1,629,165	95,902	3,644,316	5,553,352	136,858	21,640	158,498
Hospitals	140,084,875	892,795,865	52,748	3,482,131	183,666	1,628,856	95,693	3,642,397	5,550,612	136,836	21,628	158,464
Hospital units of institutions	28,982	709,652	0	0	303	309	209	1,919	2,740	22	12	34
TB and other respiratory diseases	0	310,712	0	0	55	111	64	453	683	0	10	10
Obstetrics and gynecology	213,205	1,599,417	540	51,579	89	3,898	88	6,207	10,282	24	46	70
Eye, ear, nose and throat	24,100	621,707	0	98	230	384	4	1,874	2,492	102	52	154
Rehabilitation	3	7,237,658	40	0	865	20,317	2,579	72,347	96,108	361	47	408
Orthopedic	129,427	2,014,850	0	0	650	3,927	265	11,605	16,447	66	20	86
Chronic Disease	2,140	52,816	0	5,003	9	132	10	621	772			
Surgical	267,066	1,549,451	26	0	48	4,473	236	8,437	13,194	4	8	12
Cancer	111,945	7,670,397	0	0	5,181	18,640	215	67,136	91,172	832	1,309	2,141
Heart	88,669	843,569	0	0	158	3,290	155	5,677	9,280	53	5	58
Acute long-term care hospital	122,100	1,858,543	0	0	484	18,166	4,637	49,114	72,401	141	31	172
All other	120,022	1,360,159	34	3,190	382	2,321	181	7,654	10,538	212	16	228
Federal	4,129,825	119,465,599	611	31,207	35,837	103,864	22,651	298,209	460,561	11,351	7,363	18,714
Psychiatric	0	2,572,400	0	0	363	1,243	465	5,764	7,835	39	73	112
General and other special	4,129,825	116,893,199	611	31,207	35,474	102,621	22,186	292,445	452,726	11,312	7,290	18,602
Nonfederal	137,153,254	811,269,324	52,786	3,510,794	160,157	1,634,117	87,804	3,740,986	5,623,064	127,779	16,214	143,993
Psychiatric	90,545	9,537,727	9	0	3,511	31,914	5,654	157,990	199,069	438	320	758
Hospitals	90,545	9,537,727	9	0	3,500	31,759	5,612	154,441	195,312	438	320	758
Inst. for Intellectual Disabilities	0	0	0	0	11	155	42	3,549	3,757	0	0	0
TB and other respiratory diseases	0	310,712	0	0	55	111	64	453	683	0	10	10
Long-term general and other special	93,676	1,540,894	10	7	293	6,220	901	22,304	29,718	64	32	96
Short-term general and other special	136,969,033	799,879,991	52,767	3,510,787	156,298	1,595,872	81,185	3,560,239	5,393,594	127,277	15,852	143,129
Hospital units of institutions	0	212,858	0	0	117	107	107	564	895	0	0	0
Community Hospitals	136,969,033	799,667,133	52,767	3,510,787	156,181	1,595,765	81,078	3,559,675	5,392,699	127,277	15,852	143,129
6-24 Beds	3,741,910	24,179,568	568	18,356	2,305	28,035	4,185	78,044	112,569	36	140	176
25-49	9,472,349	61,105,070	2,944	111,883	8,073	71,267	10,711	210,718	300,769	402	845	1,247
50-99	11,224,622	63,459,073	4,399	194,992	7,231	98,000	9,025	253,257	367,513	739	347	1,086
100-199	26,406,273	133,331,518	10,090	547,525	17,991	220,987	14,029	517,430	770,437	6,715	1,098	7,813
200-299	23,208,872	112,170,185	9,003	604,832	16,112	227,860	10,969	492,010	746,951	8,018	1,339	9,357
300-399	17,674,452	93,337,602	7,729	539,712	15,944	207,308	7,477	416,007	646,736	11,445	1,102	12,547
400-499	12,795,398	69,862,446	4,984	383,669	13,101	158,393	5,780	329,143	506,417	13,470	1,477	14,947
500 or more	32,445,157	242,221,671	13,050	1,109,818	75,424	583,915	18,902	1,263,066	1,941,307	86,452	9,504	95,956
Nongovernment not-for-profit	99,836,754	614,666,935	39,090	2,640,194	128,061	1,188,733	47,841	2,636,758	4,001,393	91,731	12,568	104,299
Investor-owned (for profit)	19,682,612	55,661,289	7,088	430,293	4,270	182,902	15,913	348,347	551,432	3,970	426	4,396
State and Local Government	17,449,667	129,338,909	6,589	440,300	23,850	224,130	17,324	574,570	839,874	31,576	2,858	34,434

Note: The 2021 performance data do not reflect the full impact of the COVID-19 pandemic. Please refer to the discussion in the Introduction for more information.

Tables 3–6

Table		Page
3	**Total United States**	12
4	**Bed Size Categories**	14
5	**U.S. Census Divisions**	31
6	**States**	50

Note: The 2021 performance data do not reflect the full impact of the COVID-19 pandemic. Please refer to the discussion in the Introduction for more information.

TABLE 3

TOTAL UNITED STATES

U.S. Community Hospitals
(Nonfederal, short-term general and other special hospitals)

Overview 2018–2022

	2022	2021	2020	2019	2018
TOTAL U.S. Community Hospitals	**5,129**	**5,157**	**5,139**	**5,141**	**5,198**
Bed Size Category					
6-24	780	760	754	734	709
25-49	1,274	1,274	1,250	1,257	1,273
50-99	900	912	903	897	926
100-199	901	923	938	952	976
200-299	483	502	503	515	534
300-399	308	306	311	326	316
400-499	176	164	173	163	172
500 +	307	316	307	297	292
Location					
Hospitals Urban	3,319	3,357	3,343	3,336	3,377
Hospitals Rural	1,810	1,800	1,796	1,805	1,821
Control					
State and Local Government	923	944	951	962	965
Not for Profit	2,987	2,978	2,960	2,946	2,937
Investor owned	1,219	1,235	1,228	1,233	1,296
Affiliations					
Hospitals in a System	3,510	3,514	3,483	3,453	3,491
Hospitals in a Group Purchasing Organization	3,222	3,307	3,316	3,341	3,491

Note: The 2021 performance data do not reflect the full impact of the COVID-19 pandemic. Please refer to the discussion in the Introduction for more information.

TABLE 3

TOTAL UNITED STATES

U.S. Community Hospitals
(Nonfederal, short-term general and other special hospitals)

Utilization, Personnel, Community Health Indicators 2018–2022

	2022	2021	2020	2019	2018
TOTAL FACILITY (Includes Hospital and Nursing Home Units)					
Utilization - Inpatient					
Beds	784,112	787,967	789,354	787,995	792,417
Admissions	31,555,807	31,967,073	31,393,318	34,078,100	34,251,159
Inpatient Days	188,912,326	187,599,105	177,341,078	185,149,928	185,307,228
Average Length of Stay	5.9	5.8	5.6	5.4	5.4
Inpatient Surgeries	7,641,635	7,788,190	8,003,571	8,950,559	8,999,976
Births	3,510,787	3,485,508	3,505,115	3,567,799	3,637,593
Utilization - Outpatient					
Emergency Outpatient Visits	136,969,033	126,957,429	123,267,216	143,432,284	143,454,611
Other Outpatient Visits	662,698,100	658,639,366	593,892,101	641,802,972	622,937,901
Total Outpatient Visits	799,667,133	785,596,795	717,159,317	785,235,256	766,392,512
Outpatient Surgeries	19,773,775	19,126,174	16,975,312	19,418,138	19,168,038
Personnel					
Full Time RNs	1,292,453	1,309,064	1,342,589	1,322,217	1,306,941
Full Time LPNs	68,318	62,753	62,756	63,352	63,951
Part Time RNs	606,727	580,312	573,485	575,878	559,832
Part Time LPNs	25,584	22,785	22,180	22,403	22,170
Total Full Time	4,651,219	4,615,569	4,610,279	4,600,213	4,549,056
Total Part Time	1,769,245	1,702,146	1,676,632	1,678,799	1,632,575
HOSPITAL UNIT (Excludes Separate Nursing Home Units)					
Utilization - Inpatient					
Beds	756,787	759,533	759,530	755,167	757,609
Admissions	31,485,823	31,893,717	31,306,074	33,965,386	34,130,471
Inpatient Days	181,508,006	179,742,748	168,497,152	174,701,046	174,295,886
Average Length of Stay	5.7	5.6	5.3	5.1	5.1
Personnel					
Total Full Time	4,632,587	4,594,880	4,589,364	4,576,265	4,524,517
Total Part Time	1,759,317	1,691,549	1,665,178	1,665,851	1,618,824
COMMUNITY HEALTH INDICATORS PER 1000 POPULATION					
Total Population (in thousands)	333,287	331,893	329,484	328,239	327,167
Inpatient					
Beds	2.4	2.4	2.4	2.4	2.4
Admissions	94.7	96.3	95.3	103.8	104.7
Inpatient Days	566.8	565.2	538.2	564.1	566.4
Inpatient Surgeries	22.9	23.5	24.3	27.3	27.5
Births	10.5	10.5	10.6	10.9	11.1
Outpatient					
Emergency Outpatient Visits	411	382.5	374.1	437	438.5
Other Outpatient Visits	1,988.4	1,984.5	1,802.5	1,955.3	1,904
Total Outpatient Visits	2,399.3	2,367	2,176.6	2,392.3	2,342.5
Outpatient Surgeries	59.3	57.6	51.5	59.2	58.6

Note: The 2021 performance data do not reflect the full impact of the COVID-19 pandemic. Please refer to the discussion in the Introduction for more information.

TABLE 4

BED SIZE CATEGORY 6-24

U.S. Community Hospitals
(Nonfederal, short-term general and other special hospitals)

Overview 2018–2022

	2022	2021	2020	2019	2018
Total Community Hospitals in					
Bed Size Category 6-24................................	780	760	754	734	709
Location					
Hospitals Urban	325	322	321	308	305
Hospitals Rural	455	438	433	426	404
Control					
State and Local Government.............................	236	244	237	230	218
Not for Profit...	365	342	339	324	307
Investor owned......................................	179	174	178	180	184
Affiliations					
Hospitals in a System	368	346	344	331	323
Hospitals in a Group Purchasing Organization...	439	450	447	445	438

Note: The 2021 performance data do not reflect the full impact of the COVID-19 pandemic. Please refer to the discussion in the Introduction for more information.

TABLE 4

BED SIZE CATEGORY 6-24

U.S. Community Hospitals
(Nonfederal, short-term general and other special hospitals)

Utilization, Personnel, Community Health Indicators 2018–2022

	2022	2021	2020	2019	2018
TOTAL FACILITY (Includes Hospital and Nursing Home Units)					
Utilization - Inpatient					
Beds	12,440	12,111	12,129	11,896	11,520
Admissions	297,732	289,551	287,820	328,106	300,190
Inpatient Days	1,464,202	1,394,590	1,337,915	1,364,348	1,368,699
Average Length of Stay	4.9	4.8	4.6	4.2	4.6
Inpatient Surgeries	62,058	69,354	81,919	90,819	96,125
Births	18,356	18,549	17,544	17,580	17,548
Utilization - Outpatient					
Emergency Outpatient Visits	3,741,910	3,039,051	2,831,788	3,140,643	2,874,014
Other Outpatient Visits	20,437,658	18,768,461	16,411,054	15,519,481	13,476,883
Total Outpatient Visits	24,179,568	21,807,512	19,242,842	18,660,124	16,350,897
Outpatient Surgeries	806,000	795,988	690,201	741,524	742,399
Personnel					
Full Time RNs	19,804	19,183	19,098	18,087	17,602
Full Time LPNs	3,355	3,231	3,155	2,887	2,666
Part Time RNs	16,460	14,979	14,246	13,100	11,798
Part Time LPNs	1,689	1,531	1,368	1,386	1,193
Total Full Time	87,872	83,738	80,984	76,788	73,136
Total Part Time	49,761	46,421	44,548	41,447	36,620
HOSPITAL UNIT (Excludes Separate Nursing Home Units)					
Utilization - Inpatient					
Beds	12,420	12,101	12,129	11,874	11,502
Admissions	297,728	289,547	287,820	328,085	300,172
Inpatient Days	1,459,801	1,394,464	1,337,915	1,357,228	1,347,775
Average Length of Stay	4.9	4.8	4.6	4.1	4.5
Personnel					
Total Full Time	87,843	83,719	80,748	76,654	73,092
Total Part Time	49,749	46,412	44,442	41,425	36,606

Note: The 2021 performance data do not reflect the full impact of the COVID-19 pandemic. Please refer to the discussion in the Introduction for more information.

TABLE 4

BED SIZE CATEGORY 25-49

U.S. Community Hospitals
(Nonfederal, short-term general and other special hospitals)

Overview 2018–2022

	2022	2021	2020	2019	2018
Total Community Hospitals in					
Bed Size Category 25-49..............................	**1,274**	**1,274**	**1,250**	**1,257**	**1,273**
Location					
Hospitals Urban	542	536	531	539	537
Hospitals Rural..	732	738	719	718	736
Control					
State and Local Government.............................	307	312	316	330	344
Not for Profit...	622	620	606	604	596
Investor owned...	345	342	328	323	333
Affiliations					
Hospitals in a System	779	777	761	755	751
Hospitals in a Group Purchasing Organization...	741	746	748	744	793

Note: The 2021 performance data do not reflect the full impact of the COVID-19 pandemic. Please refer to the discussion in the Introduction for more information.

TABLE 4

BED SIZE CATEGORY 25-49

U.S. Community Hospitals
(Nonfederal, short-term general and other special hospitals)

Utilization, Personnel, Community Health Indicators 2018–2022

	2022	2021	2020	2019	2018
TOTAL FACILITY (Includes Hospital and Nursing Home Units)					
Utilization - Inpatient					
Beds	41,576	41,436	40,841	41,049	41,235
Admissions	1,068,234	1,075,155	1,046,824	1,133,257	1,132,000
Inpatient Days	6,629,988	6,592,263	6,190,167	6,399,323	6,387,419
Average Length of Stay	6.2	6.1	5.9	5.6	5.6
Inpatient Surgeries	216,952	231,037	263,620	297,298	286,320
Births	111,883	108,900	112,909	111,185	111,188
Utilization - Outpatient					
Emergency Outpatient Visits	9,472,349	8,731,807	8,406,870	9,557,119	9,306,326
Other Outpatient Visits	51,632,721	50,806,995	45,685,795	48,658,996	48,273,206
Total Outpatient Visits	61,105,070	59,538,802	54,092,665	58,216,115	57,579,532
Outpatient Surgeries	1,604,328	1,534,850	1,336,889	1,510,956	1,431,257
Personnel					
Full Time RNs	52,692	52,847	52,611	52,139	51,921
Full Time LPNs	8,455	8,038	8,166	7,935	7,945
Part Time RNs	37,195	36,370	34,559	35,206	32,476
Part Time LPNs	4,549	4,150	4,001	3,768	3,644
Total Full Time	239,715	236,769	228,285	227,492	225,583
Total Part Time	124,614	122,024	117,596	119,164	109,257
HOSPITAL UNIT (Excludes Separate Nursing Home Units)					
Utilization - Inpatient					
Beds	40,648	40,669	40,089	40,112	40,232
Admissions	1,066,746	1,073,731	1,045,856	1,131,886	1,130,378
Inpatient Days	6,378,735	6,362,955	5,953,529	6,096,572	6,078,511
Average Length of Stay	6.0	5.9	5.7	5.4	5.4
Personnel					
Total Full Time	239,088	236,317	227,649	226,715	224,796
Total Part Time	124,273	121,651	117,159	118,472	108,699

Bed Size Categories

Note: The 2021 performance data do not reflect the full impact of the COVID-19 pandemic. Please refer to the discussion in the Introduction for more information.

TABLE 4

BED SIZE CATEGORY 50-99

U.S. Community Hospitals
(Nonfederal, short-term general and other special hospitals)

Overview 2018–2022

	2022	2021	2020	2019	2018
Total Community Hospitals in					
Bed Size Category 50-99...................................	900	912	903	897	926
Location					
Hospitals Urban	561	568	552	538	554
Hospitals Rural..	339	344	351	359	372
Control					
State and Local Government.............................	129	137	139	140	140
Not for Profit...	450	448	438	440	456
Investor owned..	321	327	326	317	330
Affiliations					
Hospitals in a System	643	649	633	619	642
Hospitals in a Group Purchasing Organization...	510	528	518	532	558

Note: The 2021 performance data do not reflect the full impact of the COVID-19 pandemic. Please refer to the discussion in the Introduction for more information.

TABLE 4

BED SIZE CATEGORY 50-99

U.S. Community Hospitals
(Nonfederal, short-term general and other special hospitals)

Utilization, Personnel, Community Health Indicators 2018–2022

	2022	2021	2020	2019	2018
TOTAL FACILITY (Includes Hospital and Nursing Home Units)					
Utilization - Inpatient					
Beds	63,469	63,769	63,360	63,176	65,577
Admissions	1,885,514	1,851,454	1,781,982	1,927,731	1,952,262
Inpatient Days	13,094,514	13,010,321	12,211,485	12,627,390	12,870,385
Average Length of Stay	6.9	7.0	6.9	6.6	6.6
Inpatient Surgeries	351,591	353,815	373,092	434,339	440,205
Births	194,992	188,204	189,594	190,015	198,622
Utilization - Outpatient					
Emergency Outpatient Visits	11,224,622	10,288,408	9,570,228	11,440,166	11,795,684
Other Outpatient Visits	52,234,451	52,722,105	45,996,909	49,138,538	48,671,114
Total Outpatient Visits	63,459,073	63,010,513	55,567,137	60,578,704	60,466,798
Outpatient Surgeries	1,722,626	1,639,944	1,431,571	1,636,578	1,631,225
Personnel					
Full Time RNs	75,195	74,338	74,366	74,371	74,287
Full Time LPNs	7,180	7,186	6,963	6,858	7,164
Part Time RNs	45,613	44,872	43,074	42,678	41,920
Part Time LPNs	3,657	3,695	3,402	3,196	3,075
Total Full Time	293,834	290,681	285,487	278,717	279,600
Total Part Time	149,534	146,120	142,188	139,994	138,503
HOSPITAL UNIT (Excludes Separate Nursing Home Units)					
Utilization - Inpatient					
Beds	58,335	58,153	57,617	57,123	58,952
Admissions	1,879,086	1,843,776	1,774,837	1,918,858	1,940,103
Inpatient Days	11,662,939	11,471,031	10,493,273	10,706,740	10,830,300
Average Length of Stay	6.2	6.2	5.9	5.6	5.6
Personnel					
Total Full Time	291,095	287,058	281,719	275,188	275,781
Total Part Time	147,200	143,580	139,506	137,459	135,502

Note: The 2021 performance data do not reflect the full impact of the COVID-19 pandemic. Please refer to the discussion in the Introduction for more information.

TABLE 4

BED SIZE CATEGORY 100-199

U.S. Community Hospitals
(Nonfederal, short-term general and other special hospitals)

Overview 2018–2022

	2022	2021	2020	2019	2018
Total Community Hospitals in					
Bed Size Category 100-199	901	923	938	952	976
Location					
Hospitals Urban	682	706	712	720	737
Hospitals Rural	219	217	226	232	239
Control					
State and Local Government	105	100	106	104	108
Not for Profit	601	615	623	622	618
Investor owned	195	208	209	226	250
Affiliations					
Hospitals in a System	682	707	716	727	753
Hospitals in a Group Purchasing Organization	564	590	610	631	663

Note: The 2021 performance data do not reflect the full impact of the COVID-19 pandemic. Please refer to the discussion in the Introduction for more information.

TABLE 4

BED SIZE CATEGORY 100-199

U.S. Community Hospitals
(Nonfederal, short-term general and other special hospitals)

Utilization, Personnel, Community Health Indicators 2018–2022

	2022	2021	2020	2019	2018
TOTAL FACILITY (Includes Hospital and Nursing Home Units)					
Utilization - Inpatient					
Beds	130,451	132,786	134,575	136,707	140,651
Admissions	5,029,382	5,143,867	5,062,884	5,548,899	5,681,848
Inpatient Days	28,789,120	29,134,524	27,936,206	29,492,392	30,172,662
Average Length of Stay	5.7	5.7	5.5	5.3	5.3
Inpatient Surgeries	1,064,205	1,067,560	1,123,347	1,295,666	1,327,988
Births	547,525	568,904	575,668	585,757	613,615
Utilization - Outpatient					
Emergency Outpatient Visits	26,406,273	25,465,757	24,882,574	28,888,633	29,428,234
Other Outpatient Visits	106,925,245	104,924,596	101,234,585	111,813,825	109,134,141
Total Outpatient Visits	133,331,518	130,390,353	126,117,159	140,702,458	138,562,375
Outpatient Surgeries	3,396,052	3,263,262	2,938,937	3,409,716	3,492,140
Personnel					
Full Time RNs	173,320	177,436	186,690	189,072	191,742
Full Time LPNs	11,908	10,159	11,430	11,404	11,833
Part Time RNs	95,354	90,559	93,113	94,581	94,773
Part Time LPNs	4,258	3,729	3,887	4,151	4,317
Total Full Time	633,339	634,416	648,247	658,501	667,890
Total Part Time	289,832	277,798	279,783	285,005	282,551
HOSPITAL UNIT (Excludes Separate Nursing Home Units)					
Utilization - Inpatient					
Beds	122,457	124,511	125,845	126,528	130,053
Admissions	5,013,855	5,127,100	5,038,444	5,517,976	5,649,668
Inpatient Days	26,733,086	26,839,747	25,351,070	26,336,252	26,820,362
Average Length of Stay	5.3	5.2	5.0	4.8	4.7
Personnel					
Total Full Time	628,553	629,080	642,806	651,489	661,376
Total Part Time	286,447	274,502	276,515	280,866	278,786

Bed Size Categories

Note: The 2021 performance data do not reflect the full impact of the COVID-19 pandemic. Please refer to the discussion in the Introduction for more information.

TABLE 4

BED SIZE CATEGORY 200-299

U.S. Community Hospitals
(Nonfederal, short-term general and other special hospitals)

Overview 2018–2022

	2022	2021	2020	2019	2018
Total Community Hospitals in					
Bed Size Category 200-299..........................	483	502	503	515	534
Location					
Hospitals Urban	435	459	456	465	485
Hospitals Rural.....................................	48	43	47	50	49
Control					
State and Local Government............................	47	50	50	56	54
Not for Profit..	347	355	350	356	368
Investor owned......................................	89	97	103	103	112
Affiliations					
Hospitals in a System	390	398	393	402	415
Hospitals in a Group Purchasing Organization...	338	348	347	351	384

Note: The 2021 performance data do not reflect the full impact of the COVID-19 pandemic. Please refer to the discussion in the Introduction for more information.

TABLE 4   BED SIZE CATEGORY 200-299

U.S. Community Hospitals
(Nonfederal, short-term general and other special hospitals)

Utilization, Personnel, Community Health Indicators 2018–2022

	2022	2021	2020	2019	2018
TOTAL FACILITY (Includes Hospital and Nursing Home Units)					
Utilization - Inpatient					
Beds	118,181	122,271	122,653	125,372	130,039
Admissions	5,163,725	5,346,321	5,249,192	5,813,060	6,059,101
Inpatient Days	28,173,136	28,659,048	27,032,937	28,915,694	29,818,814
Average Length of Stay	5.5	5.4	5.1	5.0	4.9
Inpatient Surgeries	1,177,969	1,250,138	1,272,211	1,459,807	1,507,119
Births	604,832	602,673	605,728	639,859	668,737
Utilization - Outpatient					
Emergency Outpatient Visits	23,208,872	22,015,308	21,031,172	25,049,922	25,763,395
Other Outpatient Visits	88,961,313	90,192,706	82,772,027	90,507,436	91,108,227
Total Outpatient Visits	112,170,185	112,208,014	103,803,199	115,557,358	116,871,622
Outpatient Surgeries	2,805,793	2,888,509	2,591,570	2,962,199	3,028,436
Personnel					
Full Time RNs	184,175	188,036	196,126	199,684	200,697
Full Time LPNs	9,165	8,717	8,424	9,095	9,017
Part Time RNs	87,372	86,312	85,139	92,587	94,255
Part Time LPNs	3,595	2,820	2,534	2,778	2,980
Total Full Time	634,207	639,524	645,284	664,859	672,784
Total Part Time	244,217	239,541	237,852	253,497	261,448
HOSPITAL UNIT (Excludes Separate Nursing Home Units)					
Utilization - Inpatient					
Beds	114,496	118,246	118,173	121,032	125,081
Admissions	5,149,717	5,331,448	5,234,208	5,794,088	6,037,697
Inpatient Days	27,180,101	27,516,931	25,721,014	27,525,745	28,272,785
Average Length of Stay	5.3	5.2	4.9	4.8	4.7
Personnel					
Total Full Time	631,496	636,131	641,738	661,108	668,565
Total Part Time	242,998	238,125	236,031	251,566	259,006

Bed Size Categories

Note: The 2021 performance data do not reflect the full impact of the COVID-19 pandemic. Please refer to the discussion in the Introduction for more information.

TABLE 4

BED SIZE CATEGORY 300-399

U.S. Community Hospitals
(Nonfederal, short-term general and other special hospitals)

Overview 2018–2022

	2022	2021	2020	2019	2018
Total Community Hospitals in					
Bed Size Category 300-399............................	308	306	311	326	316
Location					
Hospitals Urban	297	293	299	312	301
Hospitals Rural...	11	13	12	14	15
Control					
State and Local Government.............................	22	22	22	26	27
Not for Profit..	241	241	249	259	244
Investor owned..	45	43	40	41	45
Affiliations					
Hospitals in a System	257	254	256	258	247
Hospitals in a Group Purchasing Organization...	223	243	239	251	252

Note: The 2021 performance data do not reflect the full impact of the COVID-19 pandemic. Please refer to the discussion in the Introduction for more information.

TABLE 4

BED SIZE CATEGORY 300-399

U.S. Community Hospitals
(Nonfederal, short-term general and other special hospitals)

Utilization, Personnel, Community Health Indicators 2018–2022

	2022	2021	2020	2019	2018
TOTAL FACILITY (Includes Hospital and Nursing Home Units)					
Utilization - Inpatient					
Beds	106,269	105,670	107,494	113,166	109,634
Admissions	4,642,693	4,668,193	4,732,330	5,412,719	5,238,165
Inpatient Days	25,800,156	25,538,621	24,803,949	27,379,817	26,539,470
Average Length of Stay	5.6	5.5	5.2	5.1	5.1
Inpatient Surgeries	1,057,855	1,102,387	1,168,713	1,339,783	1,282,576
Births	539,712	531,849	543,807	601,183	581,720
Utilization - Outpatient					
Emergency Outpatient Visits	17,674,452	16,263,867	16,288,879	19,952,051	19,039,409
Other Outpatient Visits	75,663,150	73,942,307	69,910,400	74,883,667	68,229,543
Total Outpatient Visits	93,337,602	90,206,174	86,199,279	94,835,718	87,268,952
Outpatient Surgeries	2,366,353	2,250,933	1,971,182	2,380,600	2,227,227
Personnel					
Full Time RNs	168,904	171,452	181,667	189,507	179,100
Full Time LPNs	6,463	6,076	5,174	6,205	6,066
Part Time RNs	76,832	74,348	75,633	77,986	70,873
Part Time LPNs	2,041	1,588	1,498	1,642	1,700
Total Full Time	554,762	555,118	574,333	609,571	571,379
Total Part Time	209,039	202,558	208,499	212,430	197,569
HOSPITAL UNIT (Excludes Separate Nursing Home Units)					
Utilization - Inpatient					
Beds	104,513	103,975	106,069	110,530	106,565
Admissions	4,634,351	4,661,796	4,724,279	5,396,430	5,219,274
Inpatient Days	25,339,730	25,091,360	24,421,181	26,553,307	25,593,987
Average Length of Stay	5.5	5.4	5.2	4.9	4.9
Personnel					
Total Full Time	553,563	553,671	573,448	607,659	569,151
Total Part Time	208,665	201,969	208,173	211,718	196,540

Bed Size Categories

Note: The 2021 performance data do not reflect the full impact of the COVID-19 pandemic. Please refer to the discussion in the Introduction for more information.

TABLE 4

BED SIZE CATEGORY 400-499

U.S. Community Hospitals
(Nonfederal, short-term general and other special hospitals)

Overview 2018–2022

	2022	2021	2020	2019	2018
Total Community Hospitals in					
Bed Size Category 400-499	176	164	173	163	172
Location					
Hospitals Urban	172	159	168	159	168
Hospitals Rural	4	5	5	4	4
Control					
State and Local Government	22	23	26	25	25
Not for Profit	129	118	126	116	125
Investor owned	25	23	21	22	22
Affiliations					
Hospitals in a System	140	126	130	120	126
Hospitals in a Group Purchasing Organization	134	123	131	120	141

Note: The 2021 performance data do not reflect the full impact of the COVID-19 pandemic. Please refer to the discussion in the Introduction for more information.

TABLE 4

BED SIZE CATEGORY 400-499

U.S. Community Hospitals
(Nonfederal, short-term general and other special hospitals)

Utilization, Personnel, Community Health Indicators 2018–2022

	2022	2021	2020	2019	2018
TOTAL FACILITY (Includes Hospital and Nursing Home Units)					
Utilization - Inpatient					
Beds	77,736	72,144	76,042	72,228	76,085
Admissions	3,394,631	3,199,749	3,280,568	3,394,108	3,640,816
Inpatient Days	20,077,453	18,311,449	18,025,664	18,087,000	19,206,768
Average Length of Stay	5.9	5.7	5.5	5.3	5.3
Inpatient Surgeries	852,354	780,555	830,187	927,948	998,127
Births	383,669	366,260	382,297	352,236	391,871
Utilization - Outpatient					
Emergency Outpatient Visits	12,795,398	11,251,812	11,410,965	12,204,408	12,996,637
Other Outpatient Visits	57,067,048	52,810,354	49,033,801	58,746,995	62,225,182
Total Outpatient Visits	69,862,446	64,062,166	60,444,766	70,951,403	75,221,819
Outpatient Surgeries	1,606,159	1,413,763	1,393,566	1,570,054	1,691,233
Personnel					
Full Time RNs	127,684	121,469	132,894	125,093	133,759
Full Time LPNs	4,981	3,477	3,984	3,874	4,552
Part Time RNs	61,422	55,192	57,857	58,605	61,069
Part Time LPNs	1,601	1,159	1,293	1,376	1,329
Total Full Time	433,684	407,682	429,204	432,759	465,042
Total Part Time	175,348	161,460	162,885	164,005	166,852
HOSPITAL UNIT (Excludes Separate Nursing Home Units)					
Utilization - Inpatient					
Beds	75,956	70,579	74,358	70,517	74,451
Admissions	3,388,456	3,193,672	3,273,422	3,387,037	3,632,418
Inpatient Days	19,556,959	17,880,890	17,507,247	17,520,212	18,667,855
Average Length of Stay	5.8	5.6	5.3	5.2	5.1
Personnel					
Total Full Time	432,645	406,741	427,666	431,441	463,521
Total Part Time	174,891	161,109	162,243	163,339	166,075

Bed Size Categories

Note: The 2021 performance data do not reflect the full impact of the COVID-19 pandemic. Please refer to the discussion in the Introduction for more information.

TABLE 4

BED SIZE CATEGORY 500 +

U.S. Community Hospitals
(Nonfederal, short-term general and other special hospitals)

Overview 2018–2022

	2022	2021	2020	2019	2018
Total Community Hospitals in					
Bed Size Category 500 + ...	307	316	307	297	292
Location					
Hospitals Urban	305	314	304	295	290
Hospitals Rural..	2	2	3	2	2
Control					
State and Local Government............................	55	56	55	51	49
Not for Profit..	232	239	229	225	223
Investor owned..	20	21	23	21	20
Affiliations					
Hospitals in a System	251	257	250	241	234
Hospitals in a Group Purchasing Organization...	273	279	276	267	262

Note: The 2021 performance data do not reflect the full impact of the COVID-19 pandemic. Please refer to the discussion in the Introduction for more information.

TABLE 4

BED SIZE CATEGORY 500 +

U.S. Community Hospitals
(Nonfederal, short-term general and other special hospitals)

Utilization, Personnel, Community Health Indicators 2018–2022

	2022	2021	2020	2019	2018
TOTAL FACILITY (Includes Hospital and Nursing Home Units)					
Utilization - Inpatient					
Beds	233,990	237,780	232,260	224,401	217,676
Admissions	10,073,896	10,392,783	9,951,718	10,520,220	10,246,777
Inpatient Days	64,883,757	64,958,289	59,802,755	60,883,964	58,943,011
Average Length of Stay	6.4	6.3	6.0	5.8	5.8
Inpatient Surgeries	2,858,651	2,933,344	2,890,482	3,104,899	3,061,516
Births	1,109,818	1,100,169	1,077,568	1,069,984	1,054,292
Utilization - Outpatient					
Emergency Outpatient Visits	32,445,157	29,901,419	28,844,740	33,199,342	32,250,912
Other Outpatient Visits	209,776,514	214,471,842	182,847,530	192,534,034	181,819,605
Total Outpatient Visits	242,221,671	244,373,261	211,692,270	225,733,376	214,070,517
Outpatient Surgeries	5,466,464	5,338,925	4,621,396	5,206,511	4,924,121
Personnel					
Full Time RNs	490,679	504,303	499,137	474,264	457,833
Full Time LPNs	16,811	15,869	15,460	15,094	14,708
Part Time RNs	186,479	177,680	169,864	161,135	152,668
Part Time LPNs	4,194	4,113	4,197	4,106	3,932
Total Full Time	1,773,806	1,767,641	1,718,455	1,651,526	1,593,642
Total Part Time	526,900	506,224	483,281	463,257	439,775
HOSPITAL UNIT (Excludes Separate Nursing Home Units)					
Utilization - Inpatient					
Beds	227,962	231,299	225,250	217,451	210,773
Admissions	10,055,884	10,372,647	9,927,208	10,491,026	10,220,761
Inpatient Days	63,196,655	63,185,370	57,711,923	58,604,990	56,684,311
Average Length of Stay	6.3	6.1	5.8	5.6	5.5
Personnel					
Total Full Time	1,768,304	1,762,163	1,713,590	1,646,011	1,588,235
Total Part Time	525,094	504,201	481,109	461,006	437,610

Bed Size Categories

Note: The 2021 performance data do not reflect the full impact of the COVID-19 pandemic. Please refer to the discussion in the Introduction for more information.

AHA Hospital Statistics © 2024 Health Forum LLC, an affiliate of the American Hospital Association

Census Divisions

Census Division 1

New England
Connecticut, Maine, Massachusetts, New Hampshire, Rhode Island, Vermont

Census Division 2

Middle Atlantic
New Jersey, New York, Pennsylvania

Census Division 3

South Atlantic
Delaware, District of Columbia, Florida, Georgia, Maryland, North Carolina, South Carolina, Virginia, West Virginia

Census Division 4

East North Central
Illinois, Indiana, Michigan, Ohio, Wisconsin

Census Division 5

East South Central
Alabama, Kentucky, Mississippi, Tennessee

Census Division 6

West North Central
Iowa, Kansas, Minnesota, Missouri, Nebraska, North Dakota, South Dakota

Census Division 7

West South Central
Arkansas, Louisiana, Oklahoma, Texas

Census Division 8

Mountain
Arizona, Colorado, Idaho, Montana, Nevada, New Mexico, Utah, Wyoming

Census Division 9

Pacific
Alaska, California, Hawaii, Oregon, Washington

Note: The 2021 performance data do not reflect the full impact of the COVID-19 pandemic. Please refer to the discussion in the Introduction for more information.

TABLE 5

U.S. CENSUS DIVISION 1: NEW ENGLAND

U.S. Community Hospitals
(Nonfederal, short-term general and other special hospitals)

Overview 2018–2022

	2022	2021	2020	2019	2018
Total Community Hospitals **in Census Division 1, New England**	191	193	192	192	194
Bed Size Category					
6-24	11	11	10	10	6
25-49	41	39	39	40	43
50-99	39	40	42	41	46
100-199	48	50	51	52	49
200-299	24	21	19	20	21
300-399	12	14	14	13	13
400-499	4	7	6	7	6
500 + ...	12	11	11	9	10
Location					
Hospitals Urban	135	139	138	138	140
Hospitals Rural...	56	54	54	54	54
Control					
State and Local Government	4	4	5	5	5
Not for Profit..	164	165	164	164	165
Investor owned...	23	24	23	23	24
Affiliations					
Hospitals in a System	134	135	128	125	124
Hospitals in a Group Purchasing Organization...	122	128	125	130	130

Note: The 2021 performance data do not reflect the full impact of the COVID-19 pandemic. Please refer to the discussion in the Introduction for more information.

TABLE 5

U.S. CENSUS DIVISION 1: NEW ENGLAND

U.S. Community Hospitals
(Nonfederal, short-term general and other special hospitals)

Utilization, Personnel, Community Health Indicators 2018–2022

	2022	2021	2020	2019	2018
TOTAL FACILITY (Includes Hospital and Nursing Home Units)					
Utilization - Inpatient					
Beds	33,234	33,363	33,169	32,559	32,518
Admissions	1,461,305	1,478,509	1,456,670	1,567,740	1,568,835
Inpatient Days	9,195,363	8,919,953	8,392,111	8,682,964	8,594,184
Average Length of Stay	6.3	6.0	5.8	5.5	5.5
Inpatient Surgeries	336,661	355,161	362,626	408,843	404,164
Births	141,485	142,174	139,729	140,837	141,919
Utilization - Outpatient					
Emergency Outpatient Visits	6,975,161	6,615,842	6,365,187	7,366,120	7,232,392
Other Outpatient Visits	46,914,934	48,474,430	40,249,513	42,698,043	41,702,724
Total Outpatient Visits	53,890,095	55,090,272	46,614,700	50,064,163	48,935,116
Outpatient Surgeries	956,949	919,438	790,718	962,963	944,218
Personnel					
Full Time RNs	60,346	60,340	60,341	59,673	55,675
Full Time LPNs	2,054	1,796	1,797	1,780	1,751
Part Time RNs	44,884	44,146	43,892	44,256	43,281
Part Time LPNs	1,212	955	914	927	961
Total Full Time	263,610	262,931	256,675	257,916	250,096
Total Part Time	143,657	138,544	136,123	134,921	132,766
HOSPITAL UNIT (Excludes Separate Nursing Home Units)					
Utilization - Inpatient					
Beds	32,366	32,499	32,305	31,709	31,668
Admissions	1,459,482	1,477,164	1,455,081	1,565,910	1,566,971
Inpatient Days	8,950,300	8,690,753	8,121,139	8,418,636	8,331,410
Average Length of Stay	6.1	5.9	5.6	5.4	5.3
Personnel					
Total Full Time	263,111	262,434	255,887	257,053	249,149
Total Part Time	143,249	138,133	135,549	134,266	131,956
COMMUNITY HEALTH INDICATORS PER 1000 POPULATION					
Total Population (in thousands)	15,130	15,093	14,847	14,845	14,853
Inpatient					
Beds	2.2	2.2	2.2	2.2	2.2
Admissions	96.6	98	98.1	105.6	105.6
Inpatient Days	607.8	591	565.2	584.9	578.6
Inpatient Surgeries	22.3	23.5	24.4	27.5	27.2
Births	9.4	9.4	9.4	9.5	9.6
Outpatient					
Emergency Outpatient Visits	461	438.3	428.7	496.2	486.9
Other Outpatient Visits	3,100.9	3,211.8	2,710.9	2,876.2	2,807.6
Total Outpatient Visits	3,561.9	3,650.1	3,139.6	3,372.4	3,294.6
Outpatient Surgeries	63.3	60.9	53.3	64.9	63.6

U.S. Census Divisions

Note: The 2021 performance data do not reflect the full impact of the COVID-19 pandemic. Please refer to the discussion in the Introduction for more information.

AHA Hospital Statistics © 2024 Health Forum LLC, an affiliate of the American Hospital Association

TABLE 5 U.S. CENSUS DIVISION 2: MIDDLE ATLANTIC

U.S. Community Hospitals
(Nonfederal, short-term general and other special hospitals)

Overview 2018–2022

	2022	2021	2020	2019	2018
Total Community Hospitals					
in Census Division 2, Middle Atlantic	**424**	**426**	**429**	**435**	**447**
Bed Size Category					
6-24	28	26	24	23	20
25-49	49	46	45	46	50
50-99	66	70	70	66	70
100-199	95	98	104	115	115
200-299	65	68	65	62	72
300-399	46	43	47	48	44
400-499	18	17	18	21	24
500 + ...	57	58	56	54	52
Location					
Hospitals Urban	347	357	360	366	375
Hospitals Rural	77	69	69	69	72
Control					
State and Local Government	27	27	28	27	25
Not for Profit	343	345	344	348	355
Investor owned	54	54	57	60	67
Affiliations					
Hospitals in a System	302	301	303	301	312
Hospitals in a Group Purchasing Organization...	272	284	292	292	305

Note: The 2021 performance data do not reflect the full impact of the COVID-19 pandemic. Please refer to the discussion in the Introduction for more information.

TABLE 5

U.S. CENSUS DIVISION 2: MIDDLE ATLANTIC

U.S. Community Hospitals
(Nonfederal, short-term general and other special hospitals)

Utilization, Personnel, Community Health Indicators 2018–2022

	2022	2021	2020	2019	2018
TOTAL FACILITY (Includes Hospital and Nursing Home Units)					
Utilization - Inpatient					
Beds	106,265	106,808	108,046	108,395	109,558
Admissions	4,314,139	4,513,245	4,344,122	4,847,024	4,919,808
Inpatient Days	27,976,453	27,658,029	26,282,445	28,091,060	28,429,768
Average Length of Stay	6.5	6.1	6.1	5.8	5.8
Inpatient Surgeries	1,052,716	1,086,678	1,083,481	1,210,079	1,240,226
Births	425,696	429,428	426,512	437,062	449,748
Utilization - Outpatient					
Emergency Outpatient Visits	17,442,118	16,461,972	15,516,505	18,582,130	18,746,561
Other Outpatient Visits	102,147,671	104,889,407	89,091,153	97,478,356	95,944,515
Total Outpatient Visits	119,589,789	121,351,379	104,607,658	116,060,486	114,691,076
Outpatient Surgeries	2,732,466	2,670,791	2,379,609	2,753,593	2,651,080
Personnel					
Full Time RNs	195,190	196,554	200,526	196,433	191,768
Full Time LPNs	8,038	7,824	8,134	7,996	8,418
Part Time RNs	66,230	62,118	63,475	63,586	64,203
Part Time LPNs	2,189	2,029	2,070	2,167	2,387
Total Full Time	755,472	744,665	732,489	731,633	715,362
Total Part Time	210,002	202,795	203,798	204,982	211,260
HOSPITAL UNIT (Excludes Separate Nursing Home Units)					
Utilization - Inpatient					
Beds	101,478	101,415	102,105	102,125	102,862
Admissions	4,300,599	4,496,571	4,323,023	4,821,486	4,895,085
Inpatient Days	26,635,856	26,046,671	24,498,243	25,982,699	26,173,836
Average Length of Stay	6.2	5.8	5.7	5.4	5.3
Personnel					
Total Full Time	751,867	740,696	728,501	726,842	710,333
Total Part Time	208,366	200,879	201,341	202,385	208,325
COMMUNITY HEALTH INDICATORS PER 1000 POPULATION					
Total Population (in thousands)	41,911	42,067	41,002	41,138	41,258
Inpatient					
Beds	2.5	2.5	2.6	2.6	2.7
Admissions	102.9	107.3	105.9	117.8	119.2
Inpatient Days	667.5	657.5	641	682.9	689.1
Inpatient Surgeries	25.1	25.8	26.4	29.4	30.1
Births	10.2	10.2	10.4	10.6	10.9
Outpatient					
Emergency Outpatient Visits	416.2	391.3	378.4	451.7	454.4
Other Outpatient Visits	2,437.3	2,493.4	2,172.8	2,369.6	2,325.5
Total Outpatient Visits	2,853.4	2,884.7	2,551.3	2,821.3	2,779.9
Outpatient Surgeries	65.2	63.5	58	66.9	64.3

Note: The 2021 performance data do not reflect the full impact of the COVID-19 pandemic. Please refer to the discussion in the Introduction for more information.

TABLE 5

U.S. CENSUS DIVISION 3: SOUTH ATLANTIC

U.S. Community Hospitals
(Nonfederal, short-term general and other special hospitals)

Overview 2018–2022

	2022	2021	2020	2019	2018
Total Community Hospitals in Census Division 3, South Atlantic.............	**748**	**759**	**756**	**752**	**762**
Bed Size Category					
6-24	46	46	47	42	38
25-49	131	138	128	127	139
50-99	149	148	146	151	150
100-199	162	166	172	170	170
200-299	105	104	103	102	107
300-399	49	54	56	59	56
400-499	34	30	34	31	34
500 + ...	72	73	70	70	68
Location					
Hospitals Urban	561	580	576	571	575
Hospitals Rural...	187	179	180	181	187
Control					
State and Local Government	114	115	112	119	116
Not for Profit..	428	435	436	431	422
Investor owned...	206	209	208	202	224
Affiliations					
Hospitals in a System	625	628	621	608	609
Hospitals in a Group Purchasing Organization...	419	423	420	425	465

Note: The 2021 performance data do not reflect the full impact of the COVID-19 pandemic. Please refer to the discussion in the Introduction for more information.

TABLE 5

U.S. CENSUS DIVISION 3: SOUTH ATLANTIC

U.S. Community Hospitals
(Nonfederal, short-term general and other special hospitals)

Utilization, Personnel, Community Health Indicators 2018–2022

	2022	2021	2020	2019	2018
TOTAL FACILITY (Includes Hospital and Nursing Home Units)					
Utilization - Inpatient					
Beds	154,452	154,862	154,162	155,077	155,252
Admissions	6,660,227	6,692,136	6,535,175	7,091,809	7,048,355
Inpatient Days	39,353,416	39,418,948	36,926,714	38,487,726	38,380,244
Average Length of Stay	5.9	5.9	5.7	5.4	5.4
Inpatient Surgeries	1,594,810	1,607,536	1,692,826	1,837,512	1,818,474
Births	691,234	670,394	679,051	681,302	693,224
Utilization - Outpatient					
Emergency Outpatient Visits	27,712,049	25,532,045	25,448,326	29,444,522	29,421,949
Other Outpatient Visits	95,938,835	94,718,073	86,788,453	96,031,889	91,349,681
Total Outpatient Visits	123,650,884	120,250,118	112,236,779	125,476,411	120,771,630
Outpatient Surgeries	3,776,001	3,640,795	3,211,696	3,531,359	3,534,616
Personnel					
Full Time RNs	257,643	261,206	272,345	265,371	260,893
Full Time LPNs	12,845	11,418	10,864	10,945	11,322
Part Time RNs	91,345	87,621	84,685	86,674	84,678
Part Time LPNs	3,749	3,123	2,730	2,981	3,164
Total Full Time	883,643	874,220	879,078	873,851	853,293
Total Part Time	265,269	247,702	243,413	248,136	240,572
HOSPITAL UNIT (Excludes Separate Nursing Home Units)					
Utilization - Inpatient					
Beds	149,026	149,138	148,159	148,208	148,197
Admissions	6,646,282	6,676,715	6,515,092	7,065,484	7,022,307
Inpatient Days	37,908,639	37,860,488	35,189,743	36,367,150	36,163,691
Average Length of Stay	5.7	5.7	5.4	5.1	5.1
Personnel					
Total Full Time	880,022	869,734	874,103	868,270	847,710
Total Part Time	264,137	246,080	241,710	246,157	238,701
COMMUNITY HEALTH INDICATORS PER 1000 POPULATION					
Total Population (in thousands)	67,453	66,586	66,393	65,785	65,322
Inpatient					
Beds	2.3	2.3	2.3	2.4	2.4
Admissions	98.7	100.5	98.4	107.8	107.9
Inpatient Days	583.4	592	556.2	585.1	587.6
Inpatient Surgeries	23.6	24.1	25.5	27.9	27.8
Births	10.2	10.1	10.2	10.4	10.6
Outpatient					
Emergency Outpatient Visits	410.8	383.4	383.3	447.6	450.4
Other Outpatient Visits	1,422.3	1,422.5	1,307.2	1,459.8	1,398.4
Total Outpatient Visits	1,833.1	1,805.9	1,690.5	1,907.4	1,848.9
Outpatient Surgeries	56	54.7	48.4	53.7	54.1

U.S. Census Divisions

Note: The 2021 performance data do not reflect the full impact of the COVID-19 pandemic. Please refer to the discussion in the Introduction for more information.

AHA Hospital Statistics © 2024 Health Forum LLC, an affiliate of the American Hospital Association

TABLE 5

U.S. CENSUS DIVISION 4: EAST NORTH CENTRAL

U.S. Community Hospitals
(Nonfederal, short-term general and other special hospitals)

Overview 2018–2022

	2022	2021	2020	2019	2018
Total Community Hospitals					
in Census Division 4, East North Central	**771**	**774**	**780**	**786**	**790**
Bed Size Category					
6-24	99	94	95	91	94
25-49	215	216	217	214	204
50-99	127	123	119	127	130
100-199	137	141	151	147	153
200-299	76	85	84	93	98
300-399	47	44	44	44	39
400-499	29	29	28	29	30
500 + ...	41	42	42	41	42
Location					
Hospitals Urban	505	510	515	520	523
Hospitals Rural	266	264	265	266	267
Control					
State and Local Government	66	69	72	72	73
Not for Profit	590	591	591	594	592
Investor owned	115	114	117	120	125
Affiliations					
Hospitals in a System	563	566	568	567	563
Hospitals in a Group Purchasing Organization...	521	565	573	575	595

Note: The 2021 performance data do not reflect the full impact of the COVID-19 pandemic. Please refer to the discussion in the Introduction for more information.

TABLE 5

U.S. CENSUS DIVISION 4: EAST NORTH CENTRAL

U.S. Community Hospitals
(Nonfederal, short-term general and other special hospitals)

Utilization, Personnel, Community Health Indicators 2018–2022

	2022	2021	2020	2019	2018
TOTAL FACILITY (Includes Hospital and Nursing Home Units)					
Utilization - Inpatient					
Beds	116,292	117,782	119,113	119,505	120,431
Admissions	4,662,619	4,772,826	4,680,703	5,110,267	5,172,215
Inpatient Days	26,231,354	26,186,732	24,820,857	26,249,955	26,044,143
Average Length of Stay	5.6	5.5	5.3	5.1	5.0
Inpatient Surgeries	1,089,025	1,140,500	1,171,110	1,355,515	1,358,165
Births	469,439	475,637	477,262	494,785	509,652
Utilization - Outpatient					
Emergency Outpatient Visits	21,369,744	20,466,479	19,559,933	23,077,533	23,484,742
Other Outpatient Visits	146,138,265	143,105,238	129,002,580	142,254,069	137,450,943
Total Outpatient Visits	167,508,009	163,571,717	148,562,513	165,331,602	160,935,685
Outpatient Surgeries	3,396,511	3,334,801	3,008,160	3,475,789	3,376,611
Personnel					
Full Time RNs	190,769	198,772	210,101	207,972	210,140
Full Time LPNs	8,016	7,238	7,490	7,667	7,375
Part Time RNs	108,099	99,555	101,398	103,444	100,904
Part Time LPNs	3,958	3,286	3,378	3,528	3,300
Total Full Time	710,394	721,655	732,983	741,577	739,498
Total Part Time	339,403	315,621	317,325	330,869	313,164
HOSPITAL UNIT (Excludes Separate Nursing Home Units)					
Utilization - Inpatient					
Beds	113,798	114,764	115,838	116,132	116,940
Admissions	4,653,368	4,762,358	4,668,965	5,093,042	5,154,039
Inpatient Days	25,547,414	25,422,085	23,907,943	25,168,834	25,004,277
Average Length of Stay	5.5	5.3	5.1	4.9	4.9
Personnel					
Total Full Time	708,826	719,417	731,203	739,612	737,274
Total Part Time	338,174	314,133	316,116	329,394	311,753
COMMUNITY HEALTH INDICATORS PER 1000 POPULATION					
Total Population (in thousands)	47,098	47,204	46,835	46,902	46,932
Inpatient					
Beds	2.5	2.5	2.5	2.5	2.6
Admissions	99	101.1	99.9	109	110.2
Inpatient Days	557	554.8	530	559.7	554.9
Inpatient Surgeries	23.1	24.2	25	28.9	28.9
Births	10	10.1	10.2	10.5	10.9
Outpatient					
Emergency Outpatient Visits	453.7	433.6	417.6	492	500.4
Other Outpatient Visits	3,102.9	3,031.6	2,754.4	3,033	2,928.7
Total Outpatient Visits	3,556.6	3,465.2	3,172	3,525	3,429.1
Outpatient Surgeries	72.1	70.6	64.2	74.1	71.9

Note: The 2021 performance data do not reflect the full impact of the COVID-19 pandemic. Please refer to the discussion in the Introduction for more information.

AHA Hospital Statistics © 2024 Health Forum LLC, an affiliate of the American Hospital Association

TABLE 5

U.S. CENSUS DIVISION 5: EAST SOUTH CENTRAL

U.S. Community Hospitals
(Nonfederal, short-term general and other special hospitals)

Overview 2018–2022

	2022	2021	2020	2019	2018
Total Community Hospitals					
in Census Division 5, East South Central......	**417**	**415**	**413**	**414**	**420**
Bed Size Category					
6-24	28	26	24	26	23
25-49	137	135	128	128	129
50-99	81	80	87	87	92
100-199	87	89	84	86	87
200-299	28	30	36	33	32
300-399	22	22	19	20	23
400-499	11	10	13	12	11
500 + ...	23	23	22	22	23
Location					
Hospitals Urban	211	205	205	206	208
Hospitals Rural...	206	210	208	208	212
Control					
State and Local Government	104	105	105	107	106
Not for Profit..	187	185	184	186	187
Investor owned...	126	125	124	121	127
Affiliations					
Hospitals in a System	299	295	291	291	296
Hospitals in a Group Purchasing Organization...	203	201	217	219	234

Note: The 2021 performance data do not reflect the full impact of the COVID-19 pandemic. Please refer to the discussion in the Introduction for more information.

TABLE 5

U.S. CENSUS DIVISION 5: EAST SOUTH CENTRAL

U.S. Community Hospitals
(Nonfederal, short-term general and other special hospitals)

Utilization, Personnel, Community Health Indicators 2018–2022

	2022	2021	2020	2019	2018
TOTAL FACILITY (Includes Hospital and Nursing Home Units)					
Utilization - Inpatient					
Beds	59,997	60,128	60,615	59,389	61,065
Admissions	2,168,039	2,221,409	2,226,742	2,374,549	2,376,945
Inpatient Days	13,876,228	13,858,396	13,286,488	13,613,204	13,684,891
Average Length of Stay	6.4	6.2	6.0	5.7	5.8
Inpatient Surgeries	541,029	567,245	618,139	679,486	653,249
Births	210,306	215,745	221,308	219,009	206,549
Utilization - Outpatient					
Emergency Outpatient Visits	9,051,859	8,723,334	8,782,248	10,371,715	10,182,201
Other Outpatient Visits	36,701,799	36,557,888	33,293,462	36,956,859	35,982,640
Total Outpatient Visits	45,753,658	45,281,222	42,075,710	47,328,574	46,164,841
Outpatient Surgeries	1,487,471	1,391,079	1,291,845	1,493,309	1,441,870
Personnel					
Full Time RNs	88,023	88,805	90,818	89,609	88,794
Full Time LPNs	5,547	5,211	5,282	5,212	5,312
Part Time RNs	34,272	34,264	31,946	32,322	30,742
Part Time LPNs	2,152	1,911	1,502	1,588	1,478
Total Full Time	301,176	298,632	299,234	294,223	292,690
Total Part Time	97,337	96,157	89,302	89,322	86,272
HOSPITAL UNIT (Excludes Separate Nursing Home Units)					
Utilization - Inpatient					
Beds	57,974	57,651	57,805	56,560	57,886
Admissions	2,162,472	2,215,385	2,219,705	2,366,700	2,366,974
Inpatient Days	13,287,014	13,161,590	12,388,430	12,696,422	12,659,569
Average Length of Stay	6.1	5.9	5.6	5.4	5.3
Personnel					
Total Full Time	299,745	296,906	296,988	291,944	290,865
Total Part Time	96,762	95,522	88,578	88,576	85,582
COMMUNITY HEALTH INDICATORS PER 1000 POPULATION					
Total Population (in thousands)	19,578	19,474	19,252	19,176	19,113
Inpatient					
Beds	3.1	3.1	3.1	3.1	3.2
Admissions	110.7	114.1	115.7	123.8	124.4
Inpatient Days	708.8	711.6	690.1	709.9	716
Inpatient Surgeries	27.6	29.1	32.1	35.4	34.2
Births	10.7	11.1	11.5	11.4	10.8
Outpatient					
Emergency Outpatient Visits	462.3	447.9	456.2	540.9	532.7
Other Outpatient Visits	1,874.6	1,877.2	1,729.3	1,927.2	1,882.6
Total Outpatient Visits	2,337	2,325.2	2,185.5	2,468.1	2,415.4
Outpatient Surgeries	76	71.4	67.1	77.9	75.4

Note: The 2021 performance data do not reflect the full impact of the COVID-19 pandemic. Please refer to the discussion in the Introduction for more information.

TABLE 5

U.S. CENSUS DIVISION 6: WEST NORTH CENTRAL

U.S. Community Hospitals
(Nonfederal, short-term general and other special hospitals)

Overview 2018–2022

	2022	2021	2020	2019	2018
Total Community Hospitals					
in Census Division 6, West North Central	685	688	685	690	695
Bed Size Category					
6-24	200	189	189	184	174
25-49	195	203	200	207	217
50-99	132	137	132	131	134
100-199	80	78	81	82	83
200-299	23	26	28	31	29
300-399	18	20	20	23	25
400-499	16	12	11	9	10
500 +	21	23	24	23	23
Location					
Hospitals Urban	252	253	251	252	257
Hospitals Rural	433	435	434	438	438
Control					
State and Local Government	207	213	213	219	221
Not for Profit	410	403	404	401	402
Investor owned	68	72	68	70	72
Affiliations					
Hospitals in a System	389	386	385	393	396
Hospitals in a Group Purchasing Organization...	490	495	513	505	530

Note: The 2021 performance data do not reflect the full impact of the COVID-19 pandemic. Please refer to the discussion in the Introduction for more information.

TABLE 5

U.S. CENSUS DIVISION 6: WEST NORTH CENTRAL

U.S. Community Hospitals
(Nonfederal, short-term general and other special hospitals)

Utilization, Personnel, Community Health Indicators 2018–2022

	2022	2021	2020	2019	2018
TOTAL FACILITY (Includes Hospital and Nursing Home Units)					
Utilization - Inpatient					
Beds	63,709	64,399	65,102	65,660	65,986
Admissions	2,098,619	2,178,522	2,172,531	2,350,517	2,394,336
Inpatient Days	13,888,858	13,871,966	13,445,304	14,357,163	14,276,160
Average Length of Stay	6.6	6.4	6.2	6.1	6.0
Inpatient Surgeries	523,919	531,716	558,795	637,623	642,326
Births	235,386	233,694	240,548	248,734	254,862
Utilization - Outpatient					
Emergency Outpatient Visits	8,929,279	8,227,990	7,982,261	9,072,506	9,097,043
Other Outpatient Visits	67,531,676	66,175,621	61,126,598	63,541,419	61,459,345
Total Outpatient Visits	76,460,955	74,403,611	69,108,859	72,613,925	70,556,388
Outpatient Surgeries	1,600,152	1,555,390	1,350,764	1,546,701	1,511,307
Personnel					
Full Time RNs	86,434	92,259	93,722	92,304	89,720
Full Time LPNs	7,120	7,126	7,513	7,521	7,478
Part Time RNs	68,420	65,973	66,095	65,646	63,857
Part Time LPNs	3,705	3,650	4,113	3,924	3,932
Total Full Time	338,546	344,704	361,725	362,149	360,002
Total Part Time	198,495	195,577	192,023	188,614	184,236
HOSPITAL UNIT (Excludes Separate Nursing Home Units)					
Utilization - Inpatient					
Beds	57,617	58,426	58,871	59,187	58,686
Admissions	2,090,036	2,169,665	2,162,471	2,338,478	2,380,728
Inpatient Days	12,289,341	12,196,579	11,561,541	12,245,081	11,954,884
Average Length of Stay	5.9	5.6	5.3	5.2	5.0
Personnel					
Total Full Time	335,703	341,348	358,455	358,581	356,186
Total Part Time	195,180	192,568	188,878	185,236	180,414
COMMUNITY HEALTH INDICATORS PER 1000 POPULATION					
Total Population (in thousands)	21,690	21,637	21,482	21,427	21,377
Inpatient					
Beds	2.9	3	3	3.1	3.1
Admissions	96.8	100.7	101.1	109.7	112
Inpatient Days	640.3	641.1	625.9	670.1	667.8
Inpatient Surgeries	24.2	24.6	26	29.8	30
Births	10.9	10.8	11.2	11.6	11.9
Outpatient					
Emergency Outpatient Visits	411.7	380.3	371.6	423.4	425.6
Other Outpatient Visits	3,113.5	3,058.4	2,845.5	2,965.5	2,875
Total Outpatient Visits	3,525.2	3,438.7	3,217.1	3,389	3,300.6
Outpatient Surgeries	73.8	71.9	62.9	72.2	70.7

Note: The 2021 performance data do not reflect the full impact of the COVID-19 pandemic. Please refer to the discussion in the Introduction for more information.

AHA Hospital Statistics © 2024 Health Forum LLC, an affiliate of the American Hospital Association

TABLE 5

U.S. CENSUS DIVISION 7: WEST SOUTH CENTRAL

U.S. Community Hospitals
(Nonfederal, short-term general and other special hospitals)

Overview 2018–2022

	2022	2021	2020	2019	2018
Total Community Hospitals **in Census Division 7, West South Central**.....	**886**	**894**	**894**	**880**	**894**
Bed Size Category					
6-24	220	218	225	216	215
25-49	278	274	272	273	270
50-99	148	154	147	137	146
100-199	86	93	96	105	113
200-299	58	59	59	58	57
300-399	40	42	36	41	41
400-499	19	13	19	12	14
500 + ...	37	41	40	38	38
Location					
Hospitals Urban	605	612	612	597	609
Hospitals Rural..............................	281	282	282	283	285
Control					
State and Local Government	186	189	190	192	197
Not for Profit................................	300	300	295	283	277
Investor owned..............................	400	405	409	405	420
Affiliations					
Hospitals in a System	530	541	536	517	533
Hospitals in a Group Purchasing Organization...	673	685	683	680	687

Note: The 2021 performance data do not reflect the full impact of the COVID-19 pandemic. Please refer to the discussion in the Introduction for more information.

TABLE 5

U.S. CENSUS DIVISION 7: WEST SOUTH CENTRAL

U.S. Community Hospitals
(Nonfederal, short-term general and other special hospitals)

Utilization, Personnel, Community Health Indicators 2018–2022

	2022	2021	2020	2019	2018
TOTAL FACILITY (Includes Hospital and Nursing Home Units)					
Utilization - Inpatient					
Beds	101,418	102,242	102,343	100,863	101,604
Admissions	4,022,285	4,007,114	3,918,093	4,159,278	4,111,344
Inpatient Days	22,552,597	22,789,678	21,180,499	21,792,893	21,799,328
Average Length of Stay	5.6	5.7	5.4	5.2	5.3
Inpatient Surgeries	1,008,858	1,012,565	1,022,557	1,121,608	1,147,081
Births	525,555	504,012	507,834	517,514	524,852
Utilization - Outpatient					
Emergency Outpatient Visits	18,366,124	16,699,105	16,145,506	18,544,338	18,555,948
Other Outpatient Visits	56,593,769	54,616,454	49,479,140	56,540,198	54,642,033
Total Outpatient Visits	74,959,893	71,315,559	65,624,646	75,084,536	73,197,981
Outpatient Surgeries	2,386,922	2,311,650	2,022,827	2,296,243	2,258,979
Personnel					
Full Time RNs	160,068	157,939	164,128	163,209	160,967
Full Time LPNs	13,320	12,331	12,310	12,527	12,490
Part Time RNs	50,264	48,544	47,180	46,173	45,531
Part Time LPNs	3,615	3,557	3,208	2,998	2,975
Total Full Time	515,602	503,899	506,531	510,946	506,553
Total Part Time	138,817	135,571	132,070	127,495	128,010
HOSPITAL UNIT (Excludes Separate Nursing Home Units)					
Utilization - Inpatient					
Beds	100,435	101,228	101,300	99,373	100,186
Admissions	4,018,095	4,003,551	3,914,269	4,153,930	4,104,425
Inpatient Days	22,343,977	22,547,399	20,889,706	21,382,592	21,389,647
Average Length of Stay	5.6	5.6	5.3	5.1	5.2
Personnel					
Total Full Time	514,699	503,006	505,885	509,878	505,468
Total Part Time	138,683	135,392	131,872	127,277	127,784
COMMUNITY HEALTH INDICATORS PER 1000 POPULATION					
Total Population (in thousands)	41,685	41,165	41,017	40,619	40,319
Inpatient					
Beds	2.4	2.5	2.5	2.5	2.5
Admissions	96.5	97.3	95.5	102.4	102
Inpatient Days	541	553.6	516.4	536.5	540.7
Inpatient Surgeries	24.2	24.6	24.9	27.6	28.5
Births	12.6	12.2	12.4	12.7	13
Outpatient					
Emergency Outpatient Visits	440.6	405.7	393.6	456.5	460.2
Other Outpatient Visits	1,357.6	1,326.8	1,206.3	1,391.9	1,355.3
Total Outpatient Visits	1,798.2	1,732.5	1,599.9	1,848.5	1,815.5
Outpatient Surgeries	57.3	56.2	49.3	56.5	56

Note: The 2021 performance data do not reflect the full impact of the COVID-19 pandemic. Please refer to the discussion in the Introduction for more information.

TABLE 5   U.S. CENSUS DIVISION 8: MOUNTAIN

U.S. Community Hospitals
(Nonfederal, short-term general and other special hospitals)

Overview 2018–2022

	2022	2021	2020	2019	2018
Total Community Hospitals					
in Census Division 8, Mountain	456	454	443	439	441
Bed Size Category					
6-24	95	98	90	95	92
25-49	137	133	127	124	124
50-99	82	78	83	80	79
100-199	63	64	63	60	68
200-299	29	31	31	33	35
300-399	24	21	19	20	18
400-499	8	11	13	11	10
500 +	18	18	17	16	15
Location					
Hospitals Urban	260	255	246	240	243
Hospitals Rural	196	199	197	199	198
Control					
State and Local Government	90	93	96	94	95
Not for Profit	233	224	216	215	212
Investor owned	133	137	131	130	134
Affiliations					
Hospitals in a System	285	281	277	275	282
Hospitals in a Group Purchasing Organization...	220	232	231	228	249

Note: The 2021 performance data do not reflect the full impact of the COVID-19 pandemic. Please refer to the discussion in the Introduction for more information.

TABLE 5

U.S. CENSUS DIVISION 8: MOUNTAIN

U.S. Community Hospitals
(Nonfederal, short-term general and other special hospitals)

Utilization, Personnel, Community Health Indicators 2018–2022

	2022	2021	2020	2019	2018
TOTAL FACILITY (Includes Hospital and Nursing Home Units)					
Utilization - Inpatient					
Beds	50,822	51,250	50,731	49,513	49,444
Admissions	1,998,233	2,012,148	1,986,777	2,112,291	2,147,839
Inpatient Days	11,337,363	11,407,159	10,738,480	10,799,364	10,874,737
Average Length of Stay	5.7	5.7	5.4	5.1	5.1
Inpatient Surgeries	487,159	483,244	495,334	563,422	572,138
Births	248,784	252,956	245,101	258,112	263,794
Utilization - Outpatient					
Emergency Outpatient Visits	8,789,979	8,081,680	7,730,715	8,569,341	8,562,516
Other Outpatient Visits	39,007,305	40,048,495	36,059,996	35,478,058	35,421,848
Total Outpatient Visits	47,797,284	48,130,175	43,790,711	44,047,399	43,984,364
Outpatient Surgeries	1,221,585	1,191,487	1,021,552	1,170,024	1,211,911
Personnel					
Full Time RNs	82,573	82,767	83,961	83,816	85,140
Full Time LPNs	3,401	2,864	2,893	2,840	2,869
Part Time RNs	35,451	37,141	36,016	33,533	31,574
Part Time LPNs	1,380	1,213	1,234	1,200	1,083
Total Full Time	283,141	282,890	277,914	277,723	281,487
Total Part Time	99,196	104,114	103,421	97,673	91,042
HOSPITAL UNIT (Excludes Separate Nursing Home Units)					
Utilization - Inpatient					
Beds	49,337	49,700	49,083	47,636	47,538
Admissions	1,996,261	2,010,609	1,984,949	2,109,615	2,143,477
Inpatient Days	10,955,805	10,997,840	10,274,207	10,226,487	10,307,405
Average Length of Stay	5.5	5.5	5.2	4.8	4.8
Personnel					
Total Full Time	282,246	282,022	276,667	276,545	280,127
Total Part Time	98,681	103,677	102,720	97,007	90,271
COMMUNITY HEALTH INDICATORS PER 1000 POPULATION					
Total Population (in thousands)	25,514	25,270	25,213	24,855	24,552
Inpatient					
Beds	2	2	2	2	2
Admissions	78.3	79.6	78.8	85	87.5
Inpatient Days	444.4	451.4	425.9	434.5	442.9
Inpatient Surgeries	19.1	19.1	19.6	22.7	23.3
Births	9.8	10	9.7	10.4	10.7
Outpatient					
Emergency Outpatient Visits	344.5	319.8	306.6	344.8	348.7
Other Outpatient Visits	1,528.8	1,584.8	1,430.2	1,427.4	1,442.7
Total Outpatient Visits	1,873.4	1,904.6	1,736.8	1,772.2	1,791.4
Outpatient Surgeries	47.9	47.1	40.5	47.1	49.4

U.S. Census Divisions

Note: The 2021 performance data do not reflect the full impact of the COVID-19 pandemic. Please refer to the discussion in the Introduction for more information.

AHA Hospital Statistics © 2024 Health Forum LLC, an affiliate of the American Hospital Association

TABLE 5

U.S. CENSUS DIVISION 9: PACIFIC

U.S. Community Hospitals
(Nonfederal, short-term general and other special hospitals)

Overview 2018–2022

	2022	2021	2020	2019	2018
Total Community Hospitals					
in Census Division 9, Pacific	551	554	547	553	555
Bed Size Category					
6-24	53	52	50	47	47
25-49	91	90	94	98	97
50-99	76	82	77	77	79
100-199	143	144	136	135	138
200-299	75	78	78	83	83
300-399	50	46	56	58	57
400-499	37	35	31	31	33
500 +	26	27	25	24	21
Location					
Hospitals Urban	443	446	440	446	447
Hospitals Rural	108	108	107	107	108
Control					
State and Local Government	125	129	130	127	127
Not for Profit	332	330	326	324	325
Investor owned	94	95	91	102	103
Affiliations					
Hospitals in a System	383	381	374	376	376
Hospitals in a Group Purchasing Organization...	302	294	262	287	296

Note: The 2021 performance data do not reflect the full impact of the COVID-19 pandemic. Please refer to the discussion in the Introduction for more information.

TABLE 5

U.S. CENSUS DIVISION 9: PACIFIC

U.S. Community Hospitals
(Nonfederal, short-term general and other special hospitals)

Utilization, Personnel, Community Health Indicators 2018–2022

	2022	2021	2020	2019	2018
TOTAL FACILITY (Includes Hospital and Nursing Home Units)					
Utilization - Inpatient					
Beds	97,923	97,133	96,073	97,034	96,559
Admissions	4,170,341	4,091,164	4,072,505	4,464,625	4,511,482
Inpatient Days	24,500,694	23,488,244	22,268,180	23,075,599	23,223,773
Average Length of Stay	5.9	5.7	5.5	5.2	5.1
Inpatient Surgeries	1,007,458	1,003,545	998,703	1,136,471	1,164,153
Births	562,902	561,468	567,770	570,444	592,993
Utilization - Outpatient					
Emergency Outpatient Visits	18,332,720	16,148,982	15,736,535	18,404,079	18,171,259
Other Outpatient Visits	71,723,846	70,053,760	68,801,206	70,824,081	68,984,172
Total Outpatient Visits	90,056,566	86,202,742	84,537,741	89,228,160	87,155,431
Outpatient Surgeries	2,215,718	2,110,743	1,898,141	2,188,157	2,237,446
Personnel					
Full Time RNs	171,407	170,422	166,647	163,830	163,844
Full Time LPNs	7,977	6,945	6,473	6,864	6,936
Part Time RNs	107,762	100,950	98,798	100,244	95,062
Part Time LPNs	3,624	3,061	3,031	3,090	2,890
Total Full Time	599,635	581,973	563,650	550,195	550,075
Total Part Time	277,069	266,065	259,157	256,787	245,253
HOSPITAL UNIT (Excludes Separate Nursing Home Units)					
Utilization - Inpatient					
Beds	94,756	94,712	94,064	94,237	93,646
Admissions	4,159,228	4,081,699	4,062,519	4,450,741	4,496,465
Inpatient Days	23,589,660	22,819,343	21,666,200	22,213,145	22,311,167
Average Length of Stay	5.7	5.6	5.3	5.0	5.0
Personnel					
Total Full Time	596,368	579,317	561,675	547,540	547,405
Total Part Time	276,085	265,165	258,414	255,553	244,038
COMMUNITY HEALTH INDICATORS PER 1000 POPULATION					
Total Population (in thousands)	53,229	53,397	53,441	53,492	53,441
Inpatient					
Beds	1.8	1.8	1.8	1.8	1.8
Admissions	78.3	76.6	76.2	83.5	84.4
Inpatient Days	460.3	439.9	416.7	431.4	434.6
Inpatient Surgeries	18.9	18.8	18.7	21.2	21.8
Births	10.6	10.5	10.6	10.7	11.1
Outpatient					
Emergency Outpatient Visits	344.4	302.4	294.5	344.1	340
Other Outpatient Visits	1,347.5	1,311.9	1,287.4	1,324	1,290.8
Total Outpatient Visits	1,691.9	1,614.4	1,581.9	1,668.1	1,630.9
Outpatient Surgeries	41.6	39.5	35.5	40.9	41.9

Note: The 2021 performance data do not reflect the full impact of the COVID-19 pandemic. Please refer to the discussion in the Introduction for more information.

TABLE 6

ALABAMA

U.S. Community Hospitals
(Nonfederal, short-term general and other special hospitals)

Overview 2018–2022

	2022	2021	2020	2019	2018
Total Community Hospitals in Alabama	102	102	101	101	101
Bed Size Category					
6-24	7	5	5	5	5
25-49	27	29	28	28	27
50-99	25	25	25	25	26
100-199	20	20	20	21	22
200-299	8	9	9	7	6
300-399	7	7	6	7	7
400-499	2	1	2	2	2
500 + ...	6	6	6	6	6
Location					
Hospitals Urban	63	63	63	63	63
Hospitals Rural...	39	39	38	38	38
Control					
State and Local Government	35	35	35	36	37
Not for Profit..	33	33	33	32	30
Investor owned...	34	34	33	33	34
Affiliations					
Hospitals in a System	70	70	70	70	69
Hospitals in a Group Purchasing Organization...	29	27	30	36	39

Note: The 2021 performance data do not reflect the full impact of the COVID-19 pandemic. Please refer to the discussion in the Introduction for more information.

50 AHA Hospital Statistics © 2024 Health Forum LLC, an affiliate of the American Hospital Association

TABLE 6

ALABAMA

U.S. Community Hospitals
(Nonfederal, short-term general and other special hospitals)

Utilization, Personnel, Community Health Indicators 2018–2022

	2022	2021	2020	2019	2018
TOTAL FACILITY (Includes Hospital and Nursing Home Units)					
Utilization - Inpatient					
Beds	15,554	15,366	15,377	15,248	15,278
Admissions	602,107	601,414	589,081	637,490	628,561
Inpatient Days	3,842,006	3,790,463	3,524,600	3,633,143	3,614,731
Average Length of Stay	6.4	6.3	6.0	5.7	5.8
Inpatient Surgeries	176,756	176,827	202,040	206,790	184,009
Births	59,789	62,177	66,659	64,583	54,302
Utilization - Outpatient					
Emergency Outpatient Visits	2,064,969	2,073,805	1,956,700	2,488,864	2,340,055
Other Outpatient Visits	6,687,101	6,563,709	5,847,372	7,547,271	7,671,113
Total Outpatient Visits	8,752,070	8,637,514	7,804,072	10,036,135	10,011,168
Outpatient Surgeries	513,797	441,932	432,214	485,735	416,529
Personnel					
Full Time RNs	24,180	24,036	24,472	24,821	24,371
Full Time LPNs	1,285	1,136	1,152	1,047	1,104
Part Time RNs	10,684	11,670	8,679	8,374	7,433
Part Time LPNs	736	721	491	411	332
Total Full Time	76,519	75,583	75,332	75,955	73,116
Total Part Time	30,559	33,889	25,988	24,837	21,425
HOSPITAL UNIT (Excludes Separate Nursing Home Units)					
Utilization - Inpatient					
Beds	15,554	15,244	14,908	14,779	14,809
Admissions	602,107	601,201	587,943	636,236	627,420
Inpatient Days	3,842,006	3,758,158	3,369,092	3,478,648	3,454,326
Average Length of Stay	6.4	6.3	5.7	5.5	5.5
Personnel					
Total Full Time	76,519	75,528	74,971	75,648	72,874
Total Part Time	30,559	33,864	25,936	24,779	21,374
COMMUNITY HEALTH INDICATORS PER 1000 POPULATION					
Total Population (in thousands)	5,074	5,040	4,922	4,903	4,888
Inpatient					
Beds	3.1	3	3.1	3.1	3.1
Admissions	118.7	119.3	119.7	130	128.6
Inpatient Days	757.2	752.1	716.2	741	739.5
Inpatient Surgeries	34.8	35.1	41.1	42.2	37.6
Births	11.8	12.3	13.5	13.2	11.1
Outpatient					
Emergency Outpatient Visits	406.9	411.5	397.6	507.6	478.7
Other Outpatient Visits	1,317.8	1,302.4	1,188.1	1,539.3	1,569.4
Total Outpatient Visits	1,724.8	1,713.8	1,585.7	2,046.9	2,048.2
Outpatient Surgeries	101.3	87.7	87.8	99.1	85.2

Note: The 2021 performance data do not reflect the full impact of the COVID-19 pandemic. Please refer to the discussion in the Introduction for more information.

TABLE 6

ALASKA

U.S. Community Hospitals
(Nonfederal, short-term general and other special hospitals)

Overview 2018–2022

	2022	2021	2020	2019	2018
Total Community Hospitals in Alaska	20	20	20	20	21
Bed Size Category					
6-24	6	6	6	5	5
25-49	4	4	4	5	6
50-99	4	4	5	5	5
100-199	4	4	3	3	3
200-299	1	1	1	1	1
300-399	0	0	0	0	0
400-499	1	1	1	1	1
500 +	0	0	0	0	0
Location					
Hospitals Urban	6	6	6	6	6
Hospitals Rural	14	14	14	14	15
Control					
State and Local Government	4	5	5	6	7
Not for Profit	14	13	12	11	11
Investor owned	2	2	3	3	3
Affiliations					
Hospitals in a System	8	8	7	7	7
Hospitals in a Group Purchasing Organization	7	8	5	6	6

Note: The 2021 performance data do not reflect the full impact of the COVID-19 pandemic. Please refer to the discussion in the Introduction for more information.

TABLE 6

ALASKA

U.S. Community Hospitals
(Nonfederal, short-term general and other special hospitals)

Utilization, Personnel, Community Health Indicators 2018–2022

	2022	2021	2020	2019	2018
TOTAL FACILITY (Includes Hospital and Nursing Home Units)					
Utilization - Inpatient					
Beds	1,639	1,639	1,588	1,606	1,636
Admissions	51,306	50,367	37,004	49,888	52,846
Inpatient Days	418,838	479,686	362,513	382,686	393,049
Average Length of Stay	8.2	9.5	9.8	7.7	7.4
Inpatient Surgeries	12,194	13,197	12,950	18,415	17,193
Births	7,522	8,210	6,824	7,831	8,323
Utilization - Outpatient					
Emergency Outpatient Visits	237,702	232,400	279,979	329,868	320,990
Other Outpatient Visits	1,041,057	1,035,565	1,418,097	1,510,113	1,635,915
Total Outpatient Visits	1,278,759	1,267,965	1,698,076	1,839,981	1,956,905
Outpatient Surgeries	43,283	44,808	35,922	45,121	48,009
Personnel					
Full Time RNs	2,650	2,934	2,698	2,432	2,470
Full Time LPNs	137	121	139	155	150
Part Time RNs	1,249	1,178	1,028	986	1,074
Part Time LPNs	65	59	59	54	62
Total Full Time	10,123	10,977	10,039	8,976	9,422
Total Part Time	4,127	3,791	3,330	3,098	3,310
HOSPITAL UNIT (Excludes Separate Nursing Home Units)					
Utilization - Inpatient					
Beds	1,416	1,426	1,385	1,363	1,451
Admissions	51,017	50,143	36,721	49,587	52,542
Inpatient Days	355,482	421,701	300,183	307,241	335,047
Average Length of Stay	7.0	8.4	8.2	6.2	6.4
Personnel					
Total Full Time	9,924	10,738	9,833	8,710	9,221
Total Part Time	3,920	3,654	3,207	2,967	3,211
COMMUNITY HEALTH INDICATORS PER 1000 POPULATION					
Total Population (in thousands)	734	733	731	732	737
Inpatient					
Beds	2.2	2.2	2.2	2.2	2.2
Admissions	69.9	68.7	50.6	68.2	71.7
Inpatient Days	570.9	654.7	495.8	523.1	533
Inpatient Surgeries	16.6	18	17.7	25.2	23.3
Births	10.3	11.2	9.3	10.7	11.3
Outpatient					
Emergency Outpatient Visits	324	317.2	382.9	450.9	435.3
Other Outpatient Visits	1,419.1	1,413.4	1,939.5	2,064.3	2,218.4
Total Outpatient Visits	1,743.2	1,730.6	2,322.4	2,515.2	2,653.7
Outpatient Surgeries	59	61.2	49.1	61.7	65.1

Note: The 2021 performance data do not reflect the full impact of the COVID-19 pandemic. Please refer to the discussion in the Introduction for more information.

AHA Hospital Statistics © 2024 Health Forum LLC, an affiliate of the American Hospital Association

TABLE 6

ARIZONA

U.S. Community Hospitals
(Nonfederal, short-term general and other special hospitals)

Overview 2018–2022

	2022	2021	2020	2019	2018
Total Community Hospitals in Arizona	87	84	81	80	83
Bed Size Category					
6-24	14	12	11	13	15
25-49	14	14	15	14	14
50-99	16	15	15	14	14
100-199	17	17	15	13	14
200-299	7	7	7	8	9
300-399	7	6	4	5	6
400-499	5	6	7	6	6
500 + ...	7	7	7	7	5
Location					
Hospitals Urban	79	76	73	71	74
Hospitals Rural..	8	8	8	9	9
Control					
State and Local Government	5	4	4	4	4
Not for Profit..	44	44	43	43	43
Investor owned..	38	36	34	33	36
Affiliations					
Hospitals in a System	70	66	63	59	61
Hospitals in a Group Purchasing Organization...	35	41	33	38	47

Note: The 2021 performance data do not reflect the full impact of the COVID-19 pandemic. Please refer to the discussion in the Introduction for more information.

TABLE 6

ARIZONA

U.S. Community Hospitals
(Nonfederal, short-term general and other special hospitals)

Utilization, Personnel, Community Health Indicators 2018–2022

	2022	2021	2020	2019	2018
TOTAL FACILITY (Includes Hospital and Nursing Home Units)					
Utilization - Inpatient					
Beds	14,673	14,796	14,271	14,038	13,846
Admissions	639,833	643,759	623,204	655,961	651,618
Inpatient Days	3,424,355	3,523,322	3,217,706	3,152,127	3,112,261
Average Length of Stay	5.4	5.5	5.2	4.8	4.8
Inpatient Surgeries	164,510	158,224	153,436	174,655	171,517
Births	74,855	75,065	66,129	73,933	78,909
Utilization - Outpatient					
Emergency Outpatient Visits	2,156,190	2,179,363	1,879,268	2,403,474	2,195,768
Other Outpatient Visits	4,471,159	7,061,167	6,105,473	6,834,901	6,235,673
Total Outpatient Visits	6,627,349	9,240,530	7,984,741	9,238,375	8,431,441
Outpatient Surgeries	313,682	309,486	261,891	302,106	327,574
Personnel					
Full Time RNs	24,113	22,772	24,094	24,048	24,406
Full Time LPNs	756	425	610	545	401
Part Time RNs	7,985	8,960	8,077	7,069	6,866
Part Time LPNs	251	185	194	158	109
Total Full Time	76,113	73,520	74,764	73,448	72,235
Total Part Time	20,967	22,893	21,275	17,936	16,549
HOSPITAL UNIT (Excludes Separate Nursing Home Units)					
Utilization - Inpatient					
Beds	14,673	14,796	14,271	14,038	13,768
Admissions	639,833	643,759	623,204	655,961	650,017
Inpatient Days	3,424,355	3,523,322	3,217,706	3,152,127	3,094,745
Average Length of Stay	5.4	5.5	5.2	4.8	4.8
Personnel					
Total Full Time	76,113	73,520	74,764	73,448	72,182
Total Part Time	20,967	22,893	21,275	17,936	16,544
COMMUNITY HEALTH INDICATORS PER 1000 POPULATION					
Total Population (in thousands)	7,359	7,276	7,421	7,279	7,172
Inpatient					
Beds	2	2	1.9	1.9	1.9
Admissions	86.9	88.5	84	90.1	90.9
Inpatient Days	465.3	484.2	433.6	433.1	434
Inpatient Surgeries	22.4	21.7	20.7	24	23.9
Births	10.2	10.3	8.9	10.2	11
Outpatient					
Emergency Outpatient Visits	293	299.5	253.2	330.2	306.2
Other Outpatient Visits	607.6	970.4	822.7	939	869.5
Total Outpatient Visits	900.6	1,269.9	1,075.9	1,269.2	1,175.7
Outpatient Surgeries	42.6	42.5	35.3	41.5	45.7

Note: The 2021 performance data do not reflect the full impact of the COVID-19 pandemic. Please refer to the discussion in the Introduction for more information.

AHA Hospital Statistics © 2024 Health Forum LLC, an affiliate of the American Hospital Association

TABLE 6

ARKANSAS

U.S. Community Hospitals
(Nonfederal, short-term general and other special hospitals)

Overview 2018–2022

	2022	2021	2020	2019	2018
Total Community Hospitals in Arkansas	93	92	90	89	88
Bed Size Category					
6-24	11	11	10	11	10
25-49	41	38	37	36	33
50-99	14	15	15	13	14
100-199	11	12	12	15	16
200-299	7	7	7	6	6
300-399	6	6	6	6	7
400-499	1	1	1	0	0
500 + ...	2	2	2	2	2
Location					
Hospitals Urban	43	45	43	42	41
Hospitals Rural	50	47	47	47	47
Control					
State and Local Government	9	9	12	8	9
Not for Profit	58	56	53	55	51
Investor owned	26	27	25	26	28
Affiliations					
Hospitals in a System	54	55	53	49	47
Hospitals in a Group Purchasing Organization...	78	73	78	73	76

Note: The 2021 performance data do not reflect the full impact of the COVID-19 pandemic. Please refer to the discussion in the Introduction for more information.

56   AHA Hospital Statistics © 2024 Health Forum LLC, an affiliate of the American Hospital Association

TABLE 6

ARKANSAS

U.S. Community Hospitals
(Nonfederal, short-term general and other special hospitals)

Utilization, Personnel, Community Health Indicators 2018–2022

	2022	2021	2020	2019	2018
TOTAL FACILITY (Includes Hospital and Nursing Home Units)					
Utilization - Inpatient					
Beds	9,546	9,590	9,518	9,145	9,517
Admissions	351,584	347,411	342,864	364,291	358,222
Inpatient Days	1,933,644	1,935,306	1,791,995	1,826,976	1,828,470
Average Length of Stay	5.5	5.6	5.2	5.0	5.1
Inpatient Surgeries	81,140	79,866	83,032	92,357	94,924
Births	33,726	34,185	33,511	34,678	34,821
Utilization - Outpatient					
Emergency Outpatient Visits	1,446,356	1,410,733	1,352,491	1,556,206	1,509,448
Other Outpatient Visits	4,761,464	4,817,914	4,377,227	4,914,195	4,925,120
Total Outpatient Visits	6,207,820	6,228,647	5,729,718	6,470,401	6,434,568
Outpatient Surgeries	223,646	207,801	194,138	226,136	215,656
Personnel					
Full Time RNs	12,178	12,353	12,558	13,347	12,821
Full Time LPNs	1,548	1,374	1,450	1,349	1,504
Part Time RNs	5,785	5,584	5,947	5,410	5,533
Part Time LPNs	484	473	419	352	385
Total Full Time	40,976	40,887	41,277	42,713	42,361
Total Part Time	17,165	16,900	17,031	15,322	16,318
HOSPITAL UNIT (Excludes Separate Nursing Home Units)					
Utilization - Inpatient					
Beds	9,258	9,277	9,210	8,837	9,193
Admissions	351,421	347,299	342,678	364,093	357,700
Inpatient Days	1,867,163	1,859,360	1,704,229	1,739,783	1,732,975
Average Length of Stay	5.3	5.4	5.0	4.8	4.8
Personnel					
Total Full Time	40,805	40,713	41,085	42,523	42,133
Total Part Time	17,122	16,863	16,986	15,277	16,292
COMMUNITY HEALTH INDICATORS PER 1000 POPULATION					
Total Population (in thousands)	3,046	3,026	3,031	3,018	3,014
Inpatient					
Beds	3.1	3.2	3.1	3	3.2
Admissions	115.4	114.8	113.1	120.7	118.9
Inpatient Days	634.9	639.6	591.3	605.4	606.7
Inpatient Surgeries	26.6	26.4	27.4	30.6	31.5
Births	11.1	11.3	11.1	11.5	11.6
Outpatient					
Emergency Outpatient Visits	474.9	466.2	446.3	515.7	500.8
Other Outpatient Visits	1,563.4	1,592.2	1,444.4	1,628.4	1,634.2
Total Outpatient Visits	2,038.3	2,058.5	1,890.7	2,144.1	2,135
Outpatient Surgeries	73.4	68.7	64.1	74.9	71.6

Note: The 2021 performance data do not reflect the full impact of the COVID-19 pandemic. Please refer to the discussion in the Introduction for more information.

AHA Hospital Statistics © 2024 Health Forum LLC, an affiliate of the American Hospital Association

TABLE 6

CALIFORNIA

U.S. Community Hospitals
(Nonfederal, short-term general and other special hospitals)

Overview 2018–2022

	2022	2021	2020	2019	2018
Total Community Hospitals in California	**355**	**358**	**353**	**359**	**359**
Bed Size Category					
6-24	16	15	13	14	14
25-49	36	37	41	43	41
50-99	49	53	48	48	49
100-199	105	105	98	98	101
200-299	62	66	67	69	68
300-399	37	33	43	46	46
400-499	32	30	26	24	26
500 +	18	19	17	17	14
Location					
Hospitals Urban	325	328	323	329	329
Hospitals Rural	30	30	30	30	30
Control					
State and Local Government	62	65	67	66	64
Not for Profit	208	207	205	204	206
Investor owned	85	86	81	89	89
Affiliations					
Hospitals in a System	262	262	257	259	258
Hospitals in a Group Purchasing Organization	171	166	141	157	161

Note: The 2021 performance data do not reflect the full impact of the COVID-19 pandemic. Please refer to the discussion in the Introduction for more information.

58   AHA Hospital Statistics © 2024 Health Forum LLC, an affiliate of the American Hospital Association

Table 6

CALIFORNIA

U.S. Community Hospitals
(Nonfederal, short-term general and other special hospitals)

Utilization, Personnel, Community Health Indicators 2018–2022

	2022	2021	2020	2019	2018
TOTAL FACILITY (Includes Hospital and Nursing Home Units)					
Utilization - Inpatient					
Beds	73,877	73,235	72,622	73,109	72,511
Admissions	3,169,185	3,102,200	3,099,784	3,361,823	3,400,991
Inpatient Days	18,351,352	17,613,554	16,913,883	17,440,927	17,484,281
Average Length of Stay	5.8	5.7	5.5	5.2	5.1
Inpatient Surgeries	716,400	717,630	698,132	799,100	818,787
Births	423,912	425,643	433,491	426,158	444,730
Utilization - Outpatient					
Emergency Outpatient Visits	13,103,190	11,376,605	11,331,971	13,079,880	13,026,736
Other Outpatient Visits	42,857,091	40,285,437	41,130,147	42,786,381	42,624,149
Total Outpatient Visits	55,960,281	51,662,042	52,462,118	55,866,261	55,650,885
Outpatient Surgeries	1,479,865	1,418,187	1,272,787	1,475,806	1,545,410
Personnel					
Full Time RNs	129,664	128,557	125,670	122,686	122,839
Full Time LPNs	6,476	5,760	5,371	5,667	5,771
Part Time RNs	80,819	72,348	71,919	73,095	69,397
Part Time LPNs	2,848	2,317	2,382	2,414	2,261
Total Full Time	443,931	429,635	417,313	402,618	401,556
Total Part Time	203,074	188,646	186,619	182,281	176,220
HOSPITAL UNIT (Excludes Separate Nursing Home Units)					
Utilization - Inpatient					
Beds	71,094	71,117	70,884	70,684	70,149
Admissions	3,158,453	3,093,000	3,090,158	3,348,373	3,386,782
Inpatient Days	17,532,592	17,028,576	16,397,057	16,692,108	16,718,712
Average Length of Stay	5.6	5.5	5.3	5.0	4.9
Personnel					
Total Full Time	441,001	427,347	415,626	400,349	399,421
Total Part Time	202,349	187,928	186,097	181,330	175,267
COMMUNITY HEALTH INDICATORS PER 1000 POPULATION					
Total Population (in thousands)	39,029	39,238	39,368	39,512	39,557
Inpatient					
Beds	1.9	1.9	1.8	1.9	1.8
Admissions	81.2	79.1	78.7	85.1	86
Inpatient Days	470.2	448.9	429.6	441.4	442
Inpatient Surgeries	18.4	18.3	17.7	20.2	20.7
Births	10.9	10.8	11	10.8	11.2
Outpatient					
Emergency Outpatient Visits	335.7	289.9	287.8	331	329.3
Other Outpatient Visits	1,098.1	1,026.7	1,044.8	1,082.9	1,077.5
Total Outpatient Visits	1,433.8	1,316.6	1,332.6	1,413.9	1,406.9
Outpatient Surgeries	37.9	36.1	32.3	37.4	39.1

Note: The 2021 performance data do not reflect the full impact of the COVID-19 pandemic. Please refer to the discussion in the Introduction for more information.

TABLE 6

COLORADO

U.S. Community Hospitals
(Nonfederal, short-term general and other special hospitals)

Overview 2018–2022

	2022	2021	2020	2019	2018
Total Community Hospitals in Colorado.............	92	91	91	90	89
Bed Size Category					
6-24	17	18	17	18	18
25-49	29	26	25	26	24
50-99	18	19	19	17	17
100-199	9	8	11	10	12
200-299	6	6	6	6	7
300-399	8	8	7	8	6
400-499	2	4	4	4	3
500 + ...	3	2	2	1	2
Location					
Hospitals Urban	52	51	51	50	49
Hospitals Rural..	40	40	40	40	40
Control					
State and Local Government	25	26	27	26	27
Not for Profit..	50	48	46	46	43
Investor owned..	17	17	18	18	19
Affiliations					
Hospitals in a System	57	56	57	59	59
Hospitals in a Group Purchasing Organization...	55	53	59	53	53

Note: The 2021 performance data do not reflect the full impact of the COVID-19 pandemic. Please refer to the discussion in the Introduction for more information.

TABLE 6

COLORADO

U.S. Community Hospitals
(Nonfederal, short-term general and other special hospitals)

Utilization, Personnel, Community Health Indicators 2018–2022

	2022	2021	2020	2019	2018
TOTAL FACILITY (Includes Hospital and Nursing Home Units)					
Utilization - Inpatient					
Beds	11,192	11,187	11,069	10,665	10,574
Admissions	434,715	436,573	419,235	446,955	446,553
Inpatient Days	2,468,885	2,426,893	2,282,926	2,290,705	2,251,677
Average Length of Stay	5.7	5.6	5.4	5.1	5.0
Inpatient Surgeries	111,554	116,758	120,563	138,225	142,149
Births	59,069	59,438	59,182	53,923	57,141
Utilization - Outpatient					
Emergency Outpatient Visits	2,358,403	2,057,619	1,884,637	2,105,511	2,037,141
Other Outpatient Visits	9,525,258	7,042,142	6,809,038	8,146,582	7,357,929
Total Outpatient Visits	11,883,661	9,099,761	8,693,675	10,252,093	9,395,070
Outpatient Surgeries	267,084	263,420	230,421	260,588	263,552
Personnel					
Full Time RNs	20,063	19,539	18,933	18,907	18,705
Full Time LPNs	576	439	416	520	525
Part Time RNs	7,544	8,756	8,926	8,301	7,984
Part Time LPNs	224	211	211	250	202
Total Full Time	67,428	61,709	61,602	64,482	61,261
Total Part Time	20,795	23,593	24,812	24,538	23,875
HOSPITAL UNIT (Excludes Separate Nursing Home Units)					
Utilization - Inpatient					
Beds	10,942	11,044	10,773	10,338	10,386
Admissions	434,611	436,513	419,045	446,611	446,412
Inpatient Days	2,407,965	2,392,490	2,212,775	2,194,672	2,192,505
Average Length of Stay	5.5	5.5	5.3	4.9	4.9
Personnel					
Total Full Time	67,238	61,616	61,351	64,287	61,096
Total Part Time	20,720	23,533	24,673	24,447	23,808
COMMUNITY HEALTH INDICATORS PER 1000 POPULATION					
Total Population (in thousands)	5,840	5,812	5,808	5,759	5,696
Inpatient					
Beds	1.9	1.9	1.9	1.9	1.9
Admissions	74.4	75.1	72.2	77.6	78.4
Inpatient Days	422.8	417.6	393.1	397.8	395.3
Inpatient Surgeries	19.1	20.1	20.8	24	25
Births	10.1	10.2	10.2	9.4	10
Outpatient					
Emergency Outpatient Visits	403.8	354	324.5	365.6	357.7
Other Outpatient Visits	1,631.1	1,211.6	1,172.4	1,414.6	1,291.9
Total Outpatient Visits	2,034.9	1,565.7	1,496.9	1,780.3	1,649.5
Outpatient Surgeries	45.7	45.3	39.7	45.3	46.3

Note: The 2021 performance data do not reflect the full impact of the COVID-19 pandemic. Please refer to the discussion in the Introduction for more information.

AHA Hospital Statistics © 2024 Health Forum LLC, an affiliate of the American Hospital Association

TABLE 6

CONNECTICUT

U.S. Community Hospitals
(Nonfederal, short-term general and other special hospitals)

Overview 2018–2022

	2022	2021	2020	2019	2018
Total Community Hospitals in Connecticut........	31	31	31	31	32
Bed Size Category					
6-24	0	0	0	0	0
25-49	3	2	2	3	3
50-99	5	6	8	7	8
100-199	11	10	11	12	11
200-299	6	6	3	3	4
300-399	2	3	3	2	3
400-499	2	2	2	2	1
500 + ...	2	2	2	2	2
Location					
Hospitals Urban	28	29	29	29	30
Hospitals Rural..	3	2	2	2	2
Control					
State and Local Government	1	1	1	1	1
Not for Profit...	29	29	29	29	31
Investor owned...	1	1	1	1	0
Affiliations					
Hospitals in a System	21	21	21	21	21
Hospitals in a Group Purchasing Organization...	20	22	22	23	23

Note: The 2021 performance data do not reflect the full impact of the COVID-19 pandemic. Please refer to the discussion in the Introduction for more information.

TABLE 6

CONNECTICUT

U.S. Community Hospitals
(Nonfederal, short-term general and other special hospitals)

Utilization, Personnel, Community Health Indicators 2018–2022

	2022	2021	2020	2019	2018
TOTAL FACILITY (Includes Hospital and Nursing Home Units)					
Utilization - Inpatient					
Beds	7,473	7,558	7,539	7,246	7,194
Admissions	361,956	364,933	356,404	372,553	366,087
Inpatient Days	2,262,500	2,188,568	2,036,200	2,049,145	2,005,853
Average Length of Stay	6.3	6.0	5.7	5.5	5.5
Inpatient Surgeries	76,688	86,046	94,644	102,223	106,446
Births	35,009	34,753	34,497	34,843	35,161
Utilization - Outpatient					
Emergency Outpatient Visits	1,610,068	1,483,355	1,410,998	1,701,496	1,755,177
Other Outpatient Visits	8,605,859	9,135,688	6,447,398	6,999,551	7,293,140
Total Outpatient Visits	10,215,927	10,619,043	7,858,396	8,701,047	9,048,317
Outpatient Surgeries	202,348	203,069	176,767	228,193	222,221
Personnel					
Full Time RNs	13,590	13,959	13,168	12,631	12,465
Full Time LPNs	359	247	183	207	235
Part Time RNs	9,264	8,649	8,118	7,722	7,804
Part Time LPNs	180	128	107	111	123
Total Full Time	48,750	48,672	45,984	45,017	45,739
Total Part Time	28,718	27,259	25,117	24,128	23,785
HOSPITAL UNIT (Excludes Separate Nursing Home Units)					
Utilization - Inpatient					
Beds	7,243	7,328	7,309	7,142	7,090
Admissions	361,341	364,323	355,847	372,205	365,713
Inpatient Days	2,185,517	2,118,463	1,962,807	2,012,482	1,969,438
Average Length of Stay	6.0	5.8	5.5	5.4	5.4
Personnel					
Total Full Time	48,641	48,562	45,743	44,974	45,687
Total Part Time	28,569	27,120	24,979	24,090	23,722
COMMUNITY HEALTH INDICATORS PER 1000 POPULATION					
Total Population (in thousands)	3,626	3,606	3,557	3,565	3,573
Inpatient					
Beds	2.1	2.1	2.1	2	2
Admissions	99.8	101.2	100.2	104.5	102.5
Inpatient Days	623.9	607	572.4	574.7	561.4
Inpatient Surgeries	21.1	23.9	26.6	28.7	29.8
Births	9.7	9.6	9.7	9.8	9.8
Outpatient					
Emergency Outpatient Visits	444	411.4	396.7	477.2	491.3
Other Outpatient Visits	2,373.2	2,533.8	1,812.6	1,963.3	2,041.4
Total Outpatient Visits	2,817.3	2,945.2	2,209.3	2,440.5	2,532.7
Outpatient Surgeries	55.8	56.3	49.7	64	62.2

Note: The 2021 performance data do not reflect the full impact of the COVID-19 pandemic. Please refer to the discussion in the Introduction for more information.

AHA Hospital Statistics © 2024 Health Forum LLC, an affiliate of the American Hospital Association

TABLE 6

DELAWARE

U.S. Community Hospitals
(Nonfederal, short-term general and other special hospitals)

Overview 2018–2022

	2022	2021	2020	2019	2018
Total Community Hospitals in Delaware............	8	8	7	7	7
Bed Size Category					
6-24	0	0	0	0	0
25-49	2	2	1	1	1
50-99	1	2	1	1	1
100-199	2	1	2	2	2
200-299	1	1	1	1	1
300-399	0	1	1	1	1
400-499	1	0	0	0	0
500 + ...	1	1	1	1	1
Location					
Hospitals Urban	6	8	7	7	7
Hospitals Rural...	2	0	0	0	0
Control					
State and Local Government	0	0	0	0	0
Not for Profit..	6	6	6	6	6
Investor owned...	2	2	1	1	1
Affiliations					
Hospitals in a System	6	6	5	5	4
Hospitals in a Group Purchasing Organization...	7	6	6	6	5

Note: The 2021 performance data do not reflect the full impact of the COVID-19 pandemic. Please refer to the discussion in the Introduction for more information.

64   AHA Hospital Statistics © 2024 Health Forum LLC, an affiliate of the American Hospital Association

TABLE 6

DELAWARE

U.S. Community Hospitals
(Nonfederal, short-term general and other special hospitals)

Utilization, Personnel, Community Health Indicators 2018–2022

	2022	2021	2020	2019	2018
TOTAL FACILITY (Includes Hospital and Nursing Home Units)					
Utilization - Inpatient					
Beds	2,338	2,136	2,181	2,112	2,101
Admissions	102,143	98,351	94,889	103,328	102,324
Inpatient Days	697,248	611,064	558,260	569,518	556,545
Average Length of Stay	6.8	6.2	5.9	5.5	5.4
Inpatient Surgeries	23,317	24,900	26,370	29,522	30,357
Births	10,906	10,363	10,715	10,358	10,798
Utilization - Outpatient					
Emergency Outpatient Visits	433,317	404,564	421,618	478,571	460,493
Other Outpatient Visits	1,971,696	2,022,665	1,552,480	1,727,202	1,705,927
Total Outpatient Visits	2,405,013	2,427,229	1,974,098	2,205,773	2,166,420
Outpatient Surgeries	61,777	62,309	51,117	59,934	59,911
Personnel					
Full Time RNs	4,842	4,179	4,762	4,699	4,729
Full Time LPNs	160	122	139	145	163
Part Time RNs	1,782	2,548	2,518	1,972	1,827
Part Time LPNs	106	92	105	90	113
Total Full Time	18,683	16,465	16,969	17,221	16,743
Total Part Time	5,433	7,482	7,113	5,891	5,830
HOSPITAL UNIT (Excludes Separate Nursing Home Units)					
Utilization - Inpatient					
Beds	2,338	2,136	2,181	2,112	2,101
Admissions	102,143	98,351	94,889	103,328	102,324
Inpatient Days	697,248	611,064	558,260	569,518	556,545
Average Length of Stay	6.8	6.2	5.9	5.5	5.4
Personnel					
Total Full Time	18,683	16,465	16,969	17,221	16,743
Total Part Time	5,433	7,482	7,113	5,891	5,830
COMMUNITY HEALTH INDICATORS PER 1000 POPULATION					
Total Population (in thousands)	1,018	1,003	987	974	967
Inpatient					
Beds	2.3	2.1	2.2	2.2	2.2
Admissions	100.3	98	96.2	106.1	105.8
Inpatient Days	684.7	609	565.7	584.9	575.4
Inpatient Surgeries	22.9	24.8	26.7	30.3	31.4
Births	10.7	10.3	10.9	10.6	11.2
Outpatient					
Emergency Outpatient Visits	425.5	403.2	427.3	491.5	476.1
Other Outpatient Visits	1,936.1	2,015.8	1,573.2	1,773.7	1,763.8
Total Outpatient Visits	2,361.6	2,419	2,000.5	2,265.2	2,240
Outpatient Surgeries	60.7	62.1	51.8	61.5	61.9

Note: The 2021 performance data do not reflect the full impact of the COVID-19 pandemic. Please refer to the discussion in the Introduction for more information.

AHA Hospital Statistics © 2024 Health Forum LLC, an affiliate of the American Hospital Association

TABLE 6

DISTRICT OF COLUMBIA

U.S. Community Hospitals
(Nonfederal, short-term general and other special hospitals)

Overview 2018–2022

	2022	2021	2020	2019	2018
Total Community Hospitals in District of Columbia	10	10	10	10	10
Bed Size Category					
6-24	0	0	0	0	0
25-49	0	0	0	0	0
50-99	0	0	0	0	1
100-199	3	3	3	3	2
200-299	2	2	2	2	2
300-399	3	3	3	3	3
400-499	1	1	1	1	1
500 +	1	1	1	1	1
Location					
Hospitals Urban	10	10	10	10	10
Hospitals Rural	0	0	0	0	0
Control					
State and Local Government	0	0	0	0	0
Not for Profit	7	7	7	7	7
Investor owned	3	3	3	3	3
Affiliations					
Hospitals in a System	8	8	8	8	7
Hospitals in a Group Purchasing Organization	5	6	6	6	6

Note: The 2021 performance data do not reflect the full impact of the COVID-19 pandemic. Please refer to the discussion in the Introduction for more information.

AHA Hospital Statistics © 2024 Health Forum LLC, an affiliate of the American Hospital Association

TABLE 6

DISTRICT OF COLUMBIA

U.S. Community Hospitals
(Nonfederal, short-term general and other special hospitals)

Utilization, Personnel, Community Health Indicators 2018–2022

	2022	2021	2020	2019	2018
TOTAL FACILITY (Includes Hospital and Nursing Home Units)					
Utilization - Inpatient					
Beds	3,363	3,278	3,244	3,186	3,114
Admissions	108,392	108,022	114,485	124,261	116,149
Inpatient Days	875,234	843,025	871,654	900,757	825,717
Average Length of Stay	8.1	7.8	7.6	7.2	7.1
Inpatient Surgeries	34,095	39,329	39,615	38,447	37,776
Births	12,216	12,201	13,275	12,682	13,399
Utilization - Outpatient					
Emergency Outpatient Visits	361,541	294,185	342,802	418,267	430,067
Other Outpatient Visits	2,582,135	2,324,354	2,057,458	2,370,694	2,166,534
Total Outpatient Visits	2,943,676	2,618,539	2,400,260	2,788,961	2,596,601
Outpatient Surgeries	55,934	58,257	55,778	63,458	63,736
Personnel					
Full Time RNs	5,729	6,331	6,647	6,473	6,417
Full Time LPNs	117	111	151	130	145
Part Time RNs	2,381	2,270	2,524	2,521	2,421
Part Time LPNs	51	34	37	28	35
Total Full Time	23,127	22,722	23,626	22,981	23,385
Total Part Time	6,310	5,774	6,308	6,147	5,975
HOSPITAL UNIT (Excludes Separate Nursing Home Units)					
Utilization - Inpatient					
Beds	3,318	3,139	3,199	3,079	3,069
Admissions	108,086	107,406	113,946	123,529	115,464
Inpatient Days	868,751	799,585	861,096	867,115	813,225
Average Length of Stay	8.0	7.4	7.6	7.0	7.0
Personnel					
Total Full Time	23,016	22,468	23,517	22,591	23,218
Total Part Time	6,278	5,599	6,227	5,894	5,918
COMMUNITY HEALTH INDICATORS PER 1000 POPULATION					
Total Population (in thousands)	672	670	713	706	702
Inpatient					
Beds	5	4.9	4.6	4.5	4.4
Admissions	161.3	161.2	160.6	176.1	165.3
Inpatient Days	1302.8	1258.2	1222.8	1276.3	1175.5
Inpatient Surgeries	50.8	58.7	55.6	54.5	53.8
Births	18.2	18.2	18.6	18	19.1
Outpatient					
Emergency Outpatient Visits	538.2	439	480.9	592.7	612.2
Other Outpatient Visits	3,843.6	3,468.9	2,886.4	3,359.1	3,084.2
Total Outpatient Visits	4,381.8	3,908	3,367.3	3,951.8	3,696.5
Outpatient Surgeries	83.3	86.9	78.3	89.9	90.7

Note: The 2021 performance data do not reflect the full impact of the COVID-19 pandemic. Please refer to the discussion in the Introduction for more information.

AHA Hospital Statistics © 2024 Health Forum LLC, an affiliate of the American Hospital Association

TABLE 6

FLORIDA

U.S. Community Hospitals
(Nonfederal, short-term general and other special hospitals)

Overview 2018–2022

	2022	2021	2020	2019	2018
Total Community Hospitals in Florida	213	216	214	212	217
Bed Size Category					
6-24	8	7	7	7	8
25-49	20	21	17	16	20
50-99	42	43	44	44	45
100-199	47	47	47	49	48
200-299	38	41	38	36	39
300-399	22	23	25	23	22
400-499	12	9	12	14	12
500 +	24	25	24	23	23
Location					
Hospitals Urban	196	199	197	195	197
Hospitals Rural	17	17	17	17	20
Control					
State and Local Government	24	23	21	22	22
Not for Profit	89	90	90	88	82
Investor owned	100	103	103	102	113
Affiliations					
Hospitals in a System	185	187	185	183	187
Hospitals in a Group Purchasing Organization	96	97	106	100	100

Note: The 2021 performance data do not reflect the full impact of the COVID-19 pandemic. Please refer to the discussion in the Introduction for more information.

AHA Hospital Statistics © 2024 Health Forum LLC, an affiliate of the American Hospital Association

TABLE 6

FLORIDA

U.S. Community Hospitals
(Nonfederal, short-term general and other special hospitals)

Utilization, Personnel, Community Health Indicators 2018–2022

	2022	2021	2020	2019	2018
TOTAL FACILITY (Includes Hospital and Nursing Home Units)					
Utilization - Inpatient					
Beds	55,144	55,288	54,985	55,733	54,744
Admissions	2,545,316	2,524,963	2,434,979	2,645,062	2,629,196
Inpatient Days	13,725,366	13,709,268	12,728,527	12,940,795	13,141,776
Average Length of Stay	5.4	5.4	5.2	4.9	5.0
Inpatient Surgeries	575,429	555,515	588,444	629,691	622,351
Births	212,163	198,096	203,076	205,759	211,751
Utilization - Outpatient					
Emergency Outpatient Visits	9,944,409	9,051,457	8,773,186	10,186,649	9,399,251
Other Outpatient Visits	22,525,262	21,083,654	18,903,088	21,446,444	17,591,262
Total Outpatient Visits	32,469,671	30,135,111	27,676,274	31,633,093	26,990,513
Outpatient Surgeries	1,023,631	957,449	846,955	890,405	934,752
Personnel					
Full Time RNs	90,402	89,189	91,186	87,526	86,303
Full Time LPNs	3,673	3,207	2,602	2,442	2,535
Part Time RNs	25,371	23,917	21,746	23,805	23,697
Part Time LPNs	955	784	588	654	774
Total Full Time	289,486	286,634	280,168	269,698	260,999
Total Part Time	76,953	69,187	64,352	69,186	68,493
HOSPITAL UNIT (Excludes Separate Nursing Home Units)					
Utilization - Inpatient					
Beds	54,504	54,636	54,033	54,837	53,891
Admissions	2,542,075	2,521,753	2,429,095	2,640,157	2,625,090
Inpatient Days	13,522,812	13,507,502	12,437,625	12,654,992	12,855,377
Average Length of Stay	5.3	5.4	5.1	4.8	4.9
Personnel					
Total Full Time	288,644	285,867	278,935	268,687	259,888
Total Part Time	76,757	69,046	64,046	68,909	68,149
COMMUNITY HEALTH INDICATORS PER 1000 POPULATION					
Total Population (in thousands)	22,245	21,781	21,733	21,478	21,299
Inpatient					
Beds	2.5	2.5	2.5	2.6	2.6
Admissions	114.4	115.9	112	123.2	123.4
Inpatient Days	617	629.4	585.7	602.5	617
Inpatient Surgeries	25.9	25.5	27.1	29.3	29.2
Births	9.5	9.1	9.3	9.6	9.9
Outpatient					
Emergency Outpatient Visits	447	415.6	403.7	474.3	441.3
Other Outpatient Visits	1,012.6	968	869.8	998.5	825.9
Total Outpatient Visits	1,459.7	1,383.5	1,273.4	1,472.8	1,267.2
Outpatient Surgeries	46	44	39	41.5	43.9

Note: The 2021 performance data do not reflect the full impact of the COVID-19 pandemic. Please refer to the discussion in the Introduction for more information.

AHA Hospital Statistics © 2024 Health Forum LLC, an affiliate of the American Hospital Association

TABLE 6

GEORGIA

U.S. Community Hospitals
(Nonfederal, short-term general and other special hospitals)

Overview 2018–2022

	2022	2021	2020	2019	2018
Total Community Hospitals in Georgia...............	**141**	**142**	**144**	**143**	**145**
Bed Size Category					
6-24	11	10	9	7	6
25-49	31	33	34	35	38
50-99	26	25	25	26	26
100-199	32	32	35	33	34
200-299	15	13	13	14	13
300-399	7	10	9	10	10
400-499	7	6	5	4	4
500 + ...	12	13	14	14	14
Location					
Hospitals Urban	86	87	89	87	89
Hospitals Rural.......................................	55	55	55	56	56
Control					
State and Local Government	34	35	33	35	38
Not for Profit..	83	83	84	85	80
Investor owned.......................................	24	24	27	23	27
Affiliations					
Hospitals in a System	97	97	98	96	97
Hospitals in a Group Purchasing Organization...	63	70	73	68	78

Note: The 2021 performance data do not reflect the full impact of the COVID-19 pandemic. Please refer to the discussion in the Introduction for more information.

TABLE 6

GEORGIA

U.S. Community Hospitals
(Nonfederal, short-term general and other special hospitals)

Utilization, Personnel, Community Health Indicators 2018–2022

	2022	2021	2020	2019	2018
TOTAL FACILITY (Includes Hospital and Nursing Home Units)					
Utilization - Inpatient					
Beds	24,625	25,106	25,098	24,896	25,114
Admissions	956,736	988,149	971,269	1,035,793	1,016,445
Inpatient Days	6,471,991	6,582,402	6,374,886	6,500,916	6,425,502
Average Length of Stay	6.8	6.7	6.6	6.3	6.3
Inpatient Surgeries	211,741	223,467	234,382	258,026	246,657
Births	117,996	115,523	119,234	121,077	121,738
Utilization - Outpatient					
Emergency Outpatient Visits	4,084,147	3,945,931	4,118,157	4,629,550	4,687,842
Other Outpatient Visits	17,104,363	17,537,718	15,026,811	15,841,438	15,265,159
Total Outpatient Visits	21,188,510	21,483,649	19,144,968	20,470,988	19,953,001
Outpatient Surgeries	540,759	532,826	470,557	526,682	503,413
Personnel					
Full Time RNs	37,221	39,153	41,001	39,317	37,550
Full Time LPNs	2,510	2,294	2,334	2,322	2,424
Part Time RNs	13,529	12,642	12,330	13,149	13,138
Part Time LPNs	657	625	609	621	685
Total Full Time	131,530	128,525	133,694	131,533	126,515
Total Part Time	39,057	36,324	35,405	38,350	37,925
HOSPITAL UNIT (Excludes Separate Nursing Home Units)					
Utilization - Inpatient					
Beds	21,671	22,204	22,625	22,331	22,530
Admissions	952,933	984,792	968,101	1,029,529	1,010,305
Inpatient Days	5,679,220	5,785,221	5,598,206	5,670,304	5,597,786
Average Length of Stay	6.0	5.9	5.8	5.5	5.5
Personnel					
Total Full Time	129,997	126,761	132,035	129,680	124,759
Total Part Time	38,733	35,873	35,061	37,963	37,606
COMMUNITY HEALTH INDICATORS PER 1000 POPULATION					
Total Population (in thousands)	10,913	10,800	10,710	10,617	10,519
Inpatient					
Beds	2.3	2.3	2.3	2.3	2.4
Admissions	87.7	91.5	90.7	97.6	96.6
Inpatient Days	593.1	609.5	595.2	612.3	610.8
Inpatient Surgeries	19.4	20.7	21.9	24.3	23.4
Births	10.8	10.7	11.1	11.4	11.6
Outpatient					
Emergency Outpatient Visits	374.3	365.4	384.5	436	445.6
Other Outpatient Visits	1,567.4	1,623.9	1,403.1	1,492	1,451.1
Total Outpatient Visits	1,941.6	1,989.3	1,787.6	1,928.1	1,896.8
Outpatient Surgeries	49.6	49.3	43.9	49.6	47.9

Note: The 2021 performance data do not reflect the full impact of the COVID-19 pandemic. Please refer to the discussion in the Introduction for more information.

AHA Hospital Statistics © 2024 Health Forum LLC, an affiliate of the American Hospital Association

TABLE 6

HAWAII

U.S. Community Hospitals
(Nonfederal, short-term general and other special hospitals)

Overview 2018–2022

	2022	2021	2020	2019	2018
Total Community Hospitals in Hawaii	23	23	22	22	22
Bed Size Category					
6-24	5	5	5	5	5
25-49	3	3	3	3	3
50-99	4	4	3	3	3
100-199	6	7	8	8	8
200-299	4	3	2	2	2
300-399	0	0	0	0	0
400-499	0	0	0	0	0
500 +	1	1	1	1	1
Location					
Hospitals Urban	15	15	15	15	15
Hospitals Rural	8	8	7	7	7
Control					
State and Local Government	6	6	5	4	5
Not for Profit	17	17	17	18	17
Investor owned	0	0	0	0	0
Affiliations					
Hospitals in a System	19	19	18	18	18
Hospitals in a Group Purchasing Organization...	12	12	8	9	9

Note: The 2021 performance data do not reflect the full impact of the COVID-19 pandemic. Please refer to the discussion in the Introduction for more information.

TABLE 6

HAWAII

U.S. Community Hospitals
(Nonfederal, short-term general and other special hospitals)

Utilization, Personnel, Community Health Indicators 2018–2022

	2022	2021	2020	2019	2018
TOTAL FACILITY (Includes Hospital and Nursing Home Units)					
Utilization - Inpatient					
Beds	2,946	2,831	2,687	2,731	2,749
Admissions	105,662	105,436	107,867	113,544	108,634
Inpatient Days	726,778	699,686	681,453	706,387	710,649
Average Length of Stay	6.9	6.6	6.3	6.2	6.5
Inpatient Surgeries	31,525	32,272	31,617	25,595	30,499
Births	13,176	13,142	13,656	15,328	16,298
Utilization - Outpatient					
Emergency Outpatient Visits	460,850	394,625	443,780	497,344	462,713
Other Outpatient Visits	2,612,164	2,444,665	2,284,560	2,279,269	2,244,228
Total Outpatient Visits	3,073,014	2,839,290	2,728,340	2,776,613	2,706,941
Outpatient Surgeries	79,129	78,310	63,463	70,317	63,849
Personnel					
Full Time RNs	4,841	4,710	4,537	4,401	4,217
Full Time LPNs	375	118	152	158	152
Part Time RNs	1,301	1,539	1,535	1,475	1,556
Part Time LPNs	107	48	48	56	50
Total Full Time	15,665	16,714	15,212	14,937	14,523
Total Part Time	3,770	4,894	4,456	4,450	4,626
HOSPITAL UNIT (Excludes Separate Nursing Home Units)					
Utilization - Inpatient					
Beds	2,841	2,774	2,687	2,731	2,644
Admissions	105,597	105,409	107,867	113,544	108,556
Inpatient Days	714,555	682,782	681,453	706,387	678,989
Average Length of Stay	6.8	6.5	6.3	6.2	6.3
Personnel					
Total Full Time	15,591	16,624	15,212	14,937	14,405
Total Part Time	3,735	4,869	4,456	4,450	4,623
COMMUNITY HEALTH INDICATORS PER 1000 POPULATION					
Total Population (in thousands)	1,440	1,442	1,407	1,416	1,420
Inpatient					
Beds	2	2	1.9	1.9	1.9
Admissions	73.4	73.1	76.7	80.2	76.5
Inpatient Days	504.6	485.4	484.3	498.9	500.3
Inpatient Surgeries	21.9	22.4	22.5	18.1	21.5
Births	9.1	9.1	9.7	10.8	11.5
Outpatient					
Emergency Outpatient Visits	320	273.7	315.4	351.3	325.7
Other Outpatient Visits	1,813.8	1,695.9	1,623.7	1,609.8	1,579.9
Total Outpatient Visits	2,133.7	1,969.6	1,939.1	1,961.1	1,905.6
Outpatient Surgeries	54.9	54.3	45.1	49.7	44.9

Note: The 2021 performance data do not reflect the full impact of the COVID-19 pandemic. Please refer to the discussion in the Introduction for more information.

TABLE 6

IDAHO

U.S. Community Hospitals
(Nonfederal, short-term general and other special hospitals)

Overview 2018–2022

	2022	2021	2020	2019	2018
Total Community Hospitals in Idaho..................	47	47	46	46	45
Bed Size Category					
6-24	14	17	17	17	17
25-49	18	14	13	13	13
50-99	6	7	7	7	6
100-199	4	4	4	4	4
200-299	2	2	2	2	3
300-399	2	1	1	2	1
400-499	0	1	1	0	0
500 + ...	1	1	1	1	1
Location					
Hospitals Urban	22	23	22	22	21
Hospitals Rural	25	24	24	24	24
Control					
State and Local Government	16	16	17	17	17
Not for Profit	20	20	19	19	20
Investor owned	11	11	10	10	8
Affiliations					
Hospitals in a System	22	22	22	24	24
Hospitals in a Group Purchasing Organization...	17	19	19	22	23

Note: The 2021 performance data do not reflect the full impact of the COVID-19 pandemic. Please refer to the discussion in the Introduction for more information.

74   AHA Hospital Statistics © 2024 Health Forum LLC, an affiliate of the American Hospital Association

TABLE 6

IDAHO

U.S. Community Hospitals
(Nonfederal, short-term general and other special hospitals)

Utilization, Personnel, Community Health Indicators 2018–2022

	2022	2021	2020	2019	2018
TOTAL FACILITY (Includes Hospital and Nursing Home Units)					
Utilization - Inpatient					
Beds	3,588	3,600	3,535	3,468	3,396
Admissions	127,568	132,057	133,525	138,405	139,996
Inpatient Days	650,271	640,779	617,583	639,152	630,699
Average Length of Stay	5.1	4.9	4.6	4.6	4.5
Inpatient Surgeries	29,367	30,610	35,590	41,061	40,049
Births	18,946	19,628	18,405	19,277	19,152
Utilization - Outpatient					
Emergency Outpatient Visits	943,798	711,037	679,359	688,976	720,026
Other Outpatient Visits	5,841,917	6,355,150	5,634,604	5,744,940	5,541,913
Total Outpatient Visits	6,785,715	7,066,187	6,313,963	6,433,916	6,261,939
Outpatient Surgeries	102,326	100,434	90,961	100,924	95,034
Personnel					
Full Time RNs	6,868	6,039	5,334	5,953	6,723
Full Time LPNs	544	542	393	413	463
Part Time RNs	2,876	2,547	2,411	2,214	3,180
Part Time LPNs	191	151	153	150	176
Total Full Time	26,507	24,692	20,857	21,795	26,903
Total Part Time	8,801	7,784	8,122	7,473	10,050
HOSPITAL UNIT (Excludes Separate Nursing Home Units)					
Utilization - Inpatient					
Beds	3,485	3,524	3,470	3,331	3,291
Admissions	126,734	131,914	133,427	138,216	139,857
Inpatient Days	632,745	626,485	598,670	598,430	601,076
Average Length of Stay	5.0	4.7	4.5	4.3	4.3
Personnel					
Total Full Time	26,329	24,642	20,810	21,699	26,842
Total Part Time	8,713	7,752	8,079	7,401	9,991
COMMUNITY HEALTH INDICATORS PER 1000 POPULATION					
Total Population (in thousands)	1,939	1,901	1,827	1,787	1,754
Inpatient					
Beds	1.9	1.9	1.9	1.9	1.9
Admissions	65.8	69.5	73.1	77.4	79.8
Inpatient Days	335.4	337.1	338	357.7	359.5
Inpatient Surgeries	15.1	16.1	19.5	23	22.8
Births	9.8	10.3	10.1	10.8	10.9
Outpatient					
Emergency Outpatient Visits	486.7	374	371.9	385.5	410.5
Other Outpatient Visits	3,012.8	3,343.2	3,084.2	3,214.7	3,159.2
Total Outpatient Visits	3,499.5	3,717.2	3,456.1	3,600.3	3,569.7
Outpatient Surgeries	52.8	52.8	49.8	56.5	54.2

Note: The 2021 performance data do not reflect the full impact of the COVID-19 pandemic. Please refer to the discussion in the Introduction for more information.

AHA Hospital Statistics © 2024 Health Forum LLC, an affiliate of the American Hospital Association

TABLE 6

ILLINOIS

U.S. Community Hospitals
(Nonfederal, short-term general and other special hospitals)

Overview 2018–2022

	2022	2021	2020	2019	2018
Total Community Hospitals in Illinois	181	181	184	185	187
Bed Size Category					
6-24	14	15	15	16	16
25-49	43	41	42	38	36
50-99	25	24	22	26	27
100-199	47	48	50	47	47
200-299	20	20	23	26	28
300-399	14	15	14	15	15
400-499	10	10	10	9	10
500 +	8	8	8	8	8
Location					
Hospitals Urban	120	125	127	128	130
Hospitals Rural	61	56	57	57	57
Control					
State and Local Government	22	23	24	23	23
Not for Profit	143	144	145	146	146
Investor owned	16	14	15	16	18
Affiliations					
Hospitals in a System	122	127	126	124	123
Hospitals in a Group Purchasing Organization	118	139	139	138	139

Note: The 2021 performance data do not reflect the full impact of the COVID-19 pandemic. Please refer to the discussion in the Introduction for more information.

TABLE 6

ILLINOIS

U.S. Community Hospitals
(Nonfederal, short-term general and other special hospitals)

Utilization, Personnel, Community Health Indicators 2018–2022

	2022	2021	2020	2019	2018
TOTAL FACILITY (Includes Hospital and Nursing Home Units)					
Utilization - Inpatient					
Beds	30,671	30,889	31,803	31,262	32,066
Admissions	1,195,512	1,208,995	1,217,927	1,326,907	1,357,534
Inpatient Days	6,788,731	6,665,135	6,493,496	6,762,533	6,822,518
Average Length of Stay	5.7	5.5	5.3	5.1	5.0
Inpatient Surgeries	268,476	281,438	278,074	320,080	322,415
Births	122,734	124,084	126,572	132,191	136,669
Utilization - Outpatient					
Emergency Outpatient Visits	4,969,025	4,759,070	4,875,442	5,631,309	5,488,964
Other Outpatient Visits	34,737,772	33,349,256	29,342,648	33,589,589	32,139,739
Total Outpatient Visits	39,706,797	38,108,326	34,218,090	39,220,898	37,628,703
Outpatient Surgeries	758,833	733,814	644,843	721,407	734,668
Personnel					
Full Time RNs	51,584	53,550	55,417	54,321	53,339
Full Time LPNs	1,486	1,270	1,458	1,642	1,351
Part Time RNs	24,198	21,770	21,348	24,433	22,996
Part Time LPNs	649	467	536	680	482
Total Full Time	181,230	182,760	181,190	188,286	184,073
Total Part Time	85,913	80,095	78,592	88,987	77,898
HOSPITAL UNIT (Excludes Separate Nursing Home Units)					
Utilization - Inpatient					
Beds	30,340	30,375	31,227	30,661	31,370
Admissions	1,193,287	1,206,234	1,214,590	1,321,111	1,351,510
Inpatient Days	6,696,935	6,533,145	6,338,845	6,588,816	6,632,896
Average Length of Stay	5.6	5.4	5.2	5.0	4.9
Personnel					
Total Full Time	180,976	182,336	180,844	187,884	183,575
Total Part Time	85,791	79,815	78,314	88,658	77,592
COMMUNITY HEALTH INDICATORS PER 1000 POPULATION					
Total Population (in thousands)	12,582	12,671	12,588	12,672	12,741
Inpatient					
Beds	2.4	2.4	2.5	2.5	2.5
Admissions	95	95.4	96.8	104.7	106.5
Inpatient Days	539.6	526	515.9	533.7	535.5
Inpatient Surgeries	21.3	22.2	22.1	25.3	25.3
Births	9.8	9.8	10.1	10.4	10.7
Outpatient					
Emergency Outpatient Visits	394.9	375.6	387.3	444.4	430.8
Other Outpatient Visits	2,760.9	2,631.8	2,331.1	2,650.7	2,522.5
Total Outpatient Visits	3,155.8	3,007.4	2,718.4	3,095.1	2,953.3
Outpatient Surgeries	60.3	57.9	51.2	56.9	57.7

Note: The 2021 performance data do not reflect the full impact of the COVID-19 pandemic. Please refer to the discussion in the Introduction for more information.

States

TABLE 6

INDIANA

U.S. Community Hospitals
(Nonfederal, short-term general and other special hospitals)

Overview 2018–2022

	2022	2021	2020	2019	2018
Total Community Hospitals in Indiana...............	130	130	129	129	132
Bed Size Category					
6-24..	18	16	15	14	15
25-49..	42	44	43	42	42
50-99..	19	19	20	22	23
100-199..	20	19	21	21	22
200-299..	14	15	12	12	13
300-399..	5	5	5	6	6
400-499..	6	6	7	7	5
500 +..	6	6	6	5	6
Location					
Hospitals Urban	89	89	88	87	89
Hospitals Rural...	41	41	41	42	43
Control					
State and Local Government	25	25	26	26	25
Not for Profit...	74	74	72	72	73
Investor owned	31	31	31	31	34
Affiliations					
Hospitals in a System	94	94	95	94	94
Hospitals in a Group Purchasing Organization...	73	76	76	86	97

Note: The 2021 performance data do not reflect the full impact of the COVID-19 pandemic. Please refer to the discussion in the Introduction for more information.

TABLE 6

INDIANA

U.S. Community Hospitals
(Nonfederal, short-term general and other special hospitals)

Utilization, Personnel, Community Health Indicators 2018–2022

	2022	2021	2020	2019	2018
TOTAL FACILITY (Includes Hospital and Nursing Home Units)					
Utilization - Inpatient					
Beds	18,043	18,240	18,386	18,237	18,156
Admissions	707,815	721,516	685,954	735,348	728,676
Inpatient Days	4,028,917	3,979,619	3,710,602	3,864,788	3,707,730
Average Length of Stay	5.7	5.5	5.4	5.3	5.1
Inpatient Surgeries	172,117	168,919	180,257	206,319	196,696
Births	76,846	75,663	75,695	78,181	80,843
Utilization - Outpatient					
Emergency Outpatient Visits	3,547,567	3,300,429	3,050,366	3,379,414	3,700,024
Other Outpatient Visits	18,038,681	17,431,363	17,323,015	18,475,586	17,783,847
Total Outpatient Visits	21,586,248	20,731,792	20,373,381	21,855,000	21,483,871
Outpatient Surgeries	452,155	482,655	423,845	490,657	475,903
Personnel					
Full Time RNs	23,850	23,224	25,809	25,149	26,712
Full Time LPNs	1,227	1,070	1,102	1,194	1,255
Part Time RNs	18,354	15,792	15,910	15,693	15,140
Part Time LPNs	762	647	555	580	574
Total Full Time	92,821	89,962	92,867	92,244	96,556
Total Part Time	53,820	48,100	47,026	46,924	45,487
HOSPITAL UNIT (Excludes Separate Nursing Home Units)					
Utilization - Inpatient					
Beds	17,525	17,631	17,623	17,600	17,467
Admissions	706,767	720,218	684,879	734,134	726,794
Inpatient Days	3,884,340	3,836,775	3,529,437	3,637,267	3,532,634
Average Length of Stay	5.5	5.3	5.2	5.0	4.9
Personnel					
Total Full Time	92,516	89,643	92,506	92,053	96,100
Total Part Time	53,492	47,759	46,889	46,680	45,145
COMMUNITY HEALTH INDICATORS PER 1000 POPULATION					
Total Population (in thousands)	6,833	6,806	6,755	6,732	6,692
Inpatient					
Beds	2.6	2.7	2.7	2.7	2.7
Admissions	103.6	106	101.5	109.2	108.9
Inpatient Days	589.6	584.7	549.3	574.1	554.1
Inpatient Surgeries	25.2	24.8	26.7	30.6	29.4
Births	11.2	11.1	11.2	11.6	12.1
Outpatient					
Emergency Outpatient Visits	519.2	484.9	451.6	502	552.9
Other Outpatient Visits	2,639.9	2,561.2	2,564.5	2,744.4	2,657.5
Total Outpatient Visits	3,159.1	3,046.1	3,016.1	3,246.3	3,210.4
Outpatient Surgeries	66.2	70.9	62.7	72.9	71.1

Note: The 2021 performance data do not reflect the full impact of the COVID-19 pandemic. Please refer to the discussion in the Introduction for more information.

AHA Hospital Statistics © 2024 Health Forum LLC, an affiliate of the American Hospital Association

TABLE 6

IOWA

U.S. Community Hospitals
(Nonfederal, short-term general and other special hospitals)

Overview 2018–2022

	2022	2021	2020	2019	2018
Total Community Hospitals in Iowa	**118**	**118**	**116**	**117**	**118**
Bed Size Category					
6-24	38	32	30	28	25
25-49	42	47	47	47	49
50-99	16	18	17	20	20
100-199	12	11	11	10	11
200-299	3	3	4	6	6
300-399	4	4	4	3	4
400-499	1	1	0	0	0
500 +	2	2	3	3	3
Location					
Hospitals Urban	38	38	36	36	37
Hospitals Rural	80	80	80	81	81
Control					
State and Local Government	57	59	59	59	59
Not for Profit	55	54	54	55	56
Investor owned	6	5	3	3	3
Affiliations					
Hospitals in a System	87	87	85	88	89
Hospitals in a Group Purchasing Organization...	116	117	116	116	116

Note: The 2021 performance data do not reflect the full impact of the COVID-19 pandemic. Please refer to the discussion in the Introduction for more information.

TABLE 6

IOWA

U.S. Community Hospitals
(Nonfederal, short-term general and other special hospitals)

Utilization, Personnel, Community Health Indicators 2018–2022

	2022	2021	2020	2019	2018
TOTAL FACILITY (Includes Hospital and Nursing Home Units)					
Utilization - Inpatient					
Beds	8,698	8,768	9,090	9,459	9,423
Admissions	262,298	265,505	287,313	308,139	315,047
Inpatient Days	1,705,062	1,707,090	1,756,353	1,879,720	1,913,280
Average Length of Stay	6.5	6.4	6.1	6.1	6.1
Inpatient Surgeries	57,832	62,260	68,487	78,137	82,348
Births	34,640	34,171	36,858	37,417	37,441
Utilization - Outpatient					
Emergency Outpatient Visits	1,255,943	1,144,450	1,196,718	1,317,142	1,359,801
Other Outpatient Visits	13,647,303	11,766,218	10,819,126	10,902,397	10,134,622
Total Outpatient Visits	14,903,246	12,910,668	12,015,844	12,219,539	11,494,423
Outpatient Surgeries	252,218	244,979	224,240	260,513	248,337
Personnel					
Full Time RNs	11,942	12,445	13,636	13,120	13,490
Full Time LPNs	886	837	861	791	801
Part Time RNs	7,030	6,784	7,159	7,017	7,047
Part Time LPNs	496	480	567	420	467
Total Full Time	48,079	49,883	50,557	49,024	50,371
Total Part Time	24,138	23,275	23,668	22,987	23,162
HOSPITAL UNIT (Excludes Separate Nursing Home Units)					
Utilization - Inpatient					
Beds	7,611	7,692	8,010	8,152	8,045
Admissions	261,324	264,849	286,617	306,666	312,710
Inpatient Days	1,411,163	1,408,767	1,423,935	1,457,375	1,441,340
Average Length of Stay	5.4	5.3	5.0	4.8	4.6
Personnel					
Total Full Time	47,613	49,384	50,049	48,392	49,691
Total Part Time	23,527	22,727	23,135	22,344	22,429
COMMUNITY HEALTH INDICATORS PER 1000 POPULATION					
Total Population (in thousands)	3,201	3,193	3,164	3,155	3,156
Inpatient					
Beds	2.7	2.7	2.9	3	3
Admissions	82	83.2	90.8	97.7	99.8
Inpatient Days	532.7	534.6	555.2	595.8	606.2
Inpatient Surgeries	18.1	19.5	21.6	24.8	26.1
Births	10.8	10.7	11.7	11.9	11.9
Outpatient					
Emergency Outpatient Visits	392.4	358.4	378.3	417.5	430.8
Other Outpatient Visits	4,264.1	3,684.9	3,419.9	3,455.5	3,211.1
Total Outpatient Visits	4,656.5	4,043.3	3,798.2	3,873	3,641.9
Outpatient Surgeries	78.8	76.7	70.9	82.6	78.7

Note: The 2021 performance data do not reflect the full impact of the COVID-19 pandemic. Please refer to the discussion in the Introduction for more information.

AHA Hospital Statistics © 2024 Health Forum LLC, an affiliate of the American Hospital Association

TABLE 6

KANSAS

U.S. Community Hospitals
(Nonfederal, short-term general and other special hospitals)

Overview 2018–2022

	2022	2021	2020	2019	2018
Total Community Hospitals in Kansas...............	135	135	135	138	139
Bed Size Category					
6-24	39	39	40	38	31
25-49	53	52	50	55	60
50-99	23	24	24	23	26
100-199	11	10	11	12	12
200-299	4	5	5	5	5
300-399	0	0	0	2	2
400-499	2	2	2	0	0
500 + ...	3	3	3	3	3
Location					
Hospitals Urban	44	43	43	44	45
Hospitals Rural	91	92	92	94	94
Control					
State and Local Government	58	58	57	61	62
Not for Profit..	52	52	51	50	50
Investor owned..	25	25	27	27	27
Affiliations					
Hospitals in a System	47	47	50	54	55
Hospitals in a Group Purchasing Organization...	108	112	109	110	111

Note: The 2021 performance data do not reflect the full impact of the COVID-19 pandemic. Please refer to the discussion in the Introduction for more information.

TABLE 6

KANSAS

U.S. Community Hospitals
(Nonfederal, short-term general and other special hospitals)

Utilization, Personnel, Community Health Indicators 2018–2022

	2022	2021	2020	2019	2018
TOTAL FACILITY (Includes Hospital and Nursing Home Units)					
Utilization - Inpatient					
Beds	9,303	9,395	9,370	9,544	9,659
Admissions	286,980	295,215	298,809	316,464	318,566
Inpatient Days	1,796,247	1,816,212	1,778,977	1,936,123	1,870,624
Average Length of Stay	6.3	6.2	6.0	6.1	5.9
Inpatient Surgeries	62,108	66,596	70,315	78,814	78,271
Births	31,724	31,378	31,810	32,477	32,642
Utilization - Outpatient					
Emergency Outpatient Visits	1,255,041	1,114,923	1,065,421	1,196,829	1,196,146
Other Outpatient Visits	8,713,290	8,524,772	7,633,568	7,734,885	7,612,888
Total Outpatient Visits	9,968,331	9,639,695	8,698,989	8,931,714	8,809,034
Outpatient Surgeries	218,437	213,973	183,358	205,955	199,316
Personnel					
Full Time RNs	12,680	13,353	13,699	13,552	13,310
Full Time LPNs	1,254	1,225	1,303	1,238	1,196
Part Time RNs	6,183	6,292	6,439	5,798	5,407
Part Time LPNs	420	420	426	405	404
Total Full Time	48,931	48,955	48,690	47,489	45,894
Total Part Time	18,392	19,068	21,955	19,033	17,782
HOSPITAL UNIT (Excludes Separate Nursing Home Units)					
Utilization - Inpatient					
Beds	8,459	8,429	8,407	8,510	8,586
Admissions	286,027	294,172	297,692	314,931	316,835
Inpatient Days	1,559,760	1,534,211	1,488,321	1,541,312	1,542,998
Average Length of Stay	5.5	5.2	5.0	4.9	4.9
Personnel					
Total Full Time	48,432	48,274	47,978	46,755	45,129
Total Part Time	18,130	18,749	21,558	18,636	17,362
COMMUNITY HEALTH INDICATORS PER 1000 POPULATION					
Total Population (in thousands)	2,937	2,935	2,914	2,913	2,912
Inpatient					
Beds	3.2	3.2	3.2	3.3	3.3
Admissions	97.7	100.6	102.5	108.6	109.4
Inpatient Days	611.6	618.9	610.5	664.6	642.5
Inpatient Surgeries	21.1	22.7	24.1	27.1	26.9
Births	10.8	10.7	10.9	11.1	11.2
Outpatient					
Emergency Outpatient Visits	427.3	379.9	365.6	410.8	410.8
Other Outpatient Visits	2,966.6	2,904.9	2,619.8	2,655	2,614.8
Total Outpatient Visits	3,393.9	3,284.9	2,985.4	3,065.8	3,025.6
Outpatient Surgeries	74.4	72.9	62.9	70.7	68.5

Note: The 2021 performance data do not reflect the full impact of the COVID-19 pandemic. Please refer to the discussion in the Introduction for more information.

AHA Hospital Statistics © 2024 Health Forum LLC, an affiliate of the American Hospital Association

TABLE 6

KENTUCKY

U.S. Community Hospitals
(Nonfederal, short-term general and other special hospitals)

Overview 2018–2022

	2022	2021	2020	2019	2018
Total Community Hospitals in Kentucky	**104**	**104**	**104**	**104**	**105**
Bed Size Category					
6-24	6	5	5	5	5
25-49	44	42	41	41	40
50-99	11	13	14	14	15
100-199	23	24	22	23	23
200-299	8	7	9	8	9
300-399	5	6	6	6	7
400-499	4	4	5	4	2
500 +	3	3	2	3	4
Location					
Hospitals Urban	42	37	37	38	39
Hospitals Rural	62	67	67	66	66
Control					
State and Local Government	9	10	10	11	11
Not for Profit	71	71	72	72	72
Investor owned	24	23	22	21	22
Affiliations					
Hospitals in a System	84	82	82	81	82
Hospitals in a Group Purchasing Organization	37	37	43	39	50

Note: The 2021 performance data do not reflect the full impact of the COVID-19 pandemic. Please refer to the discussion in the Introduction for more information.

TABLE 6

KENTUCKY

U.S. Community Hospitals
(Nonfederal, short-term general and other special hospitals)

Utilization, Personnel, Community Health Indicators 2018–2022

	2022	2021	2020	2019	2018
TOTAL FACILITY (Includes Hospital and Nursing Home Units)					
Utilization - Inpatient					
Beds	13,992	14,124	14,257	14,151	14,329
Admissions	499,303	506,923	505,529	557,552	560,981
Inpatient Days	3,040,113	3,062,832	2,930,079	3,097,160	3,157,874
Average Length of Stay	6.1	6.0	5.8	5.6	5.6
Inpatient Surgeries	118,598	129,107	134,439	152,306	154,042
Births	50,917	49,013	51,851	54,340	53,245
Utilization - Outpatient					
Emergency Outpatient Visits	2,369,536	2,367,836	2,303,273	2,693,016	2,679,937
Other Outpatient Visits	12,606,775	13,359,910	12,143,942	12,781,236	12,219,136
Total Outpatient Visits	14,976,311	15,727,746	14,447,215	15,474,252	14,899,073
Outpatient Surgeries	366,644	368,126	324,194	362,945	378,009
Personnel					
Full Time RNs	21,255	21,153	22,378	22,230	22,063
Full Time LPNs	1,033	877	838	873	993
Part Time RNs	7,461	7,338	8,354	8,299	7,890
Part Time LPNs	375	315	258	247	249
Total Full Time	74,155	70,771	71,406	70,264	69,590
Total Part Time	22,137	20,936	23,265	22,126	20,882
HOSPITAL UNIT (Excludes Separate Nursing Home Units)					
Utilization - Inpatient					
Beds	13,801	13,933	14,140	13,924	13,849
Admissions	496,936	504,902	504,053	555,623	557,438
Inpatient Days	2,997,491	3,022,410	2,905,100	3,028,089	3,022,680
Average Length of Stay	6.0	6.0	5.8	5.4	5.4
Personnel					
Total Full Time	74,002	70,651	71,309	70,016	69,268
Total Part Time	22,103	20,875	23,198	21,987	20,680
COMMUNITY HEALTH INDICATORS PER 1000 POPULATION					
Total Population (in thousands)	4,512	4,509	4,477	4,468	4,468
Inpatient					
Beds	3.1	3.1	3.2	3.2	3.2
Admissions	110.7	112.4	112.9	124.8	125.5
Inpatient Days	673.7	679.2	654.4	693.2	706.7
Inpatient Surgeries	26.3	28.6	30	34.1	34.5
Births	11.3	10.9	11.6	12.2	11.9
Outpatient					
Emergency Outpatient Visits	525.1	525.1	514.4	602.8	599.8
Other Outpatient Visits	2,793.9	2,962.7	2,712.4	2,860.8	2,734.6
Total Outpatient Visits	3,319	3,487.8	3,226.8	3,463.6	3,334.3
Outpatient Surgeries	81.3	81.6	72.4	81.2	84.6

Note: The 2021 performance data do not reflect the full impact of the COVID-19 pandemic. Please refer to the discussion in the Introduction for more information.

AHA Hospital Statistics © 2024 Health Forum LLC, an affiliate of the American Hospital Association

TABLE 6

LOUISIANA

U.S. Community Hospitals
(Nonfederal, short-term general and other special hospitals)

Overview 2018–2022

	2022	2021	2020	2019	2018
Total Community Hospitals in Louisiana............	**159**	**160**	**159**	**155**	**158**
Bed Size Category					
6-24	45	44	44	41	43
25-49	56	55	55	56	57
50-99	24	25	24	21	19
100-199	12	13	14	16	18
200-299	10	10	9	9	9
300-399	6	8	6	6	6
400-499	2	1	3	2	2
500 +	4	4	4	4	4
Location					
Hospitals Urban	118	117	117	113	116
Hospitals Rural	41	43	42	42	42
Control					
State and Local Government	42	43	43	46	47
Not for Profit	51	53	52	45	45
Investor owned	66	64	64	64	66
Affiliations					
Hospitals in a System	86	87	84	81	84
Hospitals in a Group Purchasing Organization...	61	67	60	55	52

Note: The 2021 performance data do not reflect the full impact of the COVID-19 pandemic. Please refer to the discussion in the Introduction for more information.

TABLE 6

LOUISIANA

U.S. Community Hospitals
(Nonfederal, short-term general and other special hospitals)

Utilization, Personnel, Community Health Indicators 2018–2022

	2022	2021	2020	2019	2018
TOTAL FACILITY (Includes Hospital and Nursing Home Units)					
Utilization - Inpatient					
Beds	14,643	14,999	15,096	15,226	15,272
Admissions	512,575	533,635	540,736	566,912	551,844
Inpatient Days	2,965,012	3,053,219	2,990,526	3,138,996	3,143,237
Average Length of Stay	5.8	5.7	5.5	5.5	5.7
Inpatient Surgeries	121,548	129,756	130,953	147,189	155,113
Births	62,123	59,190	60,377	60,330	64,371
Utilization - Outpatient					
Emergency Outpatient Visits	2,635,771	2,471,746	2,369,527	2,806,279	2,938,738
Other Outpatient Visits	9,227,880	8,482,421	8,312,512	10,716,632	9,986,720
Total Outpatient Visits	11,863,651	10,954,167	10,682,039	13,522,911	12,925,458
Outpatient Surgeries	354,304	387,645	317,674	347,556	351,952
Personnel					
Full Time RNs	20,432	20,248	20,713	22,376	21,447
Full Time LPNs	2,783	2,882	2,865	3,232	2,941
Part Time RNs	9,029	10,760	10,739	8,137	7,928
Part Time LPNs	862	1,191	1,236	879	808
Total Full Time	76,967	75,378	73,978	80,381	77,809
Total Part Time	25,595	32,150	31,348	23,693	23,037
HOSPITAL UNIT (Excludes Separate Nursing Home Units)					
Utilization - Inpatient					
Beds	14,333	14,781	14,864	14,579	14,624
Admissions	510,516	532,406	539,795	565,132	549,898
Inpatient Days	2,919,134	3,002,971	2,922,403	2,968,018	2,970,547
Average Length of Stay	5.7	5.6	5.4	5.3	5.4
Personnel					
Total Full Time	76,685	75,149	73,859	79,897	77,393
Total Part Time	25,578	32,095	31,263	23,579	22,909
COMMUNITY HEALTH INDICATORS PER 1000 POPULATION					
Total Population (in thousands)	4,590	4,624	4,645	4,649	4,660
Inpatient					
Beds	3.2	3.2	3.2	3.3	3.3
Admissions	111.7	115.4	116.4	121.9	118.4
Inpatient Days	645.9	660.3	643.8	675.2	674.5
Inpatient Surgeries	26.5	28.1	28.2	31.7	33.3
Births	13.5	12.8	13	13	13.8
Outpatient					
Emergency Outpatient Visits	574.2	534.5	510.1	603.7	630.6
Other Outpatient Visits	2,010.3	1,834.4	1,789.4	2,305.2	2,143.1
Total Outpatient Visits	2,584.5	2,369	2,299.5	2,908.9	2,773.7
Outpatient Surgeries	77.2	83.8	68.4	74.8	75.5

Note: The 2021 performance data do not reflect the full impact of the COVID-19 pandemic. Please refer to the discussion in the Introduction for more information.

AHA Hospital Statistics © 2024 Health Forum LLC, an affiliate of the American Hospital Association

States

TABLE 6

MAINE

U.S. Community Hospitals
(Nonfederal, short-term general and other special hospitals)

Overview 2018–2022

	2022	2021	2020	2019	2018
Total Community Hospitals in Maine	34	34	34	34	34
Bed Size Category					
6-24	2	2	3	3	2
25-49	17	16	15	15	15
50-99	7	7	7	7	8
100-199	5	6	6	6	6
200-299	0	0	0	0	0
300-399	2	1	1	2	2
400-499	0	1	1	0	0
500 + ...	1	1	1	1	1
Location					
Hospitals Urban	13	13	13	13	13
Hospitals Rural	21	21	21	21	21
Control					
State and Local Government	1	1	2	2	2
Not for Profit	32	32	31	31	31
Investor owned	1	1	1	1	1
Affiliations					
Hospitals in a System	24	24	23	21	20
Hospitals in a Group Purchasing Organization...	25	25	26	27	26

Note: The 2021 performance data do not reflect the full impact of the COVID-19 pandemic. Please refer to the discussion in the Introduction for more information.

AHA Hospital Statistics © 2024 Health Forum LLC, an affiliate of the American Hospital Association

TABLE 6

MAINE

U.S. Community Hospitals
(Nonfederal, short-term general and other special hospitals)

Utilization, Personnel, Community Health Indicators 2018–2022

	2022	2021	2020	2019	2018
TOTAL FACILITY (Includes Hospital and Nursing Home Units)					
Utilization - Inpatient					
Beds	3,510	3,471	3,490	3,482	3,400
Admissions	109,409	113,202	117,237	128,560	131,750
Inpatient Days	941,674	894,887	830,038	892,731	873,078
Average Length of Stay	8.6	7.9	7.1	6.9	6.6
Inpatient Surgeries	32,782	34,837	35,909	39,044	37,817
Births	11,395	11,235	10,964	11,594	11,899
Utilization - Outpatient					
Emergency Outpatient Visits	698,707	817,990	653,257	721,184	681,465
Other Outpatient Visits	7,275,373	7,714,252	6,131,796	6,025,317	5,262,248
Total Outpatient Visits	7,974,080	8,532,242	6,785,053	6,746,501	5,943,713
Outpatient Surgeries	115,124	110,720	88,768	106,759	105,073
Personnel					
Full Time RNs	5,239	6,646	6,975	6,426	6,295
Full Time LPNs	136	190	192	181	220
Part Time RNs	3,670	3,360	3,734	3,461	3,379
Part Time LPNs	84	81	90	77	94
Total Full Time	23,790	27,670	27,601	29,945	29,223
Total Part Time	13,054	11,118	11,887	11,449	11,671
HOSPITAL UNIT (Excludes Separate Nursing Home Units)					
Utilization - Inpatient					
Beds	3,096	3,051	3,115	2,995	2,913
Admissions	108,655	112,830	116,616	127,506	130,627
Inpatient Days	829,095	790,156	708,022	745,071	725,327
Average Length of Stay	7.6	7.0	6.1	5.8	5.6
Personnel					
Total Full Time	23,541	27,457	27,271	29,360	28,475
Total Part Time	12,894	10,935	11,538	11,055	11,156
COMMUNITY HEALTH INDICATORS PER 1000 POPULATION					
Total Population (in thousands)	1,385	1,372	1,350	1,344	1,338
Inpatient					
Beds	2.5	2.5	2.6	2.6	2.5
Admissions	79	82.5	86.8	95.6	98.4
Inpatient Days	679.7	652.1	614.8	664.1	652.3
Inpatient Surgeries	23.7	25.4	26.6	29	28.3
Births	8.2	8.2	8.1	8.6	8.9
Outpatient					
Emergency Outpatient Visits	504.4	596.1	483.8	536.5	509.2
Other Outpatient Visits	5,251.7	5,621.6	4,541.6	4,482.4	3,931.7
Total Outpatient Visits	5,756	6,217.7	5,025.4	5,018.9	4,440.9
Outpatient Surgeries	83.1	80.7	65.7	79.4	78.5

Note: The 2021 performance data do not reflect the full impact of the COVID-19 pandemic. Please refer to the discussion in the Introduction for more information.

AHA Hospital Statistics © 2024 Health Forum LLC, an affiliate of the American Hospital Association

TABLE 6

MARYLAND

U.S. Community Hospitals
(Nonfederal, short-term general and other special hospitals)

Overview 2018–2022

	2022	2021	2020	2019	2018
Total Community Hospitals in Maryland.............	47	48	49	48	50
Bed Size Category					
6-24	0	0	0	0	0
25-49	2	2	2	3	3
50-99	8	8	10	10	9
100-199	13	15	11	13	12
200-299	12	11	15	11	14
300-399	4	3	3	5	4
400-499	6	7	6	4	5
500 + ...	2	2	2	2	3
Location					
Hospitals Urban	42	45	45	44	46
Hospitals Rural...	5	3	4	4	4
Control					
State and Local Government	0	0	0	0	0
Not for Profit...	46	47	48	47	49
Investor owned...	1	1	1	1	1
Affiliations					
Hospitals in a System	41	42	42	36	36
Hospitals in a Group Purchasing Organization...	38	37	33	38	36

Note: The 2021 performance data do not reflect the full impact of the COVID-19 pandemic. Please refer to the discussion in the Introduction for more information.

TABLE 6

MARYLAND

U.S. Community Hospitals
(Nonfederal, short-term general and other special hospitals)

Utilization, Personnel, Community Health Indicators 2018–2022

	2022	2021	2020	2019	2018
TOTAL FACILITY (Includes Hospital and Nursing Home Units)					
Utilization - Inpatient					
Beds	11,169	11,374	11,230	10,894	11,577
Admissions	482,892	498,521	508,655	543,185	566,730
Inpatient Days	2,956,970	2,892,738	2,770,647	2,923,810	2,974,120
Average Length of Stay	6.1	5.8	5.4	5.4	5.2
Inpatient Surgeries	126,398	133,472	139,244	150,382	155,910
Births	63,451	61,594	63,933	62,147	64,499
Utilization - Outpatient					
Emergency Outpatient Visits	1,920,902	1,675,790	1,870,421	2,206,790	2,222,930
Other Outpatient Visits	5,409,938	6,158,106	6,140,519	7,245,106	7,608,996
Total Outpatient Visits	7,330,840	7,833,896	8,010,940	9,451,896	9,831,926
Outpatient Surgeries	293,933	284,498	266,741	308,729	333,618
Personnel					
Full Time RNs	19,820	21,409	23,135	22,751	21,349
Full Time LPNs	485	409	454	362	372
Part Time RNs	9,458	9,355	10,271	9,360	9,418
Part Time LPNs	157	167	139	136	172
Total Full Time	71,789	74,542	79,381	78,454	74,694
Total Part Time	26,779	27,765	30,168	28,069	28,344
HOSPITAL UNIT (Excludes Separate Nursing Home Units)					
Utilization - Inpatient					
Beds	11,092	11,297	11,065	10,729	11,412
Admissions	481,690	497,284	506,557	541,045	564,878
Inpatient Days	2,940,887	2,875,755	2,734,158	2,876,278	2,923,945
Average Length of Stay	6.1	5.8	5.4	5.3	5.2
Personnel					
Total Full Time	71,739	74,084	79,249	78,344	74,590
Total Part Time	26,728	27,646	30,014	27,956	28,221
COMMUNITY HEALTH INDICATORS PER 1000 POPULATION					
Total Population (in thousands)	6,165	6,165	6,056	6,046	6,043
Inpatient					
Beds	1.8	1.8	1.9	1.8	1.9
Admissions	78.3	80.9	84	89.8	93.8
Inpatient Days	479.7	469.2	457.5	483.6	492.2
Inpatient Surgeries	20.5	21.6	23	24.9	25.8
Births	10.3	10	10.6	10.3	10.7
Outpatient					
Emergency Outpatient Visits	311.6	271.8	308.9	365	367.9
Other Outpatient Visits	877.6	998.9	1,014	1,198.4	1,259.2
Total Outpatient Visits	1,189.2	1,270.7	1,322.9	1,563.4	1,627.1
Outpatient Surgeries	47.7	46.1	44	51.1	55.2

Note: The 2021 performance data do not reflect the full impact of the COVID-19 pandemic. Please refer to the discussion in the Introduction for more information.

AHA Hospital Statistics © 2024 Health Forum LLC, an affiliate of the American Hospital Association

TABLE 6

MASSACHUSETTS

U.S. Community Hospitals
(Nonfederal, short-term general and other special hospitals)

Overview 2018–2022

	2022	2021	2020	2019	2018
Total Community Hospitals in Massachusetts...	**73**	**75**	**74**	**74**	**75**
Bed Size Category					
6-24	6	6	4	4	3
25-49	4	3	4	4	6
50-99	13	14	14	14	16
100-199	23	25	25	25	23
200-299	11	9	10	11	11
300-399	8	9	9	8	7
400-499	1	3	2	3	4
500 +	7	6	6	5	5
Location					
Hospitals Urban	70	73	72	72	73
Hospitals Rural	3	2	2	2	2
Control					
State and Local Government	2	2	2	2	2
Not for Profit	55	56	56	56	56
Investor owned	16	17	16	16	17
Affiliations					
Hospitals in a System	60	62	60	57	58
Hospitals in a Group Purchasing Organization...	41	46	47	47	48

Note: The 2021 performance data do not reflect the full impact of the COVID-19 pandemic. Please refer to the discussion in the Introduction for more information.

TABLE 6

MASSACHUSETTS

U.S. Community Hospitals
(Nonfederal, short-term general and other special hospitals)

Utilization, Personnel, Community Health Indicators 2018–2022

	2022	2021	2020	2019	2018
TOTAL FACILITY (Includes Hospital and Nursing Home Units)					
Utilization - Inpatient					
Beds	15,959	16,045	15,810	15,561	15,649
Admissions	730,753	729,055	716,146	777,310	780,198
Inpatient Days	4,427,563	4,317,694	4,078,483	4,222,166	4,205,986
Average Length of Stay	6.1	5.9	5.7	5.4	5.4
Inpatient Surgeries	156,380	167,400	164,082	191,744	183,251
Births	65,855	65,859	65,559	65,577	66,086
Utilization - Outpatient					
Emergency Outpatient Visits	3,225,024	3,019,907	2,909,532	3,385,519	3,306,597
Other Outpatient Visits	20,519,697	21,243,503	18,650,397	20,075,088	20,059,097
Total Outpatient Visits	23,744,721	24,263,410	21,559,929	23,460,607	23,365,694
Outpatient Surgeries	419,489	399,358	348,508	429,341	420,141
Personnel					
Full Time RNs	30,490	28,543	28,152	28,648	25,517
Full Time LPNs	1,043	845	856	852	752
Part Time RNs	23,844	23,602	23,983	24,790	23,799
Part Time LPNs	680	523	497	517	490
Total Full Time	138,306	134,265	129,870	130,455	124,637
Total Part Time	74,661	73,059	73,218	72,454	70,628
HOSPITAL UNIT (Excludes Separate Nursing Home Units)					
Utilization - Inpatient					
Beds	15,898	15,984	15,749	15,500	15,588
Admissions	730,748	729,051	716,142	777,301	780,182
Inpatient Days	4,416,917	4,304,065	4,061,546	4,203,114	4,184,868
Average Length of Stay	6.0	5.9	5.7	5.4	5.4
Personnel					
Total Full Time	138,292	134,252	129,840	130,441	124,602
Total Part Time	74,634	73,049	73,201	72,439	70,585
COMMUNITY HEALTH INDICATORS PER 1000 POPULATION					
Total Population (in thousands)	6,982	6,985	6,894	6,893	6,902
Inpatient					
Beds	2.3	2.3	2.3	2.3	2.3
Admissions	104.7	104.4	103.9	112.8	113
Inpatient Days	634.1	618.2	591.6	612.6	609.4
Inpatient Surgeries	22.4	24	23.8	27.8	26.5
Births	9.4	9.4	9.5	9.5	9.6
Outpatient					
Emergency Outpatient Visits	461.9	432.4	422.1	491.2	479.1
Other Outpatient Visits	2,939	3,041.4	2,705.5	2,912.6	2,906.2
Total Outpatient Visits	3,400.9	3,473.8	3,127.5	3,403.8	3,385.3
Outpatient Surgeries	60.1	57.2	50.6	62.3	60.9

Note: The 2021 performance data do not reflect the full impact of the COVID-19 pandemic. Please refer to the discussion in the Introduction for more information.

AHA Hospital Statistics © 2024 Health Forum LLC, an affiliate of the American Hospital Association

TABLE 6

MICHIGAN

U.S. Community Hospitals
(Nonfederal, short-term general and other special hospitals)

Overview 2018–2022

	2022	2021	2020	2019	2018
Total Community Hospitals in Michigan	140	139	141	145	144
Bed Size Category					
6-24	16	16	15	14	15
25-49	42	41	43	46	43
50-99	22	22	22	23	23
100-199	17	16	19	20	21
200-299	12	15	14	13	14
300-399	13	10	11	11	9
400-499	6	7	5	6	8
500 +	12	12	12	12	11
Location					
Hospitals Urban	89	88	90	93	92
Hospitals Rural	51	51	51	52	52
Control					
State and Local Government	4	6	6	6	6
Not for Profit	113	110	112	113	113
Investor owned	23	23	23	26	25
Affiliations					
Hospitals in a System	110	106	108	113	111
Hospitals in a Group Purchasing Organization	108	111	111	113	113

Note: The 2021 performance data do not reflect the full impact of the COVID-19 pandemic. Please refer to the discussion in the Introduction for more information.

TABLE 6

MICHIGAN

U.S. Community Hospitals
(Nonfederal, short-term general and other special hospitals)

Utilization, Personnel, Community Health Indicators 2018–2022

	2022	2021	2020	2019	2018
TOTAL FACILITY (Includes Hospital and Nursing Home Units)					
Utilization - Inpatient					
Beds	24,569	24,674	24,503	24,809	24,949
Admissions	1,004,007	1,031,313	1,012,951	1,115,500	1,134,295
Inpatient Days	5,736,102	5,691,930	5,426,162	5,744,466	5,717,822
Average Length of Stay	5.7	5.5	5.4	5.1	5.0
Inpatient Surgeries	228,954	250,620	244,327	291,580	299,602
Births	96,729	98,874	97,365	101,496	104,990
Utilization - Outpatient					
Emergency Outpatient Visits	4,493,966	4,403,544	4,128,257	4,903,345	5,008,903
Other Outpatient Visits	33,296,089	33,447,479	30,070,932	32,495,099	34,017,938
Total Outpatient Visits	37,790,055	37,851,023	34,199,189	37,398,444	39,026,841
Outpatient Surgeries	697,440	694,189	586,914	700,069	681,400
Personnel					
Full Time RNs	40,591	42,923	46,063	45,682	45,984
Full Time LPNs	1,186	961	998	1,079	1,148
Part Time RNs	18,638	18,458	19,276	19,195	19,538
Part Time LPNs	532	435	389	481	560
Total Full Time	141,237	145,294	150,714	152,788	156,339
Total Part Time	58,959	58,196	59,260	62,221	61,971
HOSPITAL UNIT (Excludes Separate Nursing Home Units)					
Utilization - Inpatient					
Beds	23,789	23,855	23,795	23,943	24,079
Admissions	1,001,576	1,029,163	1,010,709	1,111,702	1,130,879
Inpatient Days	5,523,084	5,465,076	5,196,743	5,459,489	5,437,171
Average Length of Stay	5.5	5.3	5.1	4.9	4.8
Personnel					
Total Full Time	140,771	144,787	150,299	152,244	155,719
Total Part Time	58,611	57,838	58,949	61,824	61,589
COMMUNITY HEALTH INDICATORS PER 1000 POPULATION					
Total Population (in thousands)	10,034	10,051	9,967	9,987	9,996
Inpatient					
Beds	2.4	2.5	2.5	2.5	2.5
Admissions	100.1	102.6	101.6	111.7	113.5
Inpatient Days	571.7	566.3	544.4	575.2	572
Inpatient Surgeries	22.8	24.9	24.5	29.2	30
Births	9.6	9.8	9.8	10.2	10.5
Outpatient					
Emergency Outpatient Visits	447.9	438.1	414.2	491	501.1
Other Outpatient Visits	3,318.3	3,327.8	3,017.2	3,253.8	3,403.2
Total Outpatient Visits	3,766.2	3,766	3,431.4	3,744.8	3,904.3
Outpatient Surgeries	69.5	69.1	58.9	70.1	68.2

Note: The 2021 performance data do not reflect the full impact of the COVID-19 pandemic. Please refer to the discussion in the Introduction for more information.

AHA Hospital Statistics © 2024 Health Forum LLC, an affiliate of the American Hospital Association

TABLE 6

MINNESOTA

U.S. Community Hospitals
(Nonfederal, short-term general and other special hospitals)

Overview 2018–2022

	2022	2021	2020	2019	2018
Total Community Hospitals in Minnesota...........	**124**	**123**	**125**	**125**	**127**
Bed Size Category					
6-24	37	31	31	30	31
25-49	24	28	29	30	31
50-99	28	28	28	28	29
100-199	21	22	22	22	21
200-299	1	1	2	2	2
300-399	4	4	4	5	5
400-499	6	6	6	5	5
500 + ...	3	3	3	3	3
Location					
Hospitals Urban	50	50	52	52	53
Hospitals Rural	74	73	73	73	74
Control					
State and Local Government	25	28	28	30	29
Not for Profit	99	95	97	95	98
Investor owned	0	0	0	0	0
Affiliations					
Hospitals in a System	87	85	87	86	86
Hospitals in a Group Purchasing Organization...	77	67	78	78	92

Note: The 2021 performance data do not reflect the full impact of the COVID-19 pandemic. Please refer to the discussion in the Introduction for more information.

AHA Hospital Statistics © 2024 Health Forum LLC, an affiliate of the American Hospital Association

TABLE 6

MINNESOTA

U.S. Community Hospitals
(Nonfederal, short-term general and other special hospitals)

Utilization, Personnel, Community Health Indicators 2018–2022

	2022	2021	2020	2019	2018
TOTAL FACILITY (Includes Hospital and Nursing Home Units)					
Utilization - Inpatient					
Beds	13,663	13,555	13,842	13,901	13,895
Admissions	455,125	500,066	489,205	551,113	572,213
Inpatient Days	3,151,933	3,235,739	3,085,908	3,331,744	3,337,371
Average Length of Stay	6.9	6.5	6.3	6.0	5.8
Inpatient Surgeries	146,142	135,217	148,575	174,668	174,122
Births	56,289	56,993	58,935	62,602	65,245
Utilization - Outpatient					
Emergency Outpatient Visits	1,908,898	1,775,919	1,722,954	2,028,615	2,051,970
Other Outpatient Visits	9,997,161	11,039,826	10,094,196	11,568,410	11,326,938
Total Outpatient Visits	11,906,059	12,815,745	11,817,150	13,597,025	13,378,908
Outpatient Surgeries	414,577	394,398	333,621	398,574	379,490
Personnel					
Full Time RNs	14,119	15,854	14,076	13,148	12,213
Full Time LPNs	971	931	1,131	1,162	1,261
Part Time RNs	30,994	29,363	29,374	30,040	29,707
Part Time LPNs	1,215	1,170	1,517	1,494	1,446
Total Full Time	62,223	64,352	82,565	82,823	81,418
Total Part Time	81,549	80,421	74,799	74,440	73,637
HOSPITAL UNIT (Excludes Separate Nursing Home Units)					
Utilization - Inpatient					
Beds	11,794	12,124	12,325	12,461	11,831
Admissions	452,929	497,782	486,531	548,106	568,980
Inpatient Days	2,686,000	2,832,382	2,638,887	2,874,105	2,691,360
Average Length of Stay	5.9	5.7	5.4	5.2	4.7
Personnel					
Total Full Time	61,601	63,811	81,999	82,283	80,617
Total Part Time	80,101	79,403	73,580	73,108	72,119
COMMUNITY HEALTH INDICATORS PER 1000 POPULATION					
Total Population (in thousands)	5,717	5,707	5,657	5,640	5,611
Inpatient					
Beds	2.4	2.4	2.4	2.5	2.5
Admissions	79.6	87.6	86.5	97.7	102
Inpatient Days	551.3	566.9	545.5	590.8	594.8
Inpatient Surgeries	25.6	23.7	26.3	31	31
Births	9.8	10	10.4	11.1	11.6
Outpatient					
Emergency Outpatient Visits	333.9	311.2	304.6	359.7	365.7
Other Outpatient Visits	1,748.6	1,934.3	1,784.3	2,051.3	2,018.6
Total Outpatient Visits	2,082.5	2,245.5	2,088.8	2,411	2,384.3
Outpatient Surgeries	72.5	69.1	59	70.7	67.6

Note: The 2021 performance data do not reflect the full impact of the COVID-19 pandemic. Please refer to the discussion in the Introduction for more information.

TABLE 6

MISSISSIPPI

U.S. Community Hospitals
(Nonfederal, short-term general and other special hospitals)

Overview 2018–2022

	2022	2021	2020	2019	2018
Total Community Hospitals in Mississippi.........	99	98	97	97	99
Bed Size Category					
6-24	4	4	4	6	6
25-49	40	39	36	34	35
50-99	21	18	20	21	21
100-199	19	22	21	18	20
200-299	5	6	7	10	8
300-399	4	3	3	2	3
400-499	2	2	2	2	2
500 + ...	4	4	4	4	4
Location					
Hospitals Urban	33	32	31	32	32
Hospitals Rural...	66	66	66	65	67
Control					
State and Local Government	40	40	40	39	38
Not for Profit...	34	33	33	33	35
Investor owned..	25	25	24	25	26
Affiliations					
Hospitals in a System	51	50	47	48	50
Hospitals in a Group Purchasing Organization...	85	86	92	87	93

Note: The 2021 performance data do not reflect the full impact of the COVID-19 pandemic. Please refer to the discussion in the Introduction for more information.

TABLE 6

MISSISSIPPI

U.S. Community Hospitals
(Nonfederal, short-term general and other special hospitals)

Utilization, Personnel, Community Health Indicators 2018–2022

	2022	2021	2020	2019	2018
TOTAL FACILITY (Includes Hospital and Nursing Home Units)					
Utilization - Inpatient					
Beds	11,544	11,643	11,796	11,624	12,071
Admissions	301,048	333,958	347,034	370,790	369,559
Inpatient Days	2,343,142	2,411,419	2,440,972	2,525,724	2,453,579
Average Length of Stay	7.8	7.2	7.0	6.8	6.6
Inpatient Surgeries	67,150	67,941	74,027	93,644	86,467
Births	35,087	36,095	34,992	34,622	33,643
Utilization - Outpatient					
Emergency Outpatient Visits	1,548,150	1,431,778	1,581,779	1,793,977	1,749,095
Other Outpatient Visits	6,213,283	5,890,863	5,300,548	5,367,757	5,430,498
Total Outpatient Visits	7,761,433	7,322,641	6,882,327	7,161,734	7,179,593
Outpatient Surgeries	174,238	157,123	145,110	193,380	195,664
Personnel					
Full Time RNs	12,125	12,441	12,829	13,246	13,432
Full Time LPNs	1,175	1,218	1,214	1,281	1,248
Part Time RNs	5,459	5,417	5,187	5,047	4,780
Part Time LPNs	366	328	297	359	307
Total Full Time	44,735	46,519	45,840	47,030	46,842
Total Part Time	15,283	14,897	14,194	14,039	13,265
HOSPITAL UNIT (Excludes Separate Nursing Home Units)					
Utilization - Inpatient					
Beds	10,127	9,961	10,049	9,997	10,439
Admissions	300,119	332,716	345,858	369,466	368,179
Inpatient Days	1,905,758	1,904,398	1,868,299	1,976,787	1,903,088
Average Length of Stay	6.4	5.7	5.4	5.4	5.2
Personnel					
Total Full Time	43,709	45,231	44,361	45,666	45,984
Total Part Time	14,821	14,392	13,652	13,553	12,879
COMMUNITY HEALTH INDICATORS PER 1000 POPULATION					
Total Population (in thousands)	2,940	2,950	2,967	2,976	2,987
Inpatient					
Beds	3.9	3.9	4	3.9	4
Admissions	102.4	113.2	117	124.6	123.7
Inpatient Days	797	817.4	822.8	848.7	821.5
Inpatient Surgeries	22.8	23	25	31.5	29
Births	11.9	12.2	11.8	11.6	11.3
Outpatient					
Emergency Outpatient Visits	526.6	485.4	533.2	602.8	585.7
Other Outpatient Visits	2,113.3	1,996.9	1786.6	1,803.6	1,818.3
Total Outpatient Visits	2,639.9	2,482.3	2319.8	2,406.4	2,404
Outpatient Surgeries	59.3	53.3	48.9	65	65.5

Note: The 2021 performance data do not reflect the full impact of the COVID-19 pandemic. Please refer to the discussion in the Introduction for more information.

AHA Hospital Statistics © 2024 Health Forum LLC, an affiliate of the American Hospital Association

TABLE 6

MISSOURI

U.S. Community Hospitals
(Nonfederal, short-term general and other special hospitals)

Overview 2018–2022

	2022	2021	2020	2019	2018
Total Community Hospitals in Missouri..............	**115**	**119**	**118**	**120**	**122**
Bed Size Category					
6-24	15	15	15	14	13
25-49	31	32	32	34	36
50-99	22	24	22	22	22
100-199	17	18	19	20	21
200-299	10	10	10	10	9
300-399	8	9	8	8	9
400-499	4	2	3	4	4
500 + ...	8	9	9	8	8
Location					
Hospitals Urban	68	71	70	71	73
Hospitals Rural	47	48	48	49	49
Control					
State and Local Government	29	29	30	30	31
Not for Profit	65	65	67	67	66
Investor owned	21	25	21	23	25
Affiliations					
Hospitals in a System	74	74	72	75	76
Hospitals in a Group Purchasing Organization...	112	112	113	117	118

Note: The 2021 performance data do not reflect the full impact of the COVID-19 pandemic. Please refer to the discussion in the Introduction for more information.

TABLE 6

MISSOURI

U.S. Community Hospitals
(Nonfederal, short-term general and other special hospitals)

Utilization, Personnel, Community Health Indicators 2018–2022

	2022	2021	2020	2019	2018
TOTAL FACILITY (Includes Hospital and Nursing Home Units)					
Utilization - Inpatient					
Beds	17,838	18,342	18,539	18,455	18,749
Admissions	715,424	730,570	717,521	769,249	780,377
Inpatient Days	4,244,382	4,178,401	3,987,099	4,184,603	4,143,162
Average Length of Stay	5.9	5.7	5.6	5.4	5.3
Inpatient Surgeries	163,814	170,670	171,161	192,947	190,425
Births	66,498	66,580	68,306	70,183	71,561
Utilization - Outpatient					
Emergency Outpatient Visits	2,770,889	2,677,792	2,614,512	2,927,912	2,979,022
Other Outpatient Visits	23,898,448	23,937,279	22,205,901	22,775,037	22,201,008
Total Outpatient Visits	26,669,337	26,615,071	24,820,413	25,702,949	25,180,030
Outpatient Surgeries	411,589	404,988	349,943	397,796	397,218
Personnel					
Full Time RNs	28,578	31,064	33,660	33,376	31,859
Full Time LPNs	2,278	2,359	2,384	2,458	2,341
Part Time RNs	13,295	13,236	12,106	12,073	11,458
Part Time LPNs	604	652	580	587	543
Total Full Time	108,393	110,786	113,397	114,494	113,185
Total Part Time	39,282	39,462	36,165	37,410	35,430
HOSPITAL UNIT (Excludes Separate Nursing Home Units)					
Utilization - Inpatient					
Beds	17,168	17,672	17,839	17,667	17,979
Admissions	712,764	727,987	714,449	765,769	776,718
Inpatient Days	4,098,223	4,029,887	3,803,218	3,958,285	3,921,677
Average Length of Stay	5.7	5.5	5.3	5.2	5.0
Personnel					
Total Full Time	108,043	110,365	113,096	114,085	112,882
Total Part Time	39,111	39,278	36,025	37,203	35,270
COMMUNITY HEALTH INDICATORS PER 1000 POPULATION					
Total Population (in thousands)	6,178	6,168	6,152	6,137	6,126
Inpatient					
Beds	2.9	3	3	3	3.1
Admissions	115.8	118.4	116.6	125.3	127.4
Inpatient Days	687	677.4	648.1	681.8	676.3
Inpatient Surgeries	26.5	27.7	27.8	31.4	31.1
Births	10.8	10.8	11.1	11.4	11.7
Outpatient					
Emergency Outpatient Visits	448.5	434.1	425	477.1	486.3
Other Outpatient Visits	3,868.3	3,880.8	3,609.8	3,710.8	3,623.8
Total Outpatient Visits	4,316.9	4,314.9	4,034.8	4,187.9	4,110.1
Outpatient Surgeries	66.6	65.7	56.9	64.8	64.8

Note: The 2021 performance data do not reflect the full impact of the COVID-19 pandemic. Please refer to the discussion in the Introduction for more information.

AHA Hospital Statistics © 2024 Health Forum LLC, an affiliate of the American Hospital Association

TABLE 6

MONTANA

U.S. Community Hospitals
(Nonfederal, short-term general and other special hospitals)

Overview 2018–2022

	2022	2021	2020	2019	2018
Total Community Hospitals in Montana.............	59	59	56	57	56
Bed Size Category					
6-24	16	16	14	14	12
25-49	25	26	23	23	24
50-99	8	7	9	11	11
100-199	5	5	5	5	6
200-299	4	4	3	3	2
300-399	0	0	1	0	0
400-499	1	0	0	0	0
500 + ...	0	1	1	1	1
Location					
Hospitals Urban	15	10	9	9	9
Hospitals Rural..................................	44	49	47	48	47
Control					
State and Local Government	5	8	8	6	7
Not for Profit.....................................	50	46	44	46	44
Investor owned..................................	4	5	4	5	5
Affiliations					
Hospitals in a System	14	14	14	17	19
Hospitals in a Group Purchasing Organization...	40	40	44	41	45

Note: The 2021 performance data do not reflect the full impact of the COVID-19 pandemic. Please refer to the discussion in the Introduction for more information.

TABLE 6

MONTANA

U.S. Community Hospitals
(Nonfederal, short-term general and other special hospitals)

Utilization, Personnel, Community Health Indicators 2018–2022

	2022	2021	2020	2019	2018
TOTAL FACILITY (Includes Hospital and Nursing Home Units)					
Utilization - Inpatient					
Beds	3,598	3,620	3,755	3,614	3,542
Admissions	93,985	93,750	91,431	100,441	98,467
Inpatient Days	746,527	718,061	711,445	758,902	752,407
Average Length of Stay	7.9	7.7	7.8	7.6	7.6
Inpatient Surgeries	25,643	23,299	24,958	27,217	31,005
Births	11,009	10,558	10,429	10,378	10,965
Utilization - Outpatient					
Emergency Outpatient Visits	441,258	393,918	409,295	452,994	423,628
Other Outpatient Visits	4,843,746	4,541,322	4,010,879	4,145,710	4,024,075
Total Outpatient Visits	5,285,004	4,935,240	4,420,174	4,598,704	4,447,703
Outpatient Surgeries	83,984	80,674	61,883	76,293	81,268
Personnel					
Full Time RNs	4,438	4,737	5,056	4,810	3,972
Full Time LPNs	325	337	380	349	377
Part Time RNs	3,512	3,271	2,688	2,970	2,807
Part Time LPNs	172	171	176	170	200
Total Full Time	19,617	20,357	20,205	19,294	19,182
Total Part Time	10,591	10,432	8,976	9,315	10,164
HOSPITAL UNIT (Excludes Separate Nursing Home Units)					
Utilization - Inpatient					
Beds	2,905	2,901	2,975	2,909	2,770
Admissions	93,217	92,892	90,547	99,350	97,336
Inpatient Days	558,658	533,311	487,346	542,941	523,978
Average Length of Stay	6.0	5.7	5.4	5.5	5.4
Personnel					
Total Full Time	19,306	19,994	19,672	18,830	18,592
Total Part Time	10,392	10,210	8,592	9,026	9,771
COMMUNITY HEALTH INDICATORS PER 1000 POPULATION					
Total Population (in thousands)	1,123	1,104	1,081	1,069	1,062
Inpatient					
Beds	3.2	3.3	3.5	3.4	3.3
Admissions	83.7	84.9	84.6	94	92.7
Inpatient Days	664.8	650.3	658.4	710.1	708.3
Inpatient Surgeries	22.8	21.1	23.1	25.5	29.2
Births	9.8	9.6	9.7	9.7	10.3
Outpatient					
Emergency Outpatient Visits	393	356.7	378.8	423.8	398.8
Other Outpatient Visits	4,313.7	4,112.5	3,711.8	3,878.9	3,788.1
Total Outpatient Visits	4,706.7	4,469.2	4,090.6	4,302.8	4,186.8
Outpatient Surgeries	74.8	73.1	57.3	71.4	76.5

Note: The 2021 performance data do not reflect the full impact of the COVID-19 pandemic. Please refer to the discussion in the Introduction for more information.

AHA Hospital Statistics © 2024 Health Forum LLC, an affiliate of the American Hospital Association

TABLE 6

NEBRASKA

U.S. Community Hospitals
(Nonfederal, short-term general and other special hospitals)

Overview 2018–2022

	2022	2021	2020	2019	2018
Total Community Hospitals in Nebraska	93	92	93	93	93
Bed Size Category					
6-24	41	42	43	44	41
25-49	17	16	17	16	18
50-99	18	17	15	14	15
100-199	10	9	10	10	10
200-299	2	3	3	3	3
300-399	2	2	3	4	3
400-499	1	1	0	0	1
500 + ...	2	2	2	2	2
Location					
Hospitals Urban	27	27	28	27	27
Hospitals Rural	66	65	65	66	66
Control					
State and Local Government	34	35	35	35	36
Not for Profit	54	52	51	51	50
Investor owned	5	5	7	7	7
Affiliations					
Hospitals in a System	31	30	30	31	31
Hospitals in a Group Purchasing Organization...	32	39	41	38	47

Note: The 2021 performance data do not reflect the full impact of the COVID-19 pandemic. Please refer to the discussion in the Introduction for more information.

TABLE 6

NEBRASKA

U.S. Community Hospitals
(Nonfederal, short-term general and other special hospitals)

Utilization, Personnel, Community Health Indicators 2018–2022

	2022	2021	2020	2019	2018
TOTAL FACILITY (Includes Hospital and Nursing Home Units)					
Utilization - Inpatient					
Beds	6,695	6,667	6,622	6,756	6,842
Admissions	183,713	184,485	189,322	203,201	209,821
Inpatient Days	1,301,588	1,255,170	1,274,829	1,405,254	1,400,332
Average Length of Stay	7.1	6.8	6.7	6.9	6.7
Inpatient Surgeries	50,888	52,002	54,747	61,182	61,889
Births	22,824	22,642	21,935	22,793	23,814
Utilization - Outpatient					
Emergency Outpatient Visits	947,142	840,811	785,748	923,344	817,775
Other Outpatient Visits	5,843,360	5,502,842	4,881,710	5,137,276	4,876,424
Total Outpatient Visits	6,790,502	6,343,653	5,667,458	6,060,620	5,694,199
Outpatient Surgeries	161,278	157,374	137,880	138,482	143,948
Personnel					
Full Time RNs	9,516	9,789	9,843	9,641	9,444
Full Time LPNs	742	743	684	719	760
Part Time RNs	4,622	4,158	4,659	5,055	4,441
Part Time LPNs	318	275	254	328	295
Total Full Time	34,994	34,373	33,541	33,042	32,680
Total Part Time	14,641	13,728	14,320	16,243	14,888
HOSPITAL UNIT (Excludes Separate Nursing Home Units)					
Utilization - Inpatient					
Beds	6,275	6,266	6,289	6,360	6,317
Admissions	183,158	183,970	188,982	202,578	209,097
Inpatient Days	1,195,153	1,146,117	1,175,040	1,274,442	1,236,103
Average Length of Stay	6.5	6.2	6.2	6.3	5.9
Personnel					
Total Full Time	34,815	34,126	33,329	32,796	32,341
Total Part Time	14,473	13,574	14,214	16,089	14,715
COMMUNITY HEALTH INDICATORS PER 1000 POPULATION					
Total Population (in thousands)	1,968	1,964	1,938	1,934	1,929
Inpatient					
Beds	3.4	3.4	3.4	3.5	3.5
Admissions	93.4	93.9	97.7	105	108.8
Inpatient Days	661.4	639.2	658	726.5	725.8
Inpatient Surgeries	25.9	26.5	28.3	31.6	32.1
Births	11.6	11.5	11.3	11.8	12.3
Outpatient					
Emergency Outpatient Visits	481.3	428.2	405.5	477.3	423.9
Other Outpatient Visits	2,969.3	2,802.3	2,519.5	2,655.7	2,527.6
Total Outpatient Visits	3,450.6	3,230.5	2,925.1	3,133.1	2,951.5
Outpatient Surgeries	82	80.1	71.2	71.6	74.6

Note: The 2021 performance data do not reflect the full impact of the COVID-19 pandemic. Please refer to the discussion in the Introduction for more information.

AHA Hospital Statistics © 2024 Health Forum LLC, an affiliate of the American Hospital Association

TABLE 6

NEVADA

U.S. Community Hospitals
(Nonfederal, short-term general and other special hospitals)

Overview 2018–2022

	2022	2021	2020	2019	2018
Total Community Hospitals in Nevada................	46	47	46	43	44
Bed Size Category					
6-24	8	7	7	7	5
25-49	7	9	8	7	7
50-99	11	11	11	9	11
100-199	9	10	10	10	11
200-299	3	3	3	3	4
300-399	5	4	4	4	3
400-499	0	0	1	1	1
500 + ...	3	3	2	2	2
Location					
Hospitals Urban	36	36	35	32	33
Hospitals Rural...	10	11	11	11	11
Control					
State and Local Government	6	6	6	6	6
Not for Profit..	14	15	15	14	15
Investor owned...	26	26	25	23	23
Affiliations					
Hospitals in a System	35	35	34	31	32
Hospitals in a Group Purchasing Organization...	18	18	17	12	13

Note: The 2021 performance data do not reflect the full impact of the COVID-19 pandemic. Please refer to the discussion in the Introduction for more information.

TABLE 6

NEVADA

U.S. Community Hospitals
(Nonfederal, short-term general and other special hospitals)

Utilization, Personnel, Community Health Indicators 2018–2022

	2022	2021	2020	2019	2018
TOTAL FACILITY (Includes Hospital and Nursing Home Units)					
Utilization - Inpatient					
Beds	6,476	6,507	6,490	6,309	6,493
Admissions	256,447	240,207	262,773	282,453	305,935
Inpatient Days	1,616,921	1,597,549	1,525,764	1,539,908	1,693,329
Average Length of Stay	6.3	6.7	5.8	5.5	5.5
Inpatient Surgeries	50,946	49,172	48,976	55,423	59,540
Births	22,272	21,480	23,200	29,049	26,694
Utilization - Outpatient					
Emergency Outpatient Visits	798,210	714,442	859,077	956,217	1,063,257
Other Outpatient Visits	2,146,851	2,146,071	2,185,216	2,386,454	2,597,573
Total Outpatient Visits	2,945,061	2,860,513	3,044,293	3,342,671	3,660,830
Outpatient Surgeries	94,670	89,360	71,893	85,267	95,625
Personnel					
Full Time RNs	8,440	9,867	10,157	9,864	9,901
Full Time LPNs	444	373	380	344	360
Part Time RNs	1,783	2,441	1,831	2,239	2,346
Part Time LPNs	69	76	47	75	94
Total Full Time	26,330	31,483	30,121	29,422	29,871
Total Part Time	4,948	7,311	5,657	6,365	6,651
HOSPITAL UNIT (Excludes Separate Nursing Home Units)					
Utilization - Inpatient					
Beds	6,433	6,400	6,447	6,309	6,493
Admissions	256,416	240,135	262,749	282,453	305,935
Inpatient Days	1,605,614	1,564,492	1,511,199	1,539,908	1,693,329
Average Length of Stay	6.3	6.5	5.8	5.5	5.5
Personnel					
Total Full Time	26,289	31,409	30,115	29,422	29,871
Total Part Time	4,948	7,270	5,655	6,365	6,651
COMMUNITY HEALTH INDICATORS PER 1000 POPULATION					
Total Population (in thousands)	3,178	3,144	3,138	3,080	3,034
Inpatient					
Beds	2	2.1	2.1	2	2.1
Admissions	80.7	76.4	83.7	91.7	100.8
Inpatient Days	508.8	508.1	486.2	499.9	558
Inpatient Surgeries	16	15.6	15.6	18	19.6
Births	7	6.8	7.4	9.4	8.8
Outpatient					
Emergency Outpatient Visits	251.2	227.2	273.7	310.4	350.4
Other Outpatient Visits	675.6	682.6	696.3	774.8	856
Total Outpatient Visits	926.8	909.8	970.1	1,085.2	1,206.4
Outpatient Surgeries	29.8	28.4	22.9	27.7	31.5

Note: The 2021 performance data do not reflect the full impact of the COVID-19 pandemic. Please refer to the discussion in the Introduction for more information.

AHA Hospital Statistics © 2024 Health Forum LLC, an affiliate of the American Hospital Association

TABLE 6

NEW HAMPSHIRE

U.S. Community Hospitals
(Nonfederal, short-term general and other special hospitals)

Overview 2018–2022

	2022	2021	2020	2019	2018
Total Community Hospitals in New Hampshire...	28	28	28	28	28
Bed Size Category					
6-24	2	2	2	2	1
25-49	10	10	10	10	11
50-99	7	7	7	7	7
100-199	5	5	5	5	5
200-299	3	3	3	3	3
300-399	0	0	0	0	0
400-499	1	1	1	1	1
500 +	0	0	0	0	0
Location					
Hospitals Urban	11	11	11	11	11
Hospitals Rural	17	17	17	17	17
Control					
State and Local Government	0	0	0	0	0
Not for Profit	23	23	23	23	24
Investor owned	5	5	5	5	4
Affiliations					
Hospitals in a System	17	16	13	15	14
Hospitals in a Group Purchasing Organization...	21	20	18	20	22

Note: The 2021 performance data do not reflect the full impact of the COVID-19 pandemic. Please refer to the discussion in the Introduction for more information.

TABLE 6

NEW HAMPSHIRE

U.S. Community Hospitals
(Nonfederal, short-term general and other special hospitals)

Utilization, Personnel, Community Health Indicators 2018–2022

	2022	2021	2020	2019	2018
TOTAL FACILITY (Includes Hospital and Nursing Home Units)					
Utilization - Inpatient					
Beds	2,856	2,759	2,806	2,804	2,783
Admissions	115,320	116,979	115,425	121,800	124,365
Inpatient Days	696,657	652,041	623,568	648,227	656,919
Average Length of Stay	6.0	5.6	5.4	5.3	5.3
Inpatient Surgeries	36,791	30,522	30,920	34,925	33,927
Births	12,978	12,714	12,333	11,541	12,365
Utilization - Outpatient					
Emergency Outpatient Visits	651,205	637,529	672,189	712,254	618,367
Other Outpatient Visits	5,618,096	5,618,577	4,818,587	5,113,669	4,765,795
Total Outpatient Visits	6,269,301	6,256,106	5,490,776	5,825,923	5,384,162
Outpatient Surgeries	110,062	97,426	83,166	89,419	90,592
Personnel					
Full Time RNs	5,319	5,442	6,034	5,987	5,643
Full Time LPNs	269	252	307	262	283
Part Time RNs	3,200	3,498	3,478	3,518	3,487
Part Time LPNs	101	99	94	84	78
Total Full Time	25,444	25,021	26,416	26,168	24,835
Total Part Time	11,020	11,932	11,500	12,150	11,890
HOSPITAL UNIT (Excludes Separate Nursing Home Units)					
Utilization - Inpatient					
Beds	2,846	2,759	2,761	2,759	2,738
Admissions	115,242	116,979	115,409	121,765	124,331
Inpatient Days	695,409	652,041	608,666	633,607	642,472
Average Length of Stay	6.0	5.6	5.3	5.2	5.2
Personnel					
Total Full Time	25,435	25,021	26,396	26,144	24,818
Total Part Time	11,014	11,932	11,490	12,106	11,876
COMMUNITY HEALTH INDICATORS PER 1000 POPULATION					
Total Population (in thousands)	1,395	1,389	1,366	1,360	1,356
Inpatient					
Beds	2	2	2.1	2.1	2.1
Admissions	82.7	84.2	84.5	89.6	91.7
Inpatient Days	499.3	469.4	456.4	476.7	484.3
Inpatient Surgeries	26.4	22	22.6	25.7	25
Births	9.3	9.2	9	8.5	9.1
Outpatient					
Emergency Outpatient Visits	466.7	459	492	523.8	455.9
Other Outpatient Visits	4,026.6	4,045.1	3,526.8	3,760.8	3,513.4
Total Outpatient Visits	4,493.4	4,504.1	4,018.8	4,284.7	3,969.3
Outpatient Surgeries	78.9	70.1	60.9	65.8	66.8

Note: The 2021 performance data do not reflect the full impact of the COVID-19 pandemic. Please refer to the discussion in the Introduction for more information.

AHA Hospital Statistics © 2024 Health Forum LLC, an affiliate of the American Hospital Association

TABLE 6

NEW JERSEY

U.S. Community Hospitals
(Nonfederal, short-term general and other special hospitals)

Overview 2018–2022

	2022	2021	2020	2019	2018
Total Community Hospitals in New Jersey	79	80	81	81	82
Bed Size Category					
6-24	1	1	1	1	1
25-49	6	5	5	5	6
50-99	11	12	12	13	12
100-199	20	21	23	23	23
200-299	7	9	6	8	10
300-399	16	15	17	17	16
400-499	7	6	7	5	5
500 + ...	11	11	10	9	9
Location					
Hospitals Urban	79	80	81	81	82
Hospitals Rural	0	0	0	0	0
Control					
State and Local Government	2	2	2	2	0
Not for Profit	60	63	62	62	62
Investor owned	17	15	17	17	20
Affiliations					
Hospitals in a System	60	59	59	60	60
Hospitals in a Group Purchasing Organization...	58	60	63	61	62

Note: The 2021 performance data do not reflect the full impact of the COVID-19 pandemic. Please refer to the discussion in the Introduction for more information.

TABLE 6

NEW JERSEY

U.S. Community Hospitals
(Nonfederal, short-term general and other special hospitals)

Utilization, Personnel, Community Health Indicators 2018–2022

	2022	2021	2020	2019	2018
TOTAL FACILITY (Includes Hospital and Nursing Home Units)					
Utilization - Inpatient					
Beds	21,837	21,736	21,900	20,863	20,901
Admissions	874,171	1,039,328	957,666	1,073,799	1,066,632
Inpatient Days	5,336,288	5,326,815	5,067,496	5,068,308	5,075,543
Average Length of Stay	6.1	5.1	5.3	4.7	4.8
Inpatient Surgeries	183,378	191,845	178,345	210,766	217,639
Births	99,960	99,108	95,158	94,782	97,196
Utilization - Outpatient					
Emergency Outpatient Visits	3,375,540	3,258,822	2,838,664	3,633,427	3,752,248
Other Outpatient Visits	12,709,382	14,172,145	10,470,292	11,073,241	10,201,572
Total Outpatient Visits	16,084,922	17,430,967	13,308,956	14,706,668	13,953,820
Outpatient Surgeries	384,082	373,790	310,507	365,248	353,431
Personnel					
Full Time RNs	33,759	31,396	32,965	32,827	32,323
Full Time LPNs	822	645	641	592	611
Part Time RNs	14,244	13,539	12,531	13,464	13,657
Part Time LPNs	308	263	224	197	222
Total Full Time	115,408	112,435	112,289	112,000	109,986
Total Part Time	46,154	46,202	42,212	43,486	44,038
HOSPITAL UNIT (Excludes Separate Nursing Home Units)					
Utilization - Inpatient					
Beds	21,139	20,887	20,965	20,342	20,350
Admissions	873,905	1,038,803	956,144	1,070,945	1,063,167
Inpatient Days	5,159,828	5,102,988	4,807,958	4,896,405	4,895,405
Average Length of Stay	5.9	4.9	5.0	4.6	4.6
Personnel					
Total Full Time	115,154	112,093	111,856	111,588	109,668
Total Part Time	46,053	46,060	42,031	43,367	43,894
COMMUNITY HEALTH INDICATORS PER 1000 POPULATION					
Total Population (in thousands)	9,262	9,267	8,882	8,882	8,909
Inpatient					
Beds	2.4	2.3	2.5	2.3	2.3
Admissions	94.4	112.2	107.8	120.9	119.7
Inpatient Days	576.2	574.8	570.5	570.6	569.7
Inpatient Surgeries	19.8	20.7	20.1	23.7	24.4
Births	10.8	10.7	10.7	10.7	10.9
Outpatient					
Emergency Outpatient Visits	364.5	351.7	319.6	409.1	421.2
Other Outpatient Visits	1,372.3	1,529.3	1,178.8	1,246.7	1,145.1
Total Outpatient Visits	1,736.7	1,880.9	1,498.4	1,655.7	1,566.3
Outpatient Surgeries	41.5	40.3	35	41.1	39.7

Note: The 2021 performance data do not reflect the full impact of the COVID-19 pandemic. Please refer to the discussion in the Introduction for more information.

AHA Hospital Statistics © 2024 Health Forum LLC, an affiliate of the American Hospital Association

TABLE 6

NEW MEXICO

U.S. Community Hospitals
(Nonfederal, short-term general and other special hospitals)

Overview 2018–2022

	2022	2021	2020	2019	2018
Total Community Hospitals in New Mexico........	43	44	42	42	41
Bed Size Category					
6-24	6	7	6	8	7
25-49	18	18	16	14	14
50-99	11	11	12	12	10
100-199	5	5	4	4	6
200-299	1	1	2	2	2
300-399	0	0	0	0	0
400-499	0	0	0	0	0
500 +	2	2	2	2	2
Location					
Hospitals Urban	18	19	17	17	16
Hospitals Rural	25	25	25	25	25
Control					
State and Local Government	8	8	8	9	8
Not for Profit	17	17	16	15	15
Investor owned	18	19	18	18	18
Affiliations					
Hospitals in a System	33	34	33	32	31
Hospitals in a Group Purchasing Organization...	11	15	16	21	18

Note: The 2021 performance data do not reflect the full impact of the COVID-19 pandemic. Please refer to the discussion in the Introduction for more information.

TABLE 6

NEW MEXICO

U.S. Community Hospitals
(Nonfederal, short-term general and other special hospitals)

Utilization, Personnel, Community Health Indicators 2018–2022

	2022	2021	2020	2019	2018
TOTAL FACILITY (Includes Hospital and Nursing Home Units)					
Utilization - Inpatient					
Beds	3,669	3,680	3,784	3,765	3,811
Admissions	172,571	177,356	180,702	198,127	189,362
Inpatient Days	885,056	878,214	841,386	888,056	854,720
Average Length of Stay	5.1	5.0	4.7	4.5	4.5
Inpatient Surgeries	38,012	34,602	38,878	42,943	45,914
Births	15,420	16,087	16,928	19,279	19,047
Utilization - Outpatient					
Emergency Outpatient Visits	945,647	695,779	821,586	876,730	1,055,906
Other Outpatient Visits	3,084,266	2,673,146	2,760,174	3,124,219	4,746,854
Total Outpatient Visits	4,029,913	3,368,925	3,581,760	4,000,949	5,802,760
Outpatient Surgeries	115,063	108,142	95,255	117,576	124,064
Personnel					
Full Time RNs	6,440	7,457	7,107	6,567	7,724
Full Time LPNs	300	353	273	245	340
Part Time RNs	4,156	4,343	5,655	4,624	2,909
Part Time LPNs	198	235	265	234	134
Total Full Time	22,759	26,749	24,577	23,305	26,441
Total Part Time	12,287	13,449	16,767	14,768	7,746
HOSPITAL UNIT (Excludes Separate Nursing Home Units)					
Utilization - Inpatient					
Beds	3,669	3,680	3,784	3,765	3,796
Admissions	172,571	177,356	180,702	198,127	189,246
Inpatient Days	885,056	878,214	841,386	888,056	852,656
Average Length of Stay	5.1	5.0	4.7	4.5	4.5
Personnel					
Total Full Time	22,759	26,749	24,577	23,305	26,430
Total Part Time	12,287	13,449	16,767	14,768	7,742
COMMUNITY HEALTH INDICATORS PER 1000 POPULATION					
Total Population (in thousands)	2,113	2,116	2,106	2,097	2,095
Inpatient					
Beds	1.7	1.7	1.8	1.8	1.8
Admissions	81.7	83.8	85.8	94.5	90.4
Inpatient Days	418.8	415.1	399.5	423.5	407.9
Inpatient Surgeries	18	16.4	18.5	20.5	21.9
Births	7.3	7.6	8	9.2	9.1
Outpatient					
Emergency Outpatient Visits	447.5	328.8	390.1	418.1	503.9
Other Outpatient Visits	1,459.4	1,263.4	1,310.4	1,490	2,265.3
Total Outpatient Visits	1,906.9	1,592.2	1,700.5	1,908.1	2,769.2
Outpatient Surgeries	54.4	51.1	45.2	56.1	59.2

Note: The 2021 performance data do not reflect the full impact of the COVID-19 pandemic. Please refer to the discussion in the Introduction for more information.

AHA Hospital Statistics © 2024 Health Forum LLC, an affiliate of the American Hospital Association

TABLE 6

NEW YORK

U.S. Community Hospitals
(Nonfederal, short-term general and other special hospitals)

Overview 2018–2022

	2022	2021	2020	2019	2018
Total Community Hospitals in New York	**160**	**161**	**162**	**163**	**166**
Bed Size Category					
6-24	12	12	11	10	9
25-49	11	11	12	11	10
50-99	14	16	14	12	15
100-199	36	35	38	44	45
200-299	36	35	34	29	31
300-399	12	13	14	15	14
400-499	10	10	10	13	14
500 + ...	29	29	29	29	28
Location					
Hospitals Urban	125	126	127	128	131
Hospitals Rural......................................	35	35	35	35	35
Control					
State and Local Government	23	23	25	24	24
Not for Profit..	137	138	137	139	142
Investor owned......................................	0	0	0	0	0
Affiliations					
Hospitals in a System	100	100	101	100	104
Hospitals in a Group Purchasing Organization...	101	109	117	121	123

Note: The 2021 performance data do not reflect the full impact of the COVID-19 pandemic. Please refer to the discussion in the Introduction for more information.

TABLE 6

NEW YORK

U.S. Community Hospitals
(Nonfederal, short-term general and other special hospitals)

Utilization, Personnel, Community Health Indicators 2018–2022

	2022	2021	2020	2019	2018
TOTAL FACILITY (Includes Hospital and Nursing Home Units)					
Utilization - Inpatient					
Beds	49,726	49,813	50,723	52,084	51,927
Admissions	2,030,070	2,038,218	1,970,239	2,236,457	2,268,877
Inpatient Days	14,038,591	13,860,070	13,271,875	14,681,148	14,740,138
Average Length of Stay	6.9	6.8	6.7	6.6	6.5
Inpatient Surgeries	502,950	511,615	497,516	571,170	568,405
Births	200,809	202,655	201,074	214,850	217,662
Utilization - Outpatient					
Emergency Outpatient Visits	8,233,170	7,688,123	7,212,635	8,766,573	8,729,833
Other Outpatient Visits	53,389,781	55,944,284	46,081,251	51,469,089	50,303,781
Total Outpatient Visits	61,622,951	63,632,407	53,293,886	60,235,662	59,033,614
Outpatient Surgeries	1,421,874	1,399,628	1,163,851	1,463,590	1,356,429
Personnel					
Full Time RNs	101,577	103,362	102,988	100,575	96,994
Full Time LPNs	4,455	4,624	4,883	5,158	5,201
Part Time RNs	26,058	24,926	28,028	26,787	25,934
Part Time LPNs	933	938	1,094	1,232	1,377
Total Full Time	416,748	409,327	397,729	398,754	386,206
Total Part Time	86,639	84,320	90,681	89,101	93,756
HOSPITAL UNIT (Excludes Separate Nursing Home Units)					
Utilization - Inpatient					
Beds	46,387	46,107	46,671	47,424	46,972
Admissions	2,021,905	2,028,291	1,959,075	2,221,564	2,255,980
Inpatient Days	13,031,067	12,688,054	12,002,953	13,085,402	13,022,211
Average Length of Stay	6.4	6.3	6.1	5.9	5.8
Personnel					
Total Full Time	414,022	406,215	394,953	395,272	382,299
Total Part Time	85,571	82,918	88,803	87,064	91,370
COMMUNITY HEALTH INDICATORS PER 1000 POPULATION					
Total Population (in thousands)	19,677	19,836	19,337	19,454	19,542
Inpatient					
Beds	2.5	2.5	2.6	2.7	2.7
Admissions	103.2	102.8	101.9	115	116.1
Inpatient Days	713.4	698.7	686.4	754.7	754.3
Inpatient Surgeries	25.6	25.8	25.7	29.4	29.1
Births	10.2	10.2	10.4	11	11.1
Outpatient					
Emergency Outpatient Visits	418.4	387.6	373	450.6	446.7
Other Outpatient Visits	2,713.3	2,820.4	2,383.1	2,645.7	2,574.1
Total Outpatient Visits	3,131.7	3,207.9	2,756.1	3,096.4	3,020.8
Outpatient Surgeries	72.3	70.6	60.2	75.2	69.4

Note: The 2021 performance data do not reflect the full impact of the COVID-19 pandemic. Please refer to the discussion in the Introduction for more information.

AHA Hospital Statistics © 2024 Health Forum LLC, an affiliate of the American Hospital Association

TABLE 6

NORTH CAROLINA

U.S. Community Hospitals
(Nonfederal, short-term general and other special hospitals)

Overview 2018–2022

	2022	2021	2020	2019	2018
Total Community Hospitals in North Carolina	111	113	112	111	112
Bed Size Category					
6-24	10	11	11	9	8
25-49	22	23	22	24	24
50-99	20	20	17	18	21
100-199	30	31	34	31	32
200-299	11	9	10	10	9
300-399	3	4	2	4	3
400-499	1	2	4	3	3
500 +	14	13	12	12	12
Location					
Hospitals Urban	68	72	71	70	70
Hospitals Rural	43	41	41	41	42
Control					
State and Local Government	28	27	28	31	29
Not for Profit	67	69	69	65	68
Investor owned	16	17	15	15	15
Affiliations					
Hospitals in a System	98	99	98	97	99
Hospitals in a Group Purchasing Organization...	62	60	61	59	76

Note: The 2021 performance data do not reflect the full impact of the COVID-19 pandemic. Please refer to the discussion in the Introduction for more information.

TABLE 6

NORTH CAROLINA

U.S. Community Hospitals
(Nonfederal, short-term general and other special hospitals)

Utilization, Personnel, Community Health Indicators 2018–2022

	2022	2021	2020	2019	2018
TOTAL FACILITY (Includes Hospital and Nursing Home Units)					
Utilization - Inpatient					
Beds	22,106	22,041	21,746	21,673	21,549
Admissions	976,423	984,460	970,859	1,032,683	1,024,837
Inpatient Days	5,933,571	5,840,850	5,319,998	5,596,083	5,502,157
Average Length of Stay	6.1	5.9	5.5	5.4	5.4
Inpatient Surgeries	235,258	240,195	256,988	283,748	285,426
Births	117,144	115,549	111,124	108,667	110,479
Utilization - Outpatient					
Emergency Outpatient Visits	4,215,823	3,973,127	3,832,621	4,445,970	4,793,370
Other Outpatient Visits	16,508,253	16,973,758	15,672,875	18,568,986	18,469,802
Total Outpatient Visits	20,724,076	20,946,885	19,505,496	23,014,956	23,263,172
Outpatient Surgeries	630,064	606,730	522,937	596,249	587,633
Personnel					
Full Time RNs	42,927	42,510	43,113	43,114	42,771
Full Time LPNs	1,927	1,760	1,547	1,766	1,769
Part Time RNs	16,732	16,620	15,922	15,109	14,519
Part Time LPNs	660	597	444	501	428
Total Full Time	151,590	147,382	144,764	148,535	146,313
Total Part Time	46,712	44,652	43,658	40,362	38,005
HOSPITAL UNIT (Excludes Separate Nursing Home Units)					
Utilization - Inpatient					
Beds	21,416	21,305	20,885	20,760	20,572
Admissions	973,567	981,426	966,369	1,027,961	1,020,171
Inpatient Days	5,745,142	5,634,020	5,053,276	5,326,712	5,204,818
Average Length of Stay	5.9	5.7	5.2	5.2	5.1
Personnel					
Total Full Time	151,083	146,878	143,992	147,948	145,712
Total Part Time	46,351	44,306	43,186	40,042	37,702
COMMUNITY HEALTH INDICATORS PER 1000 POPULATION					
Total Population (in thousands)	10,699	10,551	10,601	10,488	10,384
Inpatient					
Beds	2.1	2.1	2.1	2.1	2.1
Admissions	91.3	93.3	91.6	98.5	98.7
Inpatient Days	554.6	553.6	501.8	533.6	529.9
Inpatient Surgeries	22	22.8	24.2	27.1	27.5
Births	10.9	11	10.5	10.4	10.6
Outpatient					
Emergency Outpatient Visits	394	376.6	361.5	423.9	461.6
Other Outpatient Visits	1,543	1,608.7	1,478.5	1,770.5	1,778.7
Total Outpatient Visits	1,937	1,985.3	1,840	2,194.4	2,240.4
Outpatient Surgeries	58.9	57.5	49.3	56.9	56.6

Note: The 2021 performance data do not reflect the full impact of the COVID-19 pandemic. Please refer to the discussion in the Introduction for more information.

AHA Hospital Statistics © 2024 Health Forum LLC, an affiliate of the American Hospital Association

TABLE 6

NORTH DAKOTA

U.S. Community Hospitals
(Nonfederal, short-term general and other special hospitals)

Overview 2018–2022

	2022	2021	2020	2019	2018
Total Community Hospitals in North Dakota......	43	43	41	40	39
Bed Size Category					
6-24	10	10	10	10	11
25-49	15	15	13	13	12
50-99	11	11	11	10	9
100-199	3	2	2	2	2
200-299	2	3	3	3	2
300-399	0	0	0	0	1
400-499	0	0	0	0	0
500 +	2	2	2	2	2
Location					
Hospitals Urban	10	9	8	8	8
Hospitals Rural	33	34	33	32	31
Control					
State and Local Government	0	0	0	0	0
Not for Profit	40	40	39	38	37
Investor owned	3	3	2	2	2
Affiliations					
Hospitals in a System	22	22	21	19	19
Hospitals in a Group Purchasing Organization...	8	12	19	15	15

Note: The 2021 performance data do not reflect the full impact of the COVID-19 pandemic. Please refer to the discussion in the Introduction for more information.

TABLE 6

NORTH DAKOTA

U.S. Community Hospitals
(Nonfederal, short-term general and other special hospitals)

Utilization, Personnel, Community Health Indicators 2018–2022

	2022	2021	2020	2019	2018
TOTAL FACILITY (Includes Hospital and Nursing Home Units)					
Utilization - Inpatient					
Beds	3,322	3,417	3,360	3,323	3,235
Admissions	87,274	91,870	88,381	93,282	90,838
Inpatient Days	713,461	694,961	669,247	692,274	671,636
Average Length of Stay	8.2	7.6	7.6	7.4	7.4
Inpatient Surgeries	21,020	21,259	22,372	25,027	25,363
Births	11,127	9,974	11,171	10,910	11,037
Utilization - Outpatient					
Emergency Outpatient Visits	457,849	369,422	290,548	318,834	313,632
Other Outpatient Visits	2,318,415	2,375,866	2,744,594	2,649,479	2,500,361
Total Outpatient Visits	2,776,264	2,745,288	3,035,142	2,968,313	2,813,993
Outpatient Surgeries	67,136	65,097	60,338	79,926	78,829
Personnel					
Full Time RNs	4,349	4,266	3,992	4,295	3,689
Full Time LPNs	362	436	544	619	540
Part Time RNs	3,390	3,254	3,056	2,714	2,986
Part Time LPNs	379	397	486	432	534
Total Full Time	15,839	15,985	15,104	15,966	15,895
Total Part Time	10,327	9,709	9,514	8,895	9,394
HOSPITAL UNIT (Excludes Separate Nursing Home Units)					
Utilization - Inpatient					
Beds	3,262	3,139	2,897	2,882	2,813
Admissions	87,245	91,353	87,653	92,584	90,090
Inpatient Days	696,515	615,699	515,655	545,409	533,761
Average Length of Stay	8.0	6.7	5.9	5.9	5.9
Personnel					
Total Full Time	15,814	15,761	14,779	15,542	15,583
Total Part Time	10,285	9,607	9,364	8,727	9,228
COMMUNITY HEALTH INDICATORS PER 1000 POPULATION					
Total Population (in thousands)	779	775	765	762	760
Inpatient					
Beds	4.3	4.4	4.4	4.4	4.3
Admissions	112	118.5	115.5	122.4	119.5
Inpatient Days	915.6	896.8	874.5	908.4	883.6
Inpatient Surgeries	27	27.4	29.2	32.8	33.4
Births	14.3	12.9	14.6	14.3	14.5
Outpatient					
Emergency Outpatient Visits	587.5	476.7	379.6	418.4	412.6
Other Outpatient Visits	2,975.1	3,065.8	3,586.3	3,476.7	3,289.6
Total Outpatient Visits	3,562.7	3,542.5	3,965.9	3,895.1	3,702.2
Outpatient Surgeries	86.2	84	78.8	104.9	103.7

Note: The 2021 performance data do not reflect the full impact of the COVID-19 pandemic. Please refer to the discussion in the Introduction for more information.

AHA Hospital Statistics © 2024 Health Forum LLC, an affiliate of the American Hospital Association

TABLE 6

OHIO

U.S. Community Hospitals
(Nonfederal, short-term general and other special hospitals)

Overview 2018–2022

	2022	2021	2020	2019	2018
Total Community Hospitals in Ohio	187	192	193	195	194
Bed Size Category					
6-24	15	14	13	15	15
25-49	54	54	56	52	50
50-99	30	32	31	31	30
100-199	37	39	39	38	40
200-299	20	23	25	30	31
300-399	12	11	10	9	7
400-499	7	6	6	7	7
500 +	12	13	13	13	14
Location					
Hospitals Urban	133	134	135	137	136
Hospitals Rural	54	58	58	58	58
Control					
State and Local Government	14	14	15	16	17
Not for Profit	137	141	139	141	139
Investor owned	36	37	39	38	38
Affiliations					
Hospitals in a System	138	140	140	137	136
Hospitals in a Group Purchasing Organization	93	111	116	106	116

Note: The 2021 performance data do not reflect the full impact of the COVID-19 pandemic. Please refer to the discussion in the Introduction for more information.

TABLE 6

OHIO

U.S. Community Hospitals
(Nonfederal, short-term general and other special hospitals)

Utilization, Personnel, Community Health Indicators 2018–2022

	2022	2021	2020	2019	2018
TOTAL FACILITY (Includes Hospital and Nursing Home Units)					
Utilization - Inpatient					
Beds	31,519	32,390	32,194	33,303	33,157
Admissions	1,290,499	1,338,977	1,283,866	1,424,277	1,430,126
Inpatient Days	6,988,804	7,275,116	6,680,898	7,276,750	7,177,655
Average Length of Stay	5.4	5.4	5.2	5.1	5.0
Inpatient Surgeries	301,389	317,413	319,770	372,142	373,607
Births	115,910	119,684	118,119	121,829	124,524
Utilization - Outpatient					
Emergency Outpatient Visits	6,034,098	5,951,084	5,480,189	6,889,120	6,788,537
Other Outpatient Visits	41,283,182	40,221,144	35,815,870	39,185,868	36,539,086
Total Outpatient Visits	47,317,280	46,172,228	41,296,059	46,074,988	43,327,623
Outpatient Surgeries	981,819	946,785	844,419	991,010	959,629
Personnel					
Full Time RNs	55,544	59,124	62,541	63,050	64,854
Full Time LPNs	3,479	3,265	3,264	3,065	3,009
Part Time RNs	29,898	27,016	27,509	26,745	26,037
Part Time LPNs	1,484	1,232	1,261	1,141	1,083
Total Full Time	219,807	224,470	228,804	229,332	229,304
Total Part Time	91,053	80,217	81,012	80,071	77,532
HOSPITAL UNIT (Excludes Separate Nursing Home Units)					
Utilization - Inpatient					
Beds	31,190	31,895	31,703	32,813	32,653
Admissions	1,287,801	1,335,766	1,280,254	1,419,408	1,424,751
Inpatient Days	6,910,342	7,182,523	6,563,433	7,118,253	7,014,378
Average Length of Stay	5.4	5.4	5.1	5.0	4.9
Personnel					
Total Full Time	219,536	223,787	228,423	228,882	228,844
Total Part Time	90,899	79,930	80,779	79,874	77,317
COMMUNITY HEALTH INDICATORS PER 1000 POPULATION					
Total Population (in thousands)	11,756	11,780	11,693	11,689	11,689
Inpatient					
Beds	2.7	2.7	2.8	2.8	2.8
Admissions	109.8	113.7	109.8	121.8	122.3
Inpatient Days	594.5	617.6	571.3	622.5	614
Inpatient Surgeries	25.6	26.9	27.3	31.8	32
Births	9.9	10.2	10.1	10.4	10.7
Outpatient					
Emergency Outpatient Visits	513.3	505.2	468.7	589.4	580.7
Other Outpatient Visits	3,511.7	3,414.4	3,063	3,352.3	3,125.8
Total Outpatient Visits	4,024.9	3,919.5	3,531.6	3,941.7	3,706.6
Outpatient Surgeries	83.5	80.4	72.2	84.8	82.1

Note: The 2021 performance data do not reflect the full impact of the COVID-19 pandemic. Please refer to the discussion in the Introduction for more information.

AHA Hospital Statistics © 2024 Health Forum LLC, an affiliate of the American Hospital Association

TABLE 6

OKLAHOMA

U.S. Community Hospitals
(Nonfederal, short-term general and other special hospitals)

Overview 2018–2022

	2022	2021	2020	2019	2018
Total Community Hospitals in Oklahoma	**125**	**125**	**122**	**124**	**125**
Bed Size Category					
6-24	38	38	36	35	35
25-49	43	40	41	46	44
50-99	19	23	20	17	20
100-199	14	13	13	14	14
200-299	2	2	3	3	3
300-399	3	3	3	3	3
400-499	2	0	0	0	0
500 +	4	6	6	6	6
Location					
Hospitals Urban	63	65	62	63	64
Hospitals Rural	62	60	60	61	61
Control					
State and Local Government	38	38	36	38	38
Not for Profit	39	39	37	37	39
Investor owned	48	48	49	49	48
Affiliations					
Hospitals in a System	64	66	66	66	68
Hospitals in a Group Purchasing Organization	68	74	73	83	77

Note: The 2021 performance data do not reflect the full impact of the COVID-19 pandemic. Please refer to the discussion in the Introduction for more information.

122   AHA Hospital Statistics © 2024 Health Forum LLC, an affiliate of the American Hospital Association

TABLE 6

OKLAHOMA

U.S. Community Hospitals
(Nonfederal, short-term general and other special hospitals)

Utilization, Personnel, Community Health Indicators 2018–2022

	2022	2021	2020	2019	2018
TOTAL FACILITY (Includes Hospital and Nursing Home Units)					
Utilization - Inpatient					
Beds	11,155	11,280	11,120	11,305	11,144
Admissions	392,881	399,222	402,426	427,388	422,246
Inpatient Days	2,291,171	2,326,982	2,223,386	2,308,688	2,296,383
Average Length of Stay	5.8	5.8	5.5	5.4	5.4
Inpatient Surgeries	98,957	101,995	105,720	112,531	113,241
Births	45,588	43,705	47,628	49,839	48,998
Utilization - Outpatient					
Emergency Outpatient Visits	1,906,646	1,694,831	1,789,799	1,945,709	1,825,825
Other Outpatient Visits	5,960,526	5,982,051	5,713,394	6,087,737	5,781,804
Total Outpatient Visits	7,867,172	7,676,882	7,503,193	8,033,446	7,607,629
Outpatient Surgeries	316,619	321,373	262,037	297,269	299,912
Personnel					
Full Time RNs	15,670	15,788	17,545	14,765	14,366
Full Time LPNs	1,602	1,477	1,482	1,461	1,374
Part Time RNs	4,263	3,961	4,105	5,145	4,541
Part Time LPNs	443	379	309	354	325
Total Full Time	53,292	52,562	53,215	50,181	48,660
Total Part Time	13,732	11,903	11,541	14,632	12,413
HOSPITAL UNIT (Excludes Separate Nursing Home Units)					
Utilization - Inpatient					
Beds	11,009	11,074	10,914	11,099	10,938
Admissions	392,602	398,955	401,884	426,834	421,720
Inpatient Days	2,254,750	2,274,585	2,159,490	2,244,046	2,232,707
Average Length of Stay	5.7	5.7	5.4	5.3	5.3
Personnel					
Total Full Time	53,192	52,437	53,074	50,049	48,503
Total Part Time	13,728	11,888	11,516	14,622	12,383
COMMUNITY HEALTH INDICATORS PER 1000 POPULATION					
Total Population (in thousands)	4,020	3,987	3,981	3,957	3,943
Inpatient					
Beds	2.8	2.8	2.8	2.9	2.8
Admissions	97.7	100.1	101.1	108	107.1
Inpatient Days	570	583.7	558.5	583.4	582.4
Inpatient Surgeries	24.6	25.6	26.6	28.4	28.7
Births	11.3	11	12	12.6	12.4
Outpatient					
Emergency Outpatient Visits	474.3	425.1	449.6	491.7	463
Other Outpatient Visits	1,482.8	1,500.5	1,435.2	1,538.5	1,466.3
Total Outpatient Visits	1,957.1	1,925.7	1,884.9	2,030.2	1,929.4
Outpatient Surgeries	78.8	80.6	65.8	75.1	76.1

Note: The 2021 performance data do not reflect the full impact of the COVID-19 pandemic. Please refer to the discussion in the Introduction for more information.

AHA Hospital Statistics © 2024 Health Forum LLC, an affiliate of the American Hospital Association

TABLE 6

OREGON

U.S. Community Hospitals
(Nonfederal, short-term general and other special hospitals)

Overview 2018–2022

	2022	2021	2020	2019	2018
Total Community Hospitals in Oregon...............	**61**	**61**	**61**	**61**	**61**
Bed Size Category					
6-24	12	13	13	12	12
25-49	20	19	19	20	20
50-99	7	6	7	7	7
100-199	12	13	12	12	12
200-299	1	1	1	1	2
300-399	4	4	4	4	3
400-499	2	2	2	2	2
500 + ...	3	3	3	3	3
Location					
Hospitals Urban	37	35	35	35	35
Hospitals Rural...	24	26	26	26	26
Control					
State and Local Government	11	11	11	11	11
Not for Profit...	47	47	47	47	47
Investor owned...	3	3	3	3	3
Affiliations					
Hospitals in a System	44	44	44	44	44
Hospitals in a Group Purchasing Organization...	59	59	59	59	59

Note: The 2021 performance data do not reflect the full impact of the COVID-19 pandemic. Please refer to the discussion in the Introduction for more information.

AHA Hospital Statistics © 2024 Health Forum LLC, an affiliate of the American Hospital Association

TABLE 6

OREGON

U.S. Community Hospitals
(Nonfederal, short-term general and other special hospitals)

Utilization, Personnel, Community Health Indicators 2018–2022

	2022	2021	2020	2019	2018
TOTAL FACILITY (Includes Hospital and Nursing Home Units)					
Utilization - Inpatient					
Beds	7,027	7,057	6,971	6,975	6,889
Admissions	319,666	313,535	323,538	348,059	347,802
Inpatient Days	1,753,762	1,629,175	1,529,425	1,602,392	1,589,931
Average Length of Stay	5.5	5.2	4.7	4.6	4.6
Inpatient Surgeries	98,057	100,722	107,087	120,185	119,793
Births	38,760	38,446	38,269	41,043	41,999
Utilization - Outpatient					
Emergency Outpatient Visits	1,548,211	1,389,723	1,380,242	1,571,368	1,581,113
Other Outpatient Visits	10,538,209	11,393,418	10,818,419	11,245,103	10,697,576
Total Outpatient Visits	12,086,420	12,783,141	12,198,661	12,816,471	12,278,689
Outpatient Surgeries	225,550	217,963	205,664	241,546	223,416
Personnel					
Full Time RNs	12,838	12,914	13,541	13,954	13,893
Full Time LPNs	170	136	143	156	166
Part Time RNs	9,258	9,226	8,528	8,592	7,815
Part Time LPNs	82	80	70	76	73
Total Full Time	47,278	46,580	46,856	48,459	48,106
Total Part Time	21,896	21,619	21,434	22,740	21,266
HOSPITAL UNIT (Excludes Separate Nursing Home Units)					
Utilization - Inpatient					
Beds	7,006	7,036	6,950	6,935	6,849
Admissions	319,656	313,527	323,527	348,049	347,782
Inpatient Days	1,748,576	1,624,292	1,522,996	1,595,469	1,582,906
Average Length of Stay	5.5	5.2	4.7	4.6	4.6
Personnel					
Total Full Time	47,244	46,548	46,827	48,428	48,076
Total Part Time	21,890	21,607	21,417	22,733	21,260
COMMUNITY HEALTH INDICATORS PER 1000 POPULATION					
Total Population (in thousands)	4,240	4,246	4,242	4,218	4,191
Inpatient					
Beds	1.7	1.7	1.6	1.7	1.6
Admissions	75.4	73.8	76.3	82.5	83
Inpatient Days	413.6	383.7	360.6	379.9	379.4
Inpatient Surgeries	23.1	23.7	25.2	28.5	28.6
Births	9.1	9.1	9	9.7	10
Outpatient					
Emergency Outpatient Visits	365.1	327.3	325.4	372.6	377.3
Other Outpatient Visits	2,485.3	2,683.2	2,550.6	2,666.1	2,552.7
Total Outpatient Visits	2,850.5	3,010.5	2,876	3,038.7	2,930
Outpatient Surgeries	53.2	51.3	48.5	57.3	53.3

Note: The 2021 performance data do not reflect the full impact of the COVID-19 pandemic. Please refer to the discussion in the Introduction for more information.

AHA Hospital Statistics © 2024 Health Forum LLC, an affiliate of the American Hospital Association

TABLE 6

PENNSYLVANIA

U.S. Community Hospitals
(Nonfederal, short-term general and other special hospitals)

Overview 2018–2022

	2022	2021	2020	2019	2018
Total Community Hospitals in Pennsylvania	185	185	186	191	199
Bed Size Category					
6-24	15	13	12	12	10
25-49	32	30	28	30	34
50-99	41	42	44	41	43
100-199	39	42	43	48	47
200-299	22	24	25	25	31
300-399	18	15	16	16	14
400-499	1	1	1	3	5
500 + ...	17	18	17	16	15
Location					
Hospitals Urban	143	151	152	157	162
Hospitals Rural	42	34	34	34	37
Control					
State and Local Government	2	2	1	1	1
Not for Profit	146	144	145	147	151
Investor owned	37	39	40	43	47
Affiliations					
Hospitals in a System	142	142	143	141	148
Hospitals in a Group Purchasing Organization...	113	115	112	110	120

Note: The 2021 performance data do not reflect the full impact of the COVID-19 pandemic. Please refer to the discussion in the Introduction for more information.

TABLE 6

PENNSYLVANIA

U.S. Community Hospitals
(Nonfederal, short-term general and other special hospitals)

Utilization, Personnel, Community Health Indicators 2018–2022

	2022	2021	2020	2019	2018
TOTAL FACILITY (Includes Hospital and Nursing Home Units)					
Utilization - Inpatient					
Beds	34,702	35,259	35,423	35,448	36,730
Admissions	1,409,898	1,435,699	1,416,217	1,536,768	1,584,299
Inpatient Days	8,601,574	8,471,144	7,943,074	8,341,604	8,614,087
Average Length of Stay	6.1	5.9	5.6	5.4	5.4
Inpatient Surgeries	366,388	383,218	407,620	428,143	454,182
Births	124,927	127,665	130,280	127,430	134,890
Utilization - Outpatient					
Emergency Outpatient Visits	5,833,408	5,515,027	5,465,206	6,182,130	6,264,480
Other Outpatient Visits	36,048,508	34,772,978	32,539,610	34,936,026	35,439,162
Total Outpatient Visits	41,881,916	40,288,005	38,004,816	41,118,156	41,703,642
Outpatient Surgeries	926,510	897,373	905,251	924,755	941,220
Personnel					
Full Time RNs	59,854	61,796	64,573	63,031	62,451
Full Time LPNs	2,761	2,555	2,610	2,246	2,606
Part Time RNs	25,928	23,653	22,916	23,335	24,612
Part Time LPNs	948	828	752	738	788
Total Full Time	223,316	222,903	222,471	220,879	219,170
Total Part Time	77,209	72,273	70,905	72,395	73,466
HOSPITAL UNIT (Excludes Separate Nursing Home Units)					
Utilization - Inpatient					
Beds	33,952	34,421	34,469	34,359	35,540
Admissions	1,404,789	1,429,477	1,407,804	1,528,977	1,575,938
Inpatient Days	8,444,961	8,255,629	7,687,332	8,000,892	8,256,220
Average Length of Stay	6.0	5.8	5.5	5.2	5.2
Personnel					
Total Full Time	222,691	222,388	221,692	219,982	218,366
Total Part Time	76,742	71,901	70,507	71,954	73,061
COMMUNITY HEALTH INDICATORS PER 1000 POPULATION					
Total Population (in thousands)	12,972	12,964	12,783	12,802	12,807
Inpatient					
Beds	2.7	2.7	2.8	2.8	2.9
Admissions	108.7	110.7	110.8	120	123.7
Inpatient Days	663.1	653.4	621.4	651.6	672.6
Inpatient Surgeries	28.2	29.6	31.9	33.4	35.5
Births	9.6	9.8	10.2	10	10.5
Outpatient					
Emergency Outpatient Visits	449.7	425.4	427.5	482.9	489.1
Other Outpatient Visits	2,778.9	2,682.3	2,545.5	2,729	2,767.2
Total Outpatient Visits	3,228.6	3,107.7	2,973	3,211.9	3,256.3
Outpatient Surgeries	71.4	69.2	70.8	72.2	73.5

Note: The 2021 performance data do not reflect the full impact of the COVID-19 pandemic. Please refer to the discussion in the Introduction for more information.

AHA Hospital Statistics © 2024 Health Forum LLC, an affiliate of the American Hospital Association

TABLE 6

RHODE ISLAND

U.S. Community Hospitals
(Nonfederal, short-term general and other special hospitals)

Overview 2018–2022

	2022	2021	2020	2019	2018
Total Community Hospitals in Rhode Island......	11	11	11	11	11
Bed Size Category					
6-24	0	0	0	0	0
25-49	0	0	0	0	0
50-99	4	4	4	4	4
100-199	3	3	3	3	3
200-299	3	2	2	2	2
300-399	0	1	1	1	1
400-499	0	0	0	0	0
500 + ...	1	1	1	1	1
Location					
Hospitals Urban	11	11	11	11	11
Hospitals Rural...	0	0	0	0	0
Control					
State and Local Government	0	0	0	0	0
Not for Profit...	11	11	11	11	9
Investor owned..	0	0	0	0	2
Affiliations					
Hospitals in a System	9	10	10	10	10
Hospitals in a Group Purchasing Organization...	6	7	6	6	6

Note: The 2021 performance data do not reflect the full impact of the COVID-19 pandemic. Please refer to the discussion in the Introduction for more information.

AHA Hospital Statistics © 2024 Health Forum LLC, an affiliate of the American Hospital Association

TABLE 6

RHODE ISLAND

U.S. Community Hospitals
(Nonfederal, short-term general and other special hospitals)

Utilization, Personnel, Community Health Indicators 2018–2022

	2022	2021	2020	2019	2018
TOTAL FACILITY (Includes Hospital and Nursing Home Units)					
Utilization - Inpatient					
Beds	2,124	2,197	2,188	2,191	2,187
Admissions	97,630	107,355	104,595	116,276	115,483
Inpatient Days	546,235	569,985	533,634	554,916	549,531
Average Length of Stay	5.6	5.3	5.1	4.8	4.8
Inpatient Surgeries	22,772	24,601	25,506	28,588	28,498
Births	11,106	12,756	11,253	12,002	11,401
Utilization - Outpatient					
Emergency Outpatient Visits	482,421	408,461	437,283	528,353	546,514
Other Outpatient Visits	1,939,768	1,923,274	1,586,201	1,770,347	1,627,424
Total Outpatient Visits	2,422,189	2,331,735	2,023,484	2,298,700	2,173,938
Outpatient Surgeries	61,024	65,268	54,656	66,690	66,889
Personnel					
Full Time RNs	3,213	3,068	3,322	3,363	3,281
Full Time LPNs	66	49	65	77	75
Part Time RNs	2,979	3,217	2,819	2,950	2,835
Part Time LPNs	76	35	43	47	48
Total Full Time	13,929	13,624	13,779	13,562	13,401
Total Part Time	10,049	9,377	8,928	9,179	8,786
HOSPITAL UNIT (Excludes Separate Nursing Home Units)					
Utilization - Inpatient					
Beds	2,124	2,197	2,188	2,191	2,187
Admissions	97,630	107,355	104,595	116,276	115,483
Inpatient Days	546,235	569,985	533,634	554,916	549,531
Average Length of Stay	5.6	5.3	5.1	4.8	4.8
Personnel					
Total Full Time	13,929	13,624	13,779	13,562	13,401
Total Part Time	10,049	9,377	8,928	9,179	8,786
COMMUNITY HEALTH INDICATORS PER 1000 POPULATION					
Total Population (in thousands)	1,094	1,096	1,057	1,059	1,057
Inpatient					
Beds	1.9	2	2.1	2.1	2.1
Admissions	89.3	98	98.9	109.8	109.2
Inpatient Days	499.4	520.2	504.8	523.8	519.7
Inpatient Surgeries	20.8	22.5	24.1	27	27
Births	10.2	11.6	10.6	11.3	10.8
Outpatient					
Emergency Outpatient Visits	441.1	372.8	413.7	498.7	516.9
Other Outpatient Visits	1,773.5	1,755.4	1,500.5	1,671.1	1,539.2
Total Outpatient Visits	2,214.6	2,128.3	1,914.1	2,169.9	2,056.1
Outpatient Surgeries	55.8	59.6	51.7	63	63.3

Note: The 2021 performance data do not reflect the full impact of the COVID-19 pandemic. Please refer to the discussion in the Introduction for more information.

AHA Hospital Statistics © 2024 Health Forum LLC, an affiliate of the American Hospital Association

TABLE 6

SOUTH CAROLINA

U.S. Community Hospitals
(Nonfederal, short-term general and other special hospitals)

Overview 2018–2022

	2022	2021	2020	2019	2018
Total Community Hospitals in South Carolina...	70	74	73	72	69
Bed Size Category					
6-24	3	4	5	3	1
25-49	17	22	20	18	19
50-99	21	18	17	18	15
100-199	10	11	13	11	11
200-299	7	8	5	9	9
300-399	4	4	7	6	6
400-499	2	1	2	2	4
500 +	6	6	4	5	4
Location					
Hospitals Urban	55	58	57	56	54
Hospitals Rural	15	16	16	16	15
Control					
State and Local Government	19	21	20	20	14
Not for Profit	30	32	32	32	30
Investor owned	21	21	21	20	25
Affiliations					
Hospitals in a System	62	63	62	61	58
Hospitals in a Group Purchasing Organization...	67	68	57	59	64

Note: The 2021 performance data do not reflect the full impact of the COVID-19 pandemic. Please refer to the discussion in the Introduction for more information.

AHA Hospital Statistics © 2024 Health Forum LLC, an affiliate of the American Hospital Association

TABLE 6

SOUTH CAROLINA

U.S. Community Hospitals
(Nonfederal, short-term general and other special hospitals)

Utilization, Personnel, Community Health Indicators 2018–2022

	2022	2021	2020	2019	2018
TOTAL FACILITY (Includes Hospital and Nursing Home Units)					
Utilization - Inpatient					
Beds	11,798	11,567	11,231	12,055	12,120
Admissions	507,295	511,817	489,874	542,122	533,023
Inpatient Days	2,954,162	2,917,156	2,705,839	2,902,583	2,856,120
Average Length of Stay	5.8	5.7	5.5	5.4	5.4
Inpatient Surgeries	154,658	153,604	158,107	166,740	166,063
Births	51,788	51,409	50,861	52,331	51,006
Utilization - Outpatient					
Emergency Outpatient Visits	2,273,244	2,182,440	2,221,467	2,408,169	2,509,535
Other Outpatient Visits	8,008,075	8,136,118	7,812,294	7,046,024	7,065,878
Total Outpatient Visits	10,281,319	10,318,558	10,033,761	9,454,193	9,575,413
Outpatient Surgeries	396,611	369,717	324,716	357,747	336,386
Personnel					
Full Time RNs	17,756	19,346	20,091	19,467	20,302
Full Time LPNs	964	710	738	644	634
Part Time RNs	7,885	7,640	6,737	7,292	6,142
Part Time LPNs	416	233	188	207	197
Total Full Time	59,858	61,452	59,280	60,610	63,150
Total Part Time	22,883	20,056	17,723	19,064	16,482
HOSPITAL UNIT (Excludes Separate Nursing Home Units)					
Utilization - Inpatient					
Beds	11,558	11,540	11,201	11,792	11,711
Admissions	506,521	511,292	489,386	540,927	531,084
Inpatient Days	2,886,288	2,908,748	2,697,597	2,820,660	2,727,563
Average Length of Stay	5.7	5.7	5.5	5.2	5.1
Personnel					
Total Full Time	59,630	61,307	59,200	60,290	62,790
Total Part Time	22,819	19,912	17,706	18,936	16,285
COMMUNITY HEALTH INDICATORS PER 1000 POPULATION					
Total Population (in thousands)	5,283	5,191	5,218	5,149	5,084
Inpatient					
Beds	2.2	2.2	2.2	2.3	2.4
Admissions	96	98.6	93.9	105.3	104.8
Inpatient Days	559.2	562	518.6	563.7	561.8
Inpatient Surgeries	29.3	29.6	30.3	32.4	32.7
Births	9.8	9.9	9.7	10.2	10
Outpatient					
Emergency Outpatient Visits	430.3	420.5	425.7	467.7	493.6
Other Outpatient Visits	1,515.9	1,567.4	1,497.2	1,368.5	1,389.8
Total Outpatient Visits	1,946.2	1,987.9	1,922.9	1,836.2	1,883.4
Outpatient Surgeries	75.1	71.2	62.2	69.5	66.2

Note: The 2021 performance data do not reflect the full impact of the COVID-19 pandemic. Please refer to the discussion in the Introduction for more information.

TABLE 6

SOUTH DAKOTA

U.S. Community Hospitals
(Nonfederal, short-term general and other special hospitals)

Overview 2018–2022

	2022	2021	2020	2019	2018
Total Community Hospitals in South Dakota	57	58	57	57	57
Bed Size Category					
6-24	20	20	20	20	22
25-49	13	13	12	12	11
50-99	14	15	15	14	13
100-199	6	6	6	6	6
200-299	1	1	1	2	2
300-399	0	1	1	1	1
400-499	2	0	0	0	0
500 +	1	2	2	2	2
Location					
Hospitals Urban	15	15	14	14	14
Hospitals Rural	42	43	43	43	43
Control					
State and Local Government	4	4	4	4	4
Not for Profit	45	45	45	45	45
Investor owned	8	9	8	8	8
Affiliations					
Hospitals in a System	41	41	40	40	40
Hospitals in a Group Purchasing Organization	37	36	37	31	31

Note: The 2021 performance data do not reflect the full impact of the COVID-19 pandemic. Please refer to the discussion in the Introduction for more information.

TABLE 6

SOUTH DAKOTA

U.S. Community Hospitals
(Nonfederal, short-term general and other special hospitals)

Utilization, Personnel, Community Health Indicators 2018–2022

	2022	2021	2020	2019	2018
TOTAL FACILITY (Includes Hospital and Nursing Home Units)					
Utilization - Inpatient					
Beds	4,190	4,255	4,279	4,222	4,183
Admissions	107,805	110,811	101,980	109,069	107,474
Inpatient Days	976,185	984,393	892,891	927,445	939,755
Average Length of Stay	9.1	8.9	8.8	8.5	8.7
Inpatient Surgeries	22,115	23,712	23,138	26,848	29,908
Births	12,284	11,956	11,533	12,352	13,122
Utilization - Outpatient					
Emergency Outpatient Visits	333,517	304,673	306,360	359,830	378,697
Other Outpatient Visits	3,113,699	3,028,818	2,747,503	2,773,935	2,807,104
Total Outpatient Visits	3,447,216	3,333,491	3,053,863	3,133,765	3,185,801
Outpatient Surgeries	74,917	74,581	61,384	65,455	64,169
Personnel					
Full Time RNs	5,250	5,488	4,816	5,172	5,715
Full Time LPNs	627	595	606	534	579
Part Time RNs	2,906	2,886	3,302	2,949	2,811
Part Time LPNs	273	256	283	258	243
Total Full Time	20,087	20,370	17,871	19,311	20,559
Total Part Time	10,166	9,914	11,602	9,606	9,943
HOSPITAL UNIT (Excludes Separate Nursing Home Units)					
Utilization - Inpatient					
Beds	3,048	3,104	3,104	3,155	3,115
Admissions	106,589	109,552	100,547	107,844	106,298
Inpatient Days	642,527	629,516	516,485	594,153	587,645
Average Length of Stay	6.0	5.7	5.1	5.5	5.5
Personnel					
Total Full Time	19,385	19,627	17,225	18,728	19,943
Total Part Time	9,553	9,230	11,002	9,129	9,291
COMMUNITY HEALTH INDICATORS PER 1000 POPULATION					
Total Population (in thousands)	910	895	893	885	882
Inpatient					
Beds	4.6	4.8	4.8	4.8	4.7
Admissions	118.5	123.8	114.2	123.3	121.8
Inpatient Days	1072.9	1099.4	1000.2	1048.4	1065.2
Inpatient Surgeries	24.3	26.5	25.9	30.3	33.9
Births	13.5	13.4	12.9	14	14.9
Outpatient					
Emergency Outpatient Visits	366.6	340.3	343.2	406.7	429.2
Other Outpatient Visits	3,422.3	3,382.7	3,077.7	3,135.6	3,181.8
Total Outpatient Visits	3,788.9	3,723	3,420.9	3,542.3	3,611.1
Outpatient Surgeries	82.3	83.3	68.8	74	72.7

Note: The 2021 performance data do not reflect the full impact of the COVID-19 pandemic. Please refer to the discussion in the Introduction for more information.

AHA Hospital Statistics © 2024 Health Forum LLC, an affiliate of the American Hospital Association

TABLE 6

TENNESSEE

U.S. Community Hospitals
(Nonfederal, short-term general and other special hospitals)

Overview 2018–2022

	2022	2021	2020	2019	2018
Total Community Hospitals in Tennessee	**112**	**111**	**111**	**112**	**115**
Bed Size Category					
6-24	11	12	10	10	7
25-49	26	25	23	25	27
50-99	24	24	28	27	30
100-199	25	23	21	24	22
200-299	7	8	11	8	9
300-399	6	6	4	5	6
400-499	3	3	4	4	5
500 +	10	10	10	9	9
Location					
Hospitals Urban	73	73	74	73	74
Hospitals Rural	39	38	37	39	41
Control					
State and Local Government	20	20	20	21	20
Not for Profit	49	48	46	49	50
Investor owned	43	43	45	42	45
Affiliations					
Hospitals in a System	94	93	92	92	95
Hospitals in a Group Purchasing Organization	52	51	52	57	52

Note: The 2021 performance data do not reflect the full impact of the COVID-19 pandemic. Please refer to the discussion in the Introduction for more information.

134   AHA Hospital Statistics © 2024 Health Forum LLC, an affiliate of the American Hospital Association

TABLE 6

TENNESSEE

U.S. Community Hospitals
(Nonfederal, short-term general and other special hospitals)

Utilization, Personnel, Community Health Indicators 2018–2022

	2022	2021	2020	2019	2018
TOTAL FACILITY (Includes Hospital and Nursing Home Units)					
Utilization - Inpatient					
Beds	18,907	18,995	19,185	18,366	19,387
Admissions	765,581	779,114	785,098	808,717	817,844
Inpatient Days	4,650,967	4,593,682	4,390,837	4,357,177	4,458,707
Average Length of Stay	6.1	5.9	5.6	5.4	5.5
Inpatient Surgeries	178,525	193,370	207,633	226,746	228,731
Births	64,513	68,460	67,806	65,464	65,359
Utilization - Outpatient					
Emergency Outpatient Visits	3,069,204	2,849,915	2,940,496	3,395,858	3,413,114
Other Outpatient Visits	11,194,640	10,743,406	10,001,600	11,260,595	10,661,893
Total Outpatient Visits	14,263,844	13,593,321	12,942,096	14,656,453	14,075,007
Outpatient Surgeries	432,792	423,898	390,327	451,249	451,668
Personnel					
Full Time RNs	30,463	31,175	31,139	29,312	28,928
Full Time LPNs	2,054	1,980	2,078	2,011	1,967
Part Time RNs	10,668	9,839	9,726	10,602	10,639
Part Time LPNs	675	547	456	571	590
Total Full Time	105,767	105,759	106,656	100,974	103,142
Total Part Time	29,358	26,435	25,855	28,320	30,700
HOSPITAL UNIT (Excludes Separate Nursing Home Units)					
Utilization - Inpatient					
Beds	18,492	18,513	18,708	17,860	18,789
Admissions	763,310	776,566	781,851	805,375	813,937
Inpatient Days	4,541,759	4,476,624	4,245,939	4,212,898	4,279,475
Average Length of Stay	6.0	5.8	5.4	5.2	5.3
Personnel					
Total Full Time	105,515	105,496	106,347	100,614	102,739
Total Part Time	29,279	26,391	25,792	28,257	30,649
COMMUNITY HEALTH INDICATORS PER 1000 POPULATION					
Total Population (in thousands)	7,051	6,975	6,887	6,829	6,770
Inpatient					
Beds	2.7	2.7	2.8	2.7	2.9
Admissions	108.6	111.7	114	118.4	120.8
Inpatient Days	659.6	658.6	637.6	638	658.6
Inpatient Surgeries	25.3	27.7	30.1	33.2	33.8
Births	9.1	9.8	9.8	9.6	9.7
Outpatient					
Emergency Outpatient Visits	435.3	408.6	427	497.3	504.2
Other Outpatient Visits	1,587.6	1,540.2	1,452.3	1,648.9	1,574.9
Total Outpatient Visits	2,022.9	1,948.8	1,879.3	2,146.2	2,079
Outpatient Surgeries	61.4	60.8	56.7	66.1	66.7

Note: The 2021 performance data do not reflect the full impact of the COVID-19 pandemic. Please refer to the discussion in the Introduction for more information.

TABLE 6

TEXAS

U.S. Community Hospitals
(Nonfederal, short-term general and other special hospitals)

Overview 2018–2022

	2022	2021	2020	2019	2018
Total Community Hospitals in Texas	**509**	**517**	**523**	**512**	**523**
Bed Size Category					
6-24	126	125	135	129	127
25-49	138	141	139	135	136
50-99	91	91	88	86	93
100-199	49	55	57	60	65
200-299	39	40	40	40	39
300-399	25	25	21	26	25
400-499	14	11	15	10	12
500 + ...	27	29	28	26	26
Location					
Hospitals Urban	381	385	390	379	388
Hospitals Rural	128	132	133	133	135
Control					
State and Local Government	97	99	99	100	103
Not for Profit	152	152	153	146	142
Investor owned	260	266	271	266	278
Affiliations					
Hospitals in a System	326	333	333	321	334
Hospitals in a Group Purchasing Organization...	466	471	472	469	482

Note: The 2021 performance data do not reflect the full impact of the COVID-19 pandemic. Please refer to the discussion in the Introduction for more information.

TABLE 6

TEXAS

U.S. Community Hospitals
(Nonfederal, short-term general and other special hospitals)

Utilization, Personnel, Community Health Indicators 2018–2022

	2022	2021	2020	2019	2018
TOTAL FACILITY (Includes Hospital and Nursing Home Units)					
Utilization - Inpatient					
Beds	66,074	66,373	66,609	65,187	65,671
Admissions	2,765,245	2,726,846	2,632,067	2,800,687	2,779,032
Inpatient Days	15,362,770	15,474,171	14,174,592	14,518,233	14,531,238
Average Length of Stay	5.6	5.7	5.4	5.2	5.2
Inpatient Surgeries	707,213	700,948	702,852	769,531	783,803
Births	384,118	366,932	366,318	372,667	376,662
Utilization - Outpatient					
Emergency Outpatient Visits	12,377,351	11,121,795	10,633,689	12,236,144	12,281,937
Other Outpatient Visits	36,643,899	35,334,068	31,076,007	34,821,634	33,948,389
Total Outpatient Visits	49,021,250	46,455,863	41,709,696	47,057,778	46,230,326
Outpatient Surgeries	1,492,353	1,394,831	1,248,978	1,425,282	1,391,459
Personnel					
Full Time RNs	111,788	109,550	113,312	112,721	112,333
Full Time LPNs	7,387	6,598	6,513	6,485	6,671
Part Time RNs	31,187	28,239	26,389	27,481	27,529
Part Time LPNs	1,826	1,514	1,244	1,413	1,457
Total Full Time	344,367	335,072	338,061	337,671	337,723
Total Part Time	82,325	74,618	72,150	73,848	76,242
HOSPITAL UNIT (Excludes Separate Nursing Home Units)					
Utilization - Inpatient					
Beds	65,835	66,096	66,312	64,858	65,431
Admissions	2,763,556	2,724,891	2,629,912	2,797,871	2,775,107
Inpatient Days	15,302,930	15,410,483	14,103,584	14,430,745	14,453,418
Average Length of Stay	5.5	5.7	5.4	5.2	5.2
Personnel					
Total Full Time	344,017	334,707	337,867	337,409	337,439
Total Part Time	82,255	74,546	72,107	73,799	76,200
COMMUNITY HEALTH INDICATORS PER 1000 POPULATION					
Total Population (in thousands)	30,030	29,528	29,361	28,996	28,702
Inpatient					
Beds	2.2	2.2	2.3	2.2	2.3
Admissions	92.1	92.3	89.6	96.6	96.8
Inpatient Days	511.6	524.1	482.8	500.7	506.3
Inpatient Surgeries	23.6	23.7	23.9	26.5	27.3
Births	12.8	12.4	12.5	12.9	13.1
Outpatient					
Emergency Outpatient Visits	412.2	376.7	362.2	422	427.9
Other Outpatient Visits	1,220.3	1,196.6	1,058.4	1,200.9	1,182.8
Total Outpatient Visits	1,632.4	1,573.3	1,420.6	1,622.9	1,610.7
Outpatient Surgeries	49.7	47.2	42.5	49.2	48.5

Note: The 2021 performance data do not reflect the full impact of the COVID-19 pandemic. Please refer to the discussion in the Introduction for more information.

AHA Hospital Statistics © 2024 Health Forum LLC, an affiliate of the American Hospital Association

TABLE 6

UTAH

U.S. Community Hospitals
(Nonfederal, short-term general and other special hospitals)

Overview 2018–2022

	2022	2021	2020	2019	2018
Total Community Hospitals in Utah	54	54	53	53	54
Bed Size Category					
6-24	13	13	12	12	11
25-49	17	18	18	18	19
50-99	7	3	3	3	3
100-199	9	11	11	11	12
200-299	4	5	5	6	5
300-399	2	2	2	1	2
400-499	0	0	0	0	0
500 +	2	2	2	2	2
Location					
Hospitals Urban	34	36	35	35	36
Hospitals Rural	20	18	18	18	18
Control					
State and Local Government	7	7	8	7	7
Not for Profit	33	29	28	28	28
Investor owned	14	18	17	18	19
Affiliations					
Hospitals in a System	43	43	43	43	44
Hospitals in a Group Purchasing Organization	30	30	30	29	30

Note: The 2021 performance data do not reflect the full impact of the COVID-19 pandemic. Please refer to the discussion in the Introduction for more information.

TABLE 6

UTAH

U.S. Community Hospitals
(Nonfederal, short-term general and other special hospitals)

Utilization, Personnel, Community Health Indicators 2018–2022

	2022	2021	2020	2019	2018
TOTAL FACILITY (Includes Hospital and Nursing Home Units)					
Utilization - Inpatient					
Beds	5,734	5,928	5,891	5,664	5,767
Admissions	235,181	248,596	236,331	248,428	274,083
Inpatient Days	1,200,362	1,313,376	1,182,890	1,151,548	1,194,433
Average Length of Stay	5.1	5.3	5.0	4.6	4.4
Inpatient Surgeries	58,344	60,708	62,857	73,686	71,535
Births	42,053	45,223	45,635	46,849	46,147
Utilization - Outpatient					
Emergency Outpatient Visits	945,016	1,136,882	987,285	862,136	849,372
Other Outpatient Visits	8,018,937	9,090,638	7,449,809	4,027,335	3,856,761
Total Outpatient Visits	8,963,953	10,227,520	8,437,094	4,889,471	4,706,133
Outpatient Surgeries	214,527	203,673	179,872	196,250	193,340
Personnel					
Full Time RNs	10,149	10,330	11,236	11,510	11,407
Full Time LPNs	306	251	271	264	240
Part Time RNs	6,827	6,177	5,657	5,473	4,824
Part Time LPNs	219	144	124	122	122
Total Full Time	35,977	35,476	36,819	36,919	35,801
Total Part Time	18,272	16,598	15,249	15,265	13,939
HOSPITAL UNIT (Excludes Separate Nursing Home Units)					
Utilization - Inpatient					
Beds	5,674	5,853	5,805	5,561	5,648
Admissions	235,075	248,490	236,002	247,986	273,596
Inpatient Days	1,186,727	1,299,859	1,163,194	1,125,123	1,167,887
Average Length of Stay	5.0	5.2	4.9	4.5	4.3
Personnel					
Total Full Time	35,952	35,438	36,725	36,814	35,690
Total Part Time	18,198	16,572	15,185	15,175	13,845
COMMUNITY HEALTH INDICATORS PER 1000 POPULATION					
Total Population (in thousands)	3,381	3,338	3,250	3,206	3,161
Inpatient					
Beds	1.7	1.8	1.8	1.8	1.8
Admissions	69.6	74.5	72.7	77.5	86.7
Inpatient Days	355.1	393.5	364	359.2	377.9
Inpatient Surgeries	17.3	18.2	19.3	23	22.6
Births	12.4	13.5	14	14.6	14.6
Outpatient					
Emergency Outpatient Visits	279.5	340.6	303.8	268.9	268.7
Other Outpatient Visits	2,371.9	2,723.4	2,292.3	1,256.2	1,220.1
Total Outpatient Visits	2,651.4	3,064	2,596.1	1,525.1	1,488.8
Outpatient Surgeries	63.5	61	55.3	61.2	61.2

Note: The 2021 performance data do not reflect the full impact of the COVID-19 pandemic. Please refer to the discussion in the Introduction for more information.

AHA Hospital Statistics © 2024 Health Forum LLC, an affiliate of the American Hospital Association **139**

TABLE 6

VERMONT

U.S. Community Hospitals
(Nonfederal, short-term general and other special hospitals)

Overview 2018–2022

	2022	2021	2020	2019	2018
Total Community Hospitals in Vermont.............	14	14	14	14	14
Bed Size Category					
6-24	1	1	1	1	0
25-49	7	8	8	8	8
50-99	3	2	2	2	3
100-199	1	1	1	1	1
200-299	1	1	1	1	1
300-399	0	0	0	0	0
400-499	0	0	0	1	0
500 + ...	1	1	1	0	1
Location					
Hospitals Urban	2	2	2	2	2
Hospitals Rural	12	12	12	12	12
Control					
State and Local Government	0	0	0	0	0
Not for Profit...	14	14	14	14	14
Investor owned...	0	0	0	0	0
Affiliations					
Hospitals in a System	3	2	1	1	1
Hospitals in a Group Purchasing Organization...	9	8	6	7	5

Note: The 2021 performance data do not reflect the full impact of the COVID-19 pandemic. Please refer to the discussion in the Introduction for more information.

TABLE 6

VERMONT

U.S. Community Hospitals
(Nonfederal, short-term general and other special hospitals)

Utilization, Personnel, Community Health Indicators 2018–2022

	2022	2021	2020	2019	2018
TOTAL FACILITY (Includes Hospital and Nursing Home Units)					
Utilization - Inpatient					
Beds	1,312	1,333	1,336	1,275	1,305
Admissions	46,237	46,985	46,863	51,241	50,952
Inpatient Days	320,734	296,778	290,188	315,779	302,817
Average Length of Stay	6.9	6.3	6.2	6.2	5.9
Inpatient Surgeries	11,248	11,755	11,565	12,319	14,225
Births	5,142	4,857	5,123	5,280	5,007
Utilization - Outpatient					
Emergency Outpatient Visits	307,736	248,600	281,928	317,314	324,272
Other Outpatient Visits	2,956,141	2,839,136	2,615,134	2,714,071	2,695,020
Total Outpatient Visits	3,263,877	3,087,736	2,897,062	3,031,385	3,019,292
Outpatient Surgeries	48,902	43,597	38,853	42,561	39,302
Personnel					
Full Time RNs	2,495	2,682	2,690	2,618	2,474
Full Time LPNs	181	213	194	201	186
Part Time RNs	1,927	1,820	1,760	1,815	1,977
Part Time LPNs	91	89	83	91	128
Total Full Time	13,391	13,679	13,025	12,769	12,261
Total Part Time	6,155	5,799	5,473	5,561	6,006
HOSPITAL UNIT (Excludes Separate Nursing Home Units)					
Utilization - Inpatient					
Beds	1,159	1,180	1,183	1,122	1,152
Admissions	45,866	46,626	46,472	50,857	50,635
Inpatient Days	277,127	256,043	246,464	269,446	259,774
Average Length of Stay	6.0	5.5	5.3	5.3	5.1
Personnel					
Total Full Time	13,273	13,518	12,858	12,572	12,166
Total Part Time	6,089	5,720	5,413	5,397	5,831
COMMUNITY HEALTH INDICATORS PER 1000 POPULATION					
Total Population (in thousands)	647	646	623	624	626
Inpatient					
Beds	2	2.1	2.1	2	2.1
Admissions	71.5	72.8	75.2	82.1	81.4
Inpatient Days	495.7	459.7	465.5	506.1	483.5
Inpatient Surgeries	17.4	18.2	18.6	19.7	22.7
Births	7.9	7.5	8.2	8.5	8
Outpatient					
Emergency Outpatient Visits	475.6	385.1	452.3	508.5	517.8
Other Outpatient Visits	4,568.5	4,397.9	4,195.3	4,349.5	4,303.1
Total Outpatient Visits	5,044.1	4,783	4,647.6	4,858.1	4,820.8
Outpatient Surgeries	75.6	67.5	62.3	68.2	62.8

Note: The 2021 performance data do not reflect the full impact of the COVID-19 pandemic. Please refer to the discussion in the Introduction for more information.

AHA Hospital Statistics © 2024 Health Forum LLC, an affiliate of the American Hospital Association

TABLE 6

VIRGINIA

U.S. Community Hospitals
(Nonfederal, short-term general and other special hospitals)

Overview 2018–2022

	2022	2021	2020	2019	2018
Total Community Hospitals in Virginia	94	94	95	97	96
Bed Size Category					
6-24	10	10	11	12	11
25-49	16	14	13	13	15
50-99	19	20	21	22	21
100-199	17	18	18	18	17
200-299	14	14	14	14	14
300-399	4	4	4	5	5
400-499	4	4	4	3	5
500 +	10	10	10	10	8
Location					
Hospitals Urban	68	69	70	72	71
Hospitals Rural	26	25	25	25	25
Control					
State and Local Government	3	3	3	4	4
Not for Profit	66	67	67	68	67
Investor owned	25	24	25	25	25
Affiliations					
Hospitals in a System	85	85	84	87	86
Hospitals in a Group Purchasing Organization	49	43	44	50	58

Note: The 2021 performance data do not reflect the full impact of the COVID-19 pandemic. Please refer to the discussion in the Introduction for more information.

TABLE 6

VIRGINIA

U.S. Community Hospitals
(Nonfederal, short-term general and other special hospitals)

Utilization, Personnel, Community Health Indicators 2018–2022

	2022	2021	2020	2019	2018
TOTAL FACILITY (Includes Hospital and Nursing Home Units)					
Utilization - Inpatient					
Beds	17,476	17,961	18,155	18,143	18,065
Admissions	758,915	751,986	727,265	824,998	801,397
Inpatient Days	4,275,325	4,549,713	4,182,649	4,653,339	4,553,821
Average Length of Stay	5.6	6.1	5.8	5.6	5.7
Inpatient Surgeries	170,585	173,080	178,424	210,051	199,518
Births	88,129	87,561	88,975	90,519	90,839
Utilization - Outpatient					
Emergency Outpatient Visits	3,501,737	3,070,182	2,905,997	3,627,232	3,686,696
Other Outpatient Visits	15,219,353	13,901,979	13,320,549	15,079,644	14,646,870
Total Outpatient Visits	18,721,090	16,972,161	16,226,546	18,706,876	18,333,566
Outpatient Surgeries	553,616	560,982	482,254	515,142	485,832
Personnel					
Full Time RNs	29,743	29,380	31,930	31,741	31,019
Full Time LPNs	1,805	1,623	1,776	1,933	2,078
Part Time RNs	10,933	9,498	9,609	10,220	10,643
Part Time LPNs	486	338	367	494	499
Total Full Time	99,007	97,993	102,417	105,671	101,666
Total Part Time	30,665	26,395	28,948	30,937	30,033
HOSPITAL UNIT (Excludes Separate Nursing Home Units)					
Utilization - Inpatient					
Beds	17,007	17,057	17,022	16,702	16,534
Admissions	758,150	749,445	724,965	820,384	796,467
Inpatient Days	4,194,488	4,348,759	3,933,014	4,230,499	4,083,446
Average Length of Stay	5.5	5.8	5.4	5.2	5.1
Personnel					
Total Full Time	98,850	97,592	101,710	104,790	100,583
Total Part Time	30,608	26,181	28,672	30,501	29,596
COMMUNITY HEALTH INDICATORS PER 1000 POPULATION					
Total Population (in thousands)	8,684	8,642	8,591	8,536	8,518
Inpatient					
Beds	2	2.1	2.1	2.1	2.1
Admissions	87.4	87	84.7	96.7	94.1
Inpatient Days	492.3	526.4	486.9	545.2	534.6
Inpatient Surgeries	19.6	20	20.8	24.6	23.4
Births	10.1	10.1	10.4	10.6	10.7
Outpatient					
Emergency Outpatient Visits	403.3	355.3	338.3	425	432.8
Other Outpatient Visits	1,752.7	1,608.6	1,550.6	1,766.7	1,719.6
Total Outpatient Visits	2,155.9	1,963.9	1,888.9	2,191.7	2,152.4
Outpatient Surgeries	63.8	64.9	56.1	60.4	57

Note: The 2021 performance data do not reflect the full impact of the COVID-19 pandemic. Please refer to the discussion in the Introduction for more information.

AHA Hospital Statistics © 2024 Health Forum LLC, an affiliate of the American Hospital Association **143**

TABLE 6

WASHINGTON

U.S. Community Hospitals
(Nonfederal, short-term general and other special hospitals)

Overview 2018–2022

	2022	2021	2020	2019	2018
Total Community Hospitals in Washington........	**92**	**92**	**91**	**91**	**92**
Bed Size Category					
6-24	14	13	13	11	11
25-49	28	27	27	27	27
50-99	12	15	14	14	15
100-199	16	15	15	14	14
200-299	7	7	7	10	10
300-399	9	9	9	8	8
400-499	2	2	2	4	4
500 + ...	4	4	4	3	3
Location					
Hospitals Urban	60	62	61	61	62
Hospitals Rural	32	30	30	30	30
Control					
State and Local Government	42	42	42	40	40
Not for Profit	46	46	45	44	44
Investor owned	4	4	4	7	8
Affiliations					
Hospitals in a System	50	48	48	48	49
Hospitals in a Group Purchasing Organization...	53	49	49	56	61

Note: The 2021 performance data do not reflect the full impact of the COVID-19 pandemic. Please refer to the discussion in the Introduction for more information.

144 AHA Hospital Statistics © 2024 Health Forum LLC, an affiliate of the American Hospital Association

TABLE 6

WASHINGTON

U.S. Community Hospitals
(Nonfederal, short-term general and other special hospitals)

Utilization, Personnel, Community Health Indicators 2018–2022

	2022	2021	2020	2019	2018
TOTAL FACILITY (Includes Hospital and Nursing Home Units)					
Utilization - Inpatient					
Beds	12,434	12,371	12,205	12,613	12,774
Admissions	524,522	519,626	504,312	591,311	601,209
Inpatient Days	3,249,964	3,066,143	2,780,906	2,943,207	3,045,863
Average Length of Stay	6.2	5.9	5.5	5.0	5.1
Inpatient Surgeries	149,282	139,724	148,917	173,176	177,881
Births	79,532	76,027	75,530	80,084	81,643
Utilization - Outpatient					
Emergency Outpatient Visits	2,982,767	2,755,629	2,300,563	2,925,619	2,779,707
Other Outpatient Visits	14,675,325	14,894,675	13,149,983	13,003,215	11,782,304
Total Outpatient Visits	17,658,092	17,650,304	15,450,546	15,928,834	14,562,011
Outpatient Surgeries	387,891	351,475	320,305	355,367	356,762
Personnel					
Full Time RNs	21,414	21,307	20,201	20,357	20,425
Full Time LPNs	819	810	668	728	697
Part Time RNs	15,135	16,659	15,788	16,096	15,220
Part Time LPNs	522	557	472	490	444
Total Full Time	82,638	78,067	74,230	75,205	76,468
Total Part Time	44,202	47,115	43,318	44,218	39,831
HOSPITAL UNIT (Excludes Separate Nursing Home Units)					
Utilization - Inpatient					
Beds	12,399	12,359	12,158	12,524	12,553
Admissions	524,505	519,620	504,246	591,188	600,803
Inpatient Days	3,238,455	3,061,992	2,764,511	2,911,940	2,995,513
Average Length of Stay	6.2	5.9	5.5	4.9	5.0
Personnel					
Total Full Time	82,608	78,060	74,177	75,116	76,282
Total Part Time	44,191	47,107	43,237	44,073	39,677
COMMUNITY HEALTH INDICATORS PER 1000 POPULATION					
Total Population (in thousands)	7,786	7,739	7,694	7,615	7,536
Inpatient					
Beds	1.6	1.6	1.6	1.7	1.7
Admissions	67.4	67.1	65.5	77.7	79.8
Inpatient Days	417.4	396.2	361.5	386.5	404.2
Inpatient Surgeries	19.2	18.1	19.4	22.7	23.6
Births	10.2	9.8	9.8	10.5	10.8
Outpatient					
Emergency Outpatient Visits	383.1	356.1	299	384.2	368.9
Other Outpatient Visits	1,884.9	1,924.7	1,709.2	1,707.6	1,563.6
Total Outpatient Visits	2,268	2,280.8	2,008.2	2,091.8	1,932.4
Outpatient Surgeries	49.8	45.4	41.6	46.7	47.3

Note: The 2021 performance data do not reflect the full impact of the COVID-19 pandemic. Please refer to the discussion in the Introduction for more information.

AHA Hospital Statistics © 2024 Health Forum LLC, an affiliate of the American Hospital Association

TABLE 6

WEST VIRGINIA

U.S. Community Hospitals
(Nonfederal, short-term general and other special hospitals)

Overview 2018–2022

	2022	2021	2020	2019	2018
Total Community Hospitals in West Virginia	54	54	52	52	56
Bed Size Category					
6-24	4	4	4	4	4
25-49	21	21	19	17	19
50-99	12	12	11	12	11
100-199	8	8	9	10	12
200-299	5	5	5	5	6
300-399	2	2	2	2	2
400-499	0	0	0	0	0
500 +	2	2	2	2	2
Location					
Hospitals Urban	30	32	30	30	31
Hospitals Rural	24	22	22	22	25
Control					
State and Local Government	6	6	7	7	9
Not for Profit	34	34	33	33	33
Investor owned	14	14	12	12	14
Affiliations					
Hospitals in a System	43	41	39	35	35
Hospitals in a Group Purchasing Organization...	32	36	34	39	42

Note: The 2021 performance data do not reflect the full impact of the COVID-19 pandemic. Please refer to the discussion in the Introduction for more information.

TABLE 6

WEST VIRGINIA

U.S. Community Hospitals
(Nonfederal, short-term general and other special hospitals)

Utilization, Personnel, Community Health Indicators 2018–2022

	2022	2021	2020	2019	2018
TOTAL FACILITY (Includes Hospital and Nursing Home Units)					
Utilization - Inpatient					
Beds	6,433	6,111	6,292	6,385	6,868
Admissions	222,115	225,867	222,900	240,377	258,254
Inpatient Days	1,463,549	1,472,732	1,414,254	1,499,925	1,544,486
Average Length of Stay	6.6	6.5	6.3	6.2	6.0
Inpatient Surgeries	63,329	63,974	71,252	70,905	74,416
Births	17,441	18,098	17,858	17,762	18,715
Utilization - Outpatient					
Emergency Outpatient Visits	976,929	934,369	962,057	1,043,324	1,231,765
Other Outpatient Visits	6,609,760	6,579,721	6,302,379	6,706,351	6,829,253
Total Outpatient Visits	7,586,689	7,514,090	7,264,436	7,749,675	8,061,018
Outpatient Surgeries	219,676	208,027	190,641	213,013	229,335
Personnel					
Full Time RNs	9,203	9,709	10,480	10,283	10,453
Full Time LPNs	1,204	1,182	1,123	1,201	1,202
Part Time RNs	3,274	3,131	3,028	3,246	2,873
Part Time LPNs	261	253	253	250	261
Total Full Time	38,573	38,505	38,779	39,148	39,828
Total Part Time	10,477	10,067	9,738	10,130	9,485
HOSPITAL UNIT (Excludes Separate Nursing Home Units)					
Utilization - Inpatient					
Beds	6,122	5,824	5,948	5,866	6,377
Admissions	221,117	224,966	221,784	238,624	256,524
Inpatient Days	1,373,803	1,389,834	1,316,511	1,351,072	1,400,986
Average Length of Stay	6.2	6.2	5.9	5.7	5.5
Personnel					
Total Full Time	38,380	38,312	38,496	38,719	39,427
Total Part Time	10,430	10,035	9,685	10,065	9,394
COMMUNITY HEALTH INDICATORS PER 1000 POPULATION					
Total Population (in thousands)	1,775	1,783	1,785	1,792	1,806
Inpatient					
Beds	3.6	3.4	3.5	3.6	3.8
Admissions	125.1	126.7	124.9	134.1	143
Inpatient Days	824.5	826	792.4	836.9	855.3
Inpatient Surgeries	35.7	35.9	39.9	39.6	41.2
Births	9.8	10.2	10	9.9	10.4
Outpatient					
Emergency Outpatient Visits	550.3	524.1	539	582.2	682.1
Other Outpatient Visits	3,723.5	3,690.3	3,531.2	3,742.1	3,781.8
Total Outpatient Visits	4,273.8	4,214.4	4,070.2	4,324.2	4,463.9
Outpatient Surgeries	123.8	116.7	106.8	118.9	127

Note: The 2021 performance data do not reflect the full impact of the COVID-19 pandemic. Please refer to the discussion in the Introduction for more information.

AHA Hospital Statistics © 2024 Health Forum LLC, an affiliate of the American Hospital Association

TABLE 6

WISCONSIN

U.S. Community Hospitals
(Nonfederal, short-term general and other special hospitals)

Overview 2018–2022

	2022	2021	2020	2019	2018
Total Community Hospitals in Wisconsin	**133**	**132**	**133**	**132**	**133**
Bed Size Category					
6-24	36	33	37	32	33
25-49	34	36	33	36	33
50-99	31	26	24	25	27
100-199	16	19	22	21	23
200-299	10	12	10	12	12
300-399	3	3	4	3	2
400-499	0	0	0	0	0
500 + ...	3	3	3	3	3
Location					
Hospitals Urban	74	74	75	75	76
Hospitals Rural	59	58	58	57	57
Control					
State and Local Government	1	1	1	1	2
Not for Profit	123	122	123	122	121
Investor owned	9	9	9	9	10
Affiliations					
Hospitals in a System	99	99	99	99	99
Hospitals in a Group Purchasing Organization...	129	128	131	132	130

Note: The 2021 performance data do not reflect the full impact of the COVID-19 pandemic. Please refer to the discussion in the Introduction for more information.

148 AHA Hospital Statistics © 2024 Health Forum LLC, an affiliate of the American Hospital Association

TABLE 6

WISCONSIN

U.S. Community Hospitals
(Nonfederal, short-term general and other special hospitals)

Utilization, Personnel, Community Health Indicators 2018–2022

	2022	2021	2020	2019	2018
TOTAL FACILITY (Includes Hospital and Nursing Home Units)					
Utilization - Inpatient					
Beds	11,490	11,589	12,227	11,894	12,103
Admissions	464,786	472,025	480,005	508,235	521,584
Inpatient Days	2,688,800	2,574,932	2,509,699	2,601,418	2,618,418
Average Length of Stay	5.8	5.5	5.2	5.1	5.0
Inpatient Surgeries	118,089	122,110	148,682	165,394	165,845
Births	57,220	57,332	59,511	61,088	62,626
Utilization - Outpatient					
Emergency Outpatient Visits	2,325,088	2,052,352	2,025,679	2,274,345	2,498,314
Other Outpatient Visits	18,782,541	18,655,996	16,450,115	18,507,927	16,970,333
Total Outpatient Visits	21,107,629	20,708,348	18,475,794	20,782,272	19,468,647
Outpatient Surgeries	506,264	477,358	508,139	572,646	525,011
Personnel					
Full Time RNs	19,200	19,951	20,271	19,770	19,251
Full Time LPNs	638	672	668	687	612
Part Time RNs	17,011	16,519	17,355	17,378	17,193
Part Time LPNs	531	505	637	646	601
Total Full Time	75,299	79,169	79,408	78,927	73,226
Total Part Time	49,658	49,013	51,435	52,666	50,276
HOSPITAL UNIT (Excludes Separate Nursing Home Units)					
Utilization - Inpatient					
Beds	10,954	11,008	11,490	11,115	11,371
Admissions	463,937	470,977	478,533	506,687	520,105
Inpatient Days	2,532,713	2,404,566	2,279,485	2,365,009	2,387,198
Average Length of Stay	5.5	5.1	4.8	4.7	4.6
Personnel					
Total Full Time	75,027	78,864	79,131	78,549	73,036
Total Part Time	49,381	48,791	51,185	52,358	50,110
COMMUNITY HEALTH INDICATORS PER 1000 POPULATION					
Total Population (in thousands)	5,893	5,896	5,833	5,822	5,814
Inpatient					
Beds	1.9	2	2.1	2	2.1
Admissions	78.9	80.1	82.3	87.3	89.7
Inpatient Days	456.3	436.7	430.3	446.8	450.4
Inpatient Surgeries	20	20.7	25.5	28.4	28.5
Births	9.7	9.7	10.2	10.5	10.8
Outpatient					
Emergency Outpatient Visits	394.6	348.1	347.3	390.6	429.7
Other Outpatient Visits	3,187.5	3,164.2	2,820.3	3,178.7	2,919.1
Total Outpatient Visits	3,582.1	3,512.3	3,167.6	3,569.3	3,348.8
Outpatient Surgeries	85.9	81	87.1	98.4	90.3

Note: The 2021 performance data do not reflect the full impact of the COVID-19 pandemic. Please refer to the discussion in the Introduction for more information.

AHA Hospital Statistics © 2024 Health Forum LLC, an affiliate of the American Hospital Association

TABLE 6

WYOMING

U.S. Community Hospitals
(Nonfederal, short-term general and other special hospitals)

Overview 2018–2022

	2022	2021	2020	2019	2018
Total Community Hospitals in Wyoming	28	28	28	28	29
Bed Size Category					
6-24	7	8	6	6	7
25-49	9	8	9	9	9
50-99	5	5	7	7	7
100-199	5	4	3	3	3
200-299	2	3	3	3	3
300-399	0	0	0	0	0
400-499	0	0	0	0	0
500 +	0	0	0	0	0
Location					
Hospitals Urban	4	4	4	4	5
Hospitals Rural	24	24	24	24	24
Control					
State and Local Government	18	18	18	19	19
Not for Profit	5	5	5	4	4
Investor owned	5	5	5	5	6
Affiliations					
Hospitals in a System	11	11	11	10	12
Hospitals in a Group Purchasing Organization	14	16	13	12	20

Note: The 2021 performance data do not reflect the full impact of the COVID-19 pandemic. Please refer to the discussion in the Introduction for more information.

TABLE 6

WYOMING

U.S. Community Hospitals
(Nonfederal, short-term general and other special hospitals)

Utilization, Personnel, Community Health Indicators 2018–2022

	2022	2021	2020	2019	2018
TOTAL FACILITY (Includes Hospital and Nursing Home Units)					
Utilization - Inpatient					
Beds	1,892	1,932	1,936	1,990	2,015
Admissions	37,933	39,850	39,576	41,521	41,825
Inpatient Days	344,986	308,965	358,780	378,966	385,211
Average Length of Stay	9.1	7.8	9.1	9.1	9.2
Inpatient Surgeries	8,783	9,871	10,076	10,212	10,429
Births	5,160	5,477	5,193	5,424	5,739
Utilization - Outpatient					
Emergency Outpatient Visits	201,457	192,640	210,208	223,303	217,418
Other Outpatient Visits	1,075,171	1,138,859	1,104,803	1,067,917	1,061,070
Total Outpatient Visits	1,276,628	1,331,499	1,315,011	1,291,220	1,278,488
Outpatient Surgeries	30,249	36,298	29,376	31,020	31,454
Personnel					
Full Time RNs	2,062	2,026	2,044	2,157	2,302
Full Time LPNs	150	144	170	160	163
Part Time RNs	768	646	771	643	658
Part Time LPNs	56	40	64	41	46
Total Full Time	8,410	8,904	8,969	9,058	9,793
Total Part Time	2,535	2,054	2,563	2,013	2,068
HOSPITAL UNIT (Excludes Separate Nursing Home Units)					
Utilization - Inpatient					
Beds	1,556	1,502	1,558	1,385	1,386
Admissions	37,804	39,550	39,273	40,911	41,078
Inpatient Days	254,685	179,667	241,931	185,230	181,229
Average Length of Stay	6.7	4.5	6.2	4.5	4.4
Personnel					
Total Full Time	8,260	8,654	8,653	8,740	9,424
Total Part Time	2,456	1,998	2,494	1,889	1,919
COMMUNITY HEALTH INDICATORS PER 1000 POPULATION					
Total Population (in thousands)	581	579	582	579	578
Inpatient					
Beds	3.3	3.3	3.3	3.4	3.5
Admissions	65.2	68.8	68	71.7	72.4
Inpatient Days	593.4	533.8	616.1	654.8	666.8
Inpatient Surgeries	15.1	17.1	17.3	17.6	18.1
Births	8.9	9.5	8.9	9.4	9.9
Outpatient					
Emergency Outpatient Visits	346.5	332.8	361	385.8	376.3
Other Outpatient Visits	1,849.3	1,967.6	1,897.2	1,845.2	1,836.6
Total Outpatient Visits	2,195.9	2,300.4	2,258.2	2,231	2,212.9
Outpatient Surgeries	52	62.7	50.4	53.6	54.4

Note: The 2021 performance data do not reflect the full impact of the COVID-19 pandemic. Please refer to the discussion in the Introduction for more information.

AHA Hospital Statistics © 2024 Health Forum LLC, an affiliate of the American Hospital Association

Table 7

Table	Page
7 Facilities and Services in the U. S. Census Divisions and States for 2022	155

The facilities and services presented in Table 7 are listed below in alphabetical order by major heading (where applicable).

Adult Day Care Program 155
Air Ambulance Services 155
Airborne Infection Isolation Room........................... 155
Alzheimer Center... 155
Ambulance Service 155
Ambulatory Surgery Center...................................... 155
Arthritis Treatment Center 155
Auxiliary 155
Bariatric/Weight Control Services 155
Biocontainment Patient Care Unit 155
Birthing/LDR/LDRP Room 155
Blood Donor Center.. 156
Breast Cancer Screening... 156
Burn Care Units 156
Case Management.. 156
Chaplaincy/Pastoral Care Services 156
Chemotherapy... 156
Children's Wellness Program..................................... 156
Chiropractic Services.. 156
Community Outreach... 156
Complementary and Alternative Medicine
    Services 156
Computer Assisted Orthopedic Surgery (CAOS)...... 157
Crisis Prevention... 157
Diabetes Prevention Program 157
Dental Services 157
Employment Support Services 157
Enabling Services 157
Enrollment Assistance Services................................. 157
Extracorporeal Shock Wave Lithotripter (ESWL) 157
Fertility Clinic.. 157
Fitness Center 157
Freestanding Outpatient Care Center 157
Genetic Testing/Counseling 158
Geriatric Services.. 158
Health Fair 158
Community Health Education 158
Health Research 158
Health Screenings 158
Hemodialysis.. 158
HIV/AIDS Services 158
Home Health Services 158
Hospice 158
Hospital-based Outpatient Care
    Center Services 159

Immunization Program 159
Indigent Care Clinic.. 159
Linguistic/Translation Services 159
Meal Delivery Services.. 159
Mobile Health Services.. 159
Neonatal Intermediate Care Units 159
Neurological Services 159
Nutrition Programs Center.. 159
Obstetrics Inpatient Care Units................................. 159
Occupational Health Services.................................... 160
Oncology Services 160
Orthopedic Services.. 160
Other Special Care Units 160
Outpatient Surgery.. 160
Pain Management Program... 160
Palliative Care Program 160
Palliative Care Inpatient Unit 160
Patient Controlled Analgesia (PCA)......................... 160
Patient Education Center 160
Patient Representative Services 161
Physical Rehabilitation Inpatient Care Units 161
Primary Care Department 161
Robotic Surgery.. 161
Rural Health Clinic 161
Sleep Center... 161
Social Work Services 161
Sports Medicine 161
Support Groups 161
Swing Bed Services 162
Teen Outreach Services 162
Telehealth 162
Tobacco Treatment/Cessation Program 162
Transportation to Health Facilities 162
Urgent Care Center 162
Violence Prevention Program - Community 162
Violence Prevention Program - Workplace 162
Virtual Colonoscopy 162
Volunteer Services Department 162
Women's Health Services 162
Wound Management Services 162

General Medical Surgical Care
    Adult Units.. 163
    Pediatric Units.. 163

Note: The 2021 performance data do not reflect the full impact of the COVID-19 pandemic. Please refer to the discussion in the Introduction for more information.

Facilities and Services

Housing Services
Assisted Living 163
Retirement Housing 163
Supportive Housing Services 163

Intensive Care Units
Cardiac 163
Medical Surgical 163
Neonatal 163
Other 163
Pediatric 163

Long-Term Care
Acute Care 163
Skilled Nursing Care 163
Intermediate Care 163
Other Long-Term Care 163

Cardiology and Cardiac Services
Adult Cardiology Services 164
Pediatric Cardiology Services 164
Adult Diagnostic Catheterization 164
Pediatric Diagnostic Catheterization 164
Adult Interventional Cardiac Catheterization 164
Pediatric Interventional Cardiac Catheterization ... 164
Adult Cardiac Surgery 164
Pediatric Cardiac Surgery 164
Adult Cardiac Electrophysiology 164
Pediatric Cardiac Electrophysiology 164
Cardiac Rehabilitation 164

Emergency Services
Off-Campus Emergency Department 165
On-Campus Emergency Department 165
Pediatric Emergency Department 165
Trauma Center (Certified) 165

Endoscopic Services
Endoscopic Ultrasound 165
Ablation of Barrett's Esophagus 165
Esophageal Impedance Study 165
Endoscopic Retrograde
   Cholangiopancreatography 165
Optical Colonoscopy 165

Physical Rehabilitation Services
Assistive Technology Center 166
Electrodiagnostic Services 166
Physical Rehabilitation Outpatient Services 166
Prosthetic Orthotic Services 166
Robot Assisted Walking Therapy 166
Simulated Rehabilitation Environment 166

Psychiatric Services
Pediatric Care (formerly
   "Child Adolescent Services") 166
Consultation/Liaison Services 166
Education Services 166
Emergency Services 166

Forensic Psychiatry Services
Forensic Psychiatry Services 167
Geriatric Services 167
Outpatient Services 167
Partial Hospitalization Program 167
Prenatal and Postpartum Psychiatric Services 167
Psychiatric Inpatient Care Units 167
Psychiatric Intensive Outpatient Services 167
Residential Treatment 167
Social and Community Psychiatry 167
Suicide Prevention Services 167

Radiology, Diagnostic
CT Scanner 167
Diagnostic Radioisotope Facility 167
Electron Beam Computed Tomography
   (EBCT) 168
Full-Field Digital Mammography (FFDM) 168
Magnetic Resonance Imaging (MRI) 168
Intraoperative Magnetic Imaging 168
Magnetoencephalography 168
Multi-slice Spiral Computed Tomography
   (<64 slice CT) 168
Multi-slice Spiral Computed Tomography
   (64+ slice CT) 168
Positron Emission Tomography (PET) 168
Positron Emission Tomography/CT (PET/CT) 168
Single Photon Emission Computerized
   Tomography (SPECT) 168
Ultrasound 169

Radiology, Therapeutic
Basic Interventional Radiology 169
Image-Guided Radiation Therapy (IGRT) 169
Intensity-Modulated Radiation Therapy
   (IMRT) 169
Proton Beam Therapy 169
Shaped Beam Radiation System 169
Stereotactic Radiosurgery 169

Substance Use Disorder Services
Medication Assisted Treatment for Other
   Substance Use Disorders 169
Medication Assisted Treatment for Opioid
   Use Disorder 169
Substance Use Disorder Inpatient Care Units 170
Substance Use Disorder Pediatric Services 170
Substance Use Disorder Outpatient Services 170
Substance Use Disorder Partial
   Hospitalization Services 170

Transplant Services
Bone Marrow 170
Heart 170
Kidney 170
Liver 170
Lung 170
Tissue 170
Other 170

Note: The 2021 performance data do not reflect the full impact of the COVID-19 pandemic. Please refer to the discussion in the Introduction for more information.

154   AHA Hospital Statistics © 2024 Health Forum LLC, an affiliate of the American Hospital Association

Table 7

2022 Facilities and Services in the U.S. Census Divisions and States

These data include only hospital-based facilities and services as reported by responding hospitals in Section C of the 2022 AHA Annual Survey, beginning on page 215. Census divisions represent all U.S. hospitals. Community hospitals are listed separately under United States. No estimates have been made for nonresponding hospitals. Definitions of facilities and services are listed in the Glossary, page 203.

CLASSIFICATION	HOSPITALS REPORTING	ADULT DAY CARE PROGRAM No.	%	AIR AMBULANCE SERVICES No.	%	AIRBORNE INFECTION ISOLATION ROOM No.	%	ALZHEIMER CENTER No.	%	AMBULANCE SERVICE No.	%	AMBULATORY SURGERY CENTER No.	%	ARTHRITIS TREATMENT CENTER No.	%	AUXILIARY No.	%	BARIATRIC/WEIGHT CONTROL SERVICES No.	%	BIOCONTAINMENT PATIENT CARE UNIT No.	%	BIRTHING/LDR/LDRP ROOM No.	%
UNITED STATES	4,097	95	2.3	161	3.9	3,386	82.6	202	4.9	600	14.6	888	21.7	325	7.9	2,067	50.5	1,201	29.3	149	3.6	2,075	50.6
COMMUNITY HOSPITALS	3,682	83	2.3	160	4.3	3,263	88.6	193	5.2	588	16.0	868	23.6	315	8.6	2,030	55.1	1,172	31.8	145	3.9	2,070	56.2
CENSUS DIVISION 1, NEW ENGLAND	148	6	4.1	6	4.1	127	85.8	17	11.5	29	19.6	45	30.4	23	15.5	70	47.3	62	41.9	9	6.1	87	58.8
Connecticut	24	3	12.5	3	12.5	20	83.3	6	25.0	7	29.2	11	45.8	6	25.0	13	54.2	18	75.0	1	4.2	19	79.2
Maine	29	0	0	0	0	27	93.1	2	6.9	8	27.6	4	13.8	1	3.4	15	51.7	7	24.1	2	6.9	20	69.0
Massachusetts	50	3	6.0	1	2.0	40	80.0	6	12.0	10	20.0	17	34.0	8	16.0	18	36.0	24	48.0	2	4.0	25	50.0
New Hampshire	26	0	0	1	3.8	25	96.2	1	3.8	1	3.8	7	26.9	4	15.4	14	53.8	9	34.6	2	7.7	13	50.0
Rhode Island	9	0	0	0	0	7	77.8	1	11.1	1	11.1	4	44.4	3	33.3	5	55.6	3	33.3	2	22.2	3	33.3
Vermont	10	0	0	1	10.0	8	80.0	1	10.0	1	10.0	2	20.0	1	10.0	5	50.0	1	10.0	0	0	7	70.0
CENSUS DIVISION 2, MIDDLE ATLANTIC	357	10	2.8	18	5.0	299	83.8	35	9.8	60	16.8	129	36.1	51	14.3	190	53.2	170	47.6	19	5.3	187	52.4
New Jersey	71	1	1.4	6	8.5	59	83.1	11	15.5	16	22.5	19	26.8	11	15.5	38	53.5	45	63.4	1	1.4	41	57.7
New York	122	7	5.7	1	0.8	107	87.7	13	10.7	24	19.7	63	51.6	25	20.5	77	63.1	67	54.9	12	9.8	80	65.6
Pennsylvania	164	2	1.2	11	6.7	133	81.1	11	6.7	20	12.2	47	28.7	15	9.1	75	45.7	58	35.4	6	3.7	66	40.2
CENSUS DIVISION 3, SOUTH ATLANTIC	541	13	2.4	38	7.0	475	87.8	30	5.5	68	12.6	131	24.2	50	9.2	291	53.8	184	34.0	27	5.0	298	55.1
Delaware	8	1	12.5	1	12.5	7	87.5	1	12.5	2	25.0	2	25.0	0	0	2	25.0	5	62.5	0	0	5	62.5
District of Columbia	9	0	0	0	0	8	88.9	2	22.2	1	11.1	4	44.4	2	22.2	3	33.3	1	11.1	1	11.1	5	55.6
Florida	154	3	1.9	10	6.5	134	87.0	9	5.8	12	7.8	37	24.0	12	7.8	76	49.4	58	37.7	2	1.3	70	45.5
Georgia	88	2	2.3	2	2.3	70	79.5	3	3.4	13	14.8	18	20.5	7	8.0	57	64.8	26	29.5	5	5.7	45	51.1
Maryland	40	4	10.0	5	12.5	38	95.0	6	15.0	3	7.5	11	27.5	10	25.0	28	70.0	22	55.0	3	7.5	30	75.0
North Carolina	68	1	1.5	7	10.3	65	95.6	6	8.8	15	22.1	22	32.4	7	10.3	34	50.0	23	33.8	1	1.5	52	76.5
South Carolina	78	0	0	1	1.3	64	82.1	1	1.3	11	14.1	11	14.1	3	3.8	35	44.9	15	19.2	5	6.4	38	48.7
Virginia	59	2	3.4	9	15.3	56	94.9	1	1.7	7	11.9	19	32.2	6	10.2	30	50.8	23	39.0	7	11.9	35	59.3
West Virginia	37	0	0	2	5.4	33	89.2	1	2.7	4	10.8	7	18.9	3	8.1	26	70.3	7	18.9	3	8.1	18	48.6
CENSUS DIVISION 4, EAST NORTH CENTRAL	621	9	1.4	17	2.7	488	78.6	50	8.1	85	13.7	150	24.2	67	10.8	363	58.5	199	32.0	16	2.6	359	57.8
Illinois	138	2	1.4	2	1.4	124	89.9	8	5.8	17	12.3	28	20.3	18	13.0	87	63.0	43	31.2	3	2.2	77	55.8
Indiana	108	0	0	3	2.8	94	87.0	2	1.9	26	24.1	25	23.1	4	3.7	48	44.4	25	23.1	1	0.9	67	62.0
Michigan	120	4	3.3	2	1.7	105	87.5	7	5.8	13	10.8	31	25.8	12	10.0	81	67.5	55	45.8	4	3.3	71	59.2
Ohio	108	1	0.9	10	9.3	95	88.0	5	4.6	16	14.8	35	32.4	13	12.0	69	63.9	43	39.8	6	5.6	55	50.9
Wisconsin	147	2	1.4	0	0	70	47.6	28	19.0	13	8.8	31	21.1	20	13.6	78	53.1	33	22.4	2	1.4	89	60.5
CENSUS DIVISION 5, EAST SOUTH CENTRAL	285	4	1.4	10	3.5	220	77.2	10	3.5	43	15.1	43	15.1	15	5.3	126	44.2	66	23.2	6	2.1	119	41.8
Alabama	52	0	0	3	5.8	37	71.2	2	3.8	8	15.4	8	15.4	4	7.7	27	51.9	14	26.9	1	1.9	24	46.2
Kentucky	72	1	1.4	2	2.8	57	79.2	2	2.8	10	13.9	12	16.7	5	6.9	39	54.2	21	29.2	1	1.4	32	44.4
Mississippi	96	3	3.1	3	3.1	69	71.9	3	3.1	13	13.5	10	10.4	3	3.1	29	30.2	12	12.5	1	1.0	34	35.4
Tennessee	65	0	0	2	3.1	57	87.7	3	4.6	12	18.5	13	20.0	3	4.6	31	47.7	19	29.2	3	4.6	29	44.6
CENSUS DIVISION 6, WEST NORTH CENTRAL	556	21	3.8	27	4.9	460	82.7	21	3.8	128	23.0	93	16.7	31	5.6	317	57.0	123	22.1	25	4.5	263	47.3
Iowa	122	2	1.6	2	1.6	99	81.1	5	4.1	50	41.0	24	19.7	3	2.5	93	76.2	24	19.7	2	1.6	54	44.3
Kansas	94	8	8.5	3	3.2	85	90.4	2	1.7	17	14.2	15	16.0	3	3.2	65	54.2	23	24.5	7	7.4	47	39.2
Minnesota	94	3	3.2	3	3.2	84	89.4	6	6.4	23	24.5	13	13.8	10	10.6	44	46.8	22	23.4	5	5.3	59	62.8
Missouri	130	1	0.8	11	8.5	104	80.0	4	3.1	20	15.4	21	16.2	9	6.9	82	63.1	35	26.9	4	3.1	57	43.8
Nebraska	39	2	5.1	2	5.1	35	89.7	1	2.6	7	17.9	9	23.1	1	2.6	15	38.5	5	12.8	2	5.1	24	61.5
North Dakota	12	1	8.3	1	8.3	9	75.0	0	0	5	41.7	5	41.7	4	33.3	9	75.0	4	33.3	2	16.7	7	58.3
South Dakota	39	5	12.8	4	10.3	30	76.9	3	7.7	6	15.4	6	15.4	1	2.6	9	23.1	5	12.8	3	7.7	15	38.5
CENSUS DIVISION 7, WEST SOUTH CENTRAL	842	4	0.5	20	2.4	686	81.5	11	1.3	92	10.9	113	13.4	15	1.8	325	38.6	186	22.1	16	1.9	309	36.7
Arkansas	98	1	1.0	1	1.0	85	86.7	1	1.0	11	11.2	10	10.2	2	2.0	51	52.0	17	17.3	4	4.1	34	34.7
Louisiana	79	0	0	3	3.8	60	75.9	1	1.3	7	8.9	17	21.5	3	3.8	26	32.9	21	26.6	2	2.5	30	38.0
Oklahoma	99	0	0	3	3.2	76	76.8	3	3.0	14	14.1	15	15.2	1	1.0	46	46.5	14	14.1	0	0	39	39.4
Texas	566	3	0.5	14	2.5	465	82.2	6	1.1	60	10.6	71	12.5	9	1.6	202	35.7	134	23.7	10	1.8	206	36.4
CENSUS DIVISION 8, MOUNTAIN	336	14	4.2	16	4.2	268	79.8	12	3.6	64	19.0	56	16.7	40	11.9	149	44.3	79	23.5	7	2.1	193	57.4
Arizona	70	1	1.4	1	1.4	54	77.1	4	5.7	4	5.7	12	17.1	6	8.6	24	34.3	19	27.1	0	0	30	42.9
Colorado	74	1	1.4	5	6.8	68	91.9	3	4.1	19	25.7	14	18.9	10	13.5	43	58.1	19	25.7	2	2.7	46	62.2
Idaho	26	3	11.5	3	11.5	20	76.9	0	0	9	34.6	0	0	4	15.4	18	69.2	8	30.8	0	0	19	73.1
Montana	45	8	17.8	3	6.7	34	75.6	2	4.4	12	26.7	5	11.1	3	6.7	18	40.0	6	13.3	3	6.7	25	55.6
Nevada	32	0	0	0	0	20	62.5	1	3.1	3	9.4	5	15.6	1	3.1	5	15.6	8	25.0	0	0	7	21.9
New Mexico	31	0	0	2	6.5	23	74.2	0	0	6	19.4	7	22.6	1	3.2	15	48.4	4	12.9	1	3.2	20	64.5
Utah	36	1	2.8	2	5.6	32	88.9	2	5.6	4	11.1	6	16.7	15	41.7	14	38.9	11	30.6	1	2.8	31	86.1
Wyoming	22	0	0	0	0	17	77.3	0	0	7	31.8	3	13.6	0	0	12	54.5	4	18.2	0	0	15	68.2
CENSUS DIVISION 9, PACIFIC	411	14	3.4	9	2.2	363	88.3	16	3.9	31	7.5	128	31.1	33	8.0	236	57.4	132	32.1	24	5.8	260	63.3
Alaska	9	0	0	0	0	8	88.9	0	0	0	0	0	0	0	0	3	33.3	1	11.1	0	0	7	77.8
California	268	10	3.7	8	3.0	233	86.9	14	5.2	20	7.5	101	37.7	24	9.0	162	60.4	95	35.4	15	5.6	160	59.7
Hawaii	15	0	0	0	0	13	86.7	0	0	0	0	3	20.0	1	6.7	3	20.0	5	33.3	0	0	8	53.3
Oregon	60	1	1.7	1	1.7	60	100	1	1.7	9	15.0	8	13.3	5	8.3	39	65.0	15	25.0	6	10.0	46	76.7
Washington	59	3	5.1	0	0	49	83.1	1	1.7	2	3.4	16	27.1	3	5.1	29	49.2	16	27.1	3	5.1	39	66.1

Note: The 2021 performance data do not reflect the full impact of the COVID-19 pandemic. Please refer to the discussion in the Introduction for more information.

Table 7 (Continued)

These data include only hospital-based facilities and services as reported by responding hospitals in Section C of the 2022 AHA Annual Survey, beginning on page 215. Census divisions represent all U.S. hospitals. Community hospitals are listed separately under United States. No estimates have been made for nonresponding hospitals. Definitions of facilities and services are listed in the Glossary, page 203.

CLASSIFICATION	HOSPITALS REPORTING	BLOOD DONOR CENTER Number	Percent	BREAST CANCER SCREENING Number	Percent	BURN CARE UNITS Number	Percent	CASE MANAGEMENT Number	Percent	CHAPLAINCY/PASTORAL CARE SERVICES Number	Percent	CHEMOTHERAPY Number	Percent	CHILDREN'S WELLNESS PROGRAM Number	Percent	CHIROPRACTIC SERVICES Number	Percent	COMMUNITY OUTREACH Number	Percent	COMPLEMENTARY AND ALTERNATIVE MEDICINE SERVICES Number	Percent
UNITED STATES	4,097	195	4.8	2,774	67.7	136	3.3	3,661	89.4	2,591	63.2	1,990	48.6	800	19.5	160	3.9	2,869	70	892	21.8
COMMUNITY HOSPITALS	3,682	191	5.2	2,746	74.6	134	3.6	3,419	92.9	2,448	66.5	1,954	53.1	783	21.3	128	3.5	2,735	74.3	849	23.1
CENSUS DIVISION 1, NEW ENGLAND	148	21	14.2	118	79.7	7	4.7	142	95.9	108	73	92	62.2	49	33.1	6	4.1	124	83.8	67	45.3
Connecticut	24	4	16.7	20	83.3	1	4.2	23	95.8	22	91.7	18	75	7	29.2	0	0	21	87.5	16	66.7
Maine	29	0	0	26	89.7	1	3.4	28	96.6	18	62.1	18	62.1	11	37.9	1	3.4	24	82.8	14	48.3
Massachusetts	50	11	22	35	70	2	4	46	92	38	76	28	56	16	32	2	4	39	78	19	38
New Hampshire	26	6	23.1	23	88.5	2	7.7	26	100	16	61.5	16	61.5	11	42.3	2	7.7	23	88.5	14	53.8
Rhode Island	9	0	0	6	66.7	1	11.1	9	100	6	88.9	7	77.8	1	11.1	1	11.1	8	88.9	2	22.2
Vermont	10	0	0	8	80	0	0	10	100	6	60	5	50	3	30	0	0	9	90	2	20
CENSUS DIVISION 2, MIDDLE ATLANTIC	357	39	10.9	261	73.1	16	4.5	333	93.3	273	76.5	220	61.6	110	30.8	18	5	284	79.6	128	35.9
New Jersey	71	8	11.3	49	69	2	2.8	64	90.1	58	81.7	44	62	31	43.7	4	5.6	55	77.5	30	42.3
New York	122	18	14.8	100	82	8	6.6	117	95.9	104	85.2	88	72.1	49	40.2	10	8.2	109	89.3	58	47.5
Pennsylvania	164	13	7.9	112	68.3	6	3.7	152	92.7	111	67.7	88	53.7	30	18.3	4	2.4	120	73.2	40	24.4
CENSUS DIVISION 3, SOUTH ATLANTIC	541	33	6.1	402	74.3	25	4.6	509	94.1	425	78.6	307	56.7	98	18.1	19	3.5	417	77.1	128	23.7
Delaware	8	1	12.5	5	62.5	1		8	100	5	62.5	6	75	3	37.5	0	0	5	62.5	1	12.5
District of Columbia	9	1	11.1	5	55.6	1	11.1	9	100	9	100	6	66.7	3	33.3	1	11.1	7	77.8	4	44.4
Florida	154	9	5.8	106	68.8	8	5.2	145	94.2	118	76.6	87	56.5	24	15.6	4	2.6	107	69.5	33	21.4
Georgia	88	4	4.5	69	78.4	2	2.3	80	90.9	67	76.1	43	48.9	8	9.1	4	4.5	65	73.9	20	22.7
Maryland	40	5	12.5	29	72.5	2	5	40	100	40	100	29	72.5	13	32.5	0	0	35	87.5	14	35
North Carolina	68	4	5.9	54	79.4	3	2.9	68	88.2	60	88.2	50	73.5	17	25	2	2.9	61	89.7	21	30.9
South Carolina	78	2	2.6	54	69.2	3	3.8	68	87.2	46	59	29	37.2	13	16.7	0	0	55	70.5	5	6.4
Virginia	59	7	11.9	49	83.1	6	10.2	58	98.3	52	88.1	38	64.4	7	11.9	6	10.2	52	88.1	25	42.4
West Virginia	37	0	0	31	83.8	1		33	89.2	28	75.7	20	54.1	10	27	2	5.4	30	81.1	5	13.5
CENSUS DIVISION 4, EAST NORTH CENTRAL	621	18	2.9	504	81.2	23	3.7	570	91.8	426	68.6	342	55.1	146	23.5	34	5.5	449	72.3	213	34.3
Illinois	138	8	5.8	117	84.8	5	3.6	128	92.8	111	80.4	79	57.2	34	24.6	8	5.8	108	78.3	33	23.9
Indiana	108	1	0.9	83	76.9	4	3.7	102	94.4	78	72.2	59	54.6	25	23.1	2	1.9	92	85.2	28	25.9
Michigan	120	4	3.3	105	87.5	4	3.3	111	92.5	90	75	87	72.5	39	32.5	6	5	105	87.5	50	41.7
Ohio	108	5	4.6	85	78.7	6	5.6	99	91.7	85	78.7	70	64.8	25	23.1	15	13.9	91	84.3	49	45.4
Wisconsin	147	0	0	114	77.6	4	2.7	130	88.4	62	42.2	47	32	23	15.6	3	2	53	36.1	53	36.1
CENSUS DIVISION 5, EAST SOUTH CENTRAL	285	6	2.1	195	68.4	8	2.8	243	85.3	168	58.9	93	32.6	33	11.6	4	1.4	193	67.7	26	9.1
Alabama	52	1	1.9	34	65.4	3	5.8	46	88.5	32	61.5	23	44.2	2	3.8	3	5.8	36	69.2	4	7.7
Kentucky	72	3	4.2	57	79.2	3	4.2	65	90.3	55	76.4	32	44.4	14	19.4	0	0	54	75	12	16.7
Mississippi	96	0	0	56	58.3	0	0	71	74	32	33.3	13	13.5	11	11.5	1	1	55	57.3	1	1
Tennessee	65	2	3.1	48	73.8	2	3.1	61	93.8	49	75.4	25	38.5	6	9.2	0	0	48	73.8	9	13.8
CENSUS DIVISION 6, WEST NORTH CENTRAL	556	15	2.7	409	73.6	18	3.2	469	84.4	286	51.4	291	52.3	127	22.8	33	5.9	385	69.2	97	17.4
Iowa	122	2	1.6	110	90.2	2	1.6	111	91	55	45.1	72	59	28	23	4	3.3	94	77	25	20.5
Kansas	120	0	0	65	54.2	2	1.7	92	76.7	44	36.7	29	24.2	15	12.5	2	1.7	59	49.2	9	7.5
Minnesota	94	3	3.2	79	84	2	2.1	79	84	52	55.3	67	71.3	35	37.2	14	14.9	77	81.9	27	28.7
Missouri	130	9	6.9	91	70	10	7.7	114	87.7	90	69.2	69	53.1	24	18.5	7	5.4	89	68.5	21	16.2
Nebraska	39	0	0	31	79.5	1	2.6	34	87.2	26	66.7	29	74.4	11	28.2	3	7.7	30	76.9	8	20.5
North Dakota	12	0	0	9	75	1	8.3	10	83.3	5	41.7	4	33.3	6	50	0	0	9	75	3	25
South Dakota	39	1	2.6	24	61.5	0	0	29	74.4	14	35.9	21	53.8	8	20.5	1	2.5	27	69.2	4	10.3
CENSUS DIVISION 7, WEST SOUTH CENTRAL	842	20	2.4	384	45.6	16	1.9	733	87.1	390	46.3	213	25.3	87	10.3	15	1.8	465	55.2	47	5.6
Arkansas	98	2	2	55	56.1	1	1	87	88.8	44	44.9	26	26.5	9	9.2	1	1	64	65.3	4	4.1
Louisiana	79	4	5.1	48	60.8	6	7.6	72	91.1	39	49.4	36	45.6	20	25.3	1	1.3	50	63.3	5	6.3
Oklahoma	99	0	0	58	58.6	3	3	89	89.9	51	51.5	24	24.2	11	11.1	4	4	56	56.6	9	9.1
Texas	566	14	2.5	223	39.4	6	1.1	485	85.7	256	45.2	127	22.4	47	8.3	8	1.4	295	52.1	29	5.1
CENSUS DIVISION 8, MOUNTAIN	336	19	5.7	205	61	8	2.3	296	88.1	186	55.4	166	49.4	65	19.3	16	4.8	240	71.4	73	21.7
Arizona	70	1	1.4	25	35.7	3	4.3	67	95.7	49	70	33	47.1	10	14.3	4	5.7	49	70	18	25.7
Colorado	74	13	17.6	56	75.7	2	2.7	69	93.2	56	75.7	48	64.9	15	20.3	4	5.4	62	83.8	27	36.5
Idaho	26	2	7.7	18	69.2	0	0	23	88.5	15	50	14	53.8	13	50	2	7.7	21	80.8	6	23.1
Montana	45	0	0	30	66.7	0	0	35	77.8	21	46.7	22	48.9	8	17.8	4	8.9	33	73.3	7	15.6
Nevada	32	1	3.1	10	31.3	0	0	23	71.9	10	31.3	8	25	5	15.6	2	6.3	12	37.5	3	9.4
New Mexico	31	0	0	20	64.5	2	6.5	24	77.4	19	61.3	11	35.5	5	16.1	0	0	16	51.6	1	3.2
Utah	36	1	2.8	30	83.3	1	2.8	34	94.4	19	27.8	21	58.3	4	11.1	0	0	31	86.1	7	19.4
Wyoming	22	1	4.5	16	72.7	0	0	21	95.5	8	36.4	9	40.9	5	22.7	0	0	16	72.7	4	18.2
CENSUS DIVISION 9, PACIFIC	411	24	5.8	296	72	15	3.6	366	89.1	329	80	266	64.7	85	20.7	15	3.6	312	75.9	113	27.5
Alaska	9	0	0	6	66.7	0	0	9	100	5	55.6	5	55.6	2	22.2	0	0	6	66.7	3	33.3
California	268	23	8.6	187	69.8	11	4.1	229	85.4	217	81	169	63.1	56	20.9	11	4.1	190	70.9	72	26.9
Hawaii	15	0	0	11	73.3	1	6.7	14	93.3	9	40	12	80	3	20	0	0	13	86.7	6	40
Oregon	60	0	0	53	88.3	2	3.3	59	98.3	50	83.3	41	68.3	13	21.7	3	5	53	88.3	16	26.7
Washington	59	1	1.7	39	66.1	1	1.7	55	93.2	51	86.4	39	66.1	11	18.6	1	1.7	50	84.7	16	27.1

Note: The 2021 performance data do not reflect the full impact of the COVID-19 pandemic. Please refer to the discussion in the Introduction for more information.

Table 7 (Continued)

These data include only hospital-based facilities and services as reported by responding hospitals in Section C of the 2022 AHA Annual Survey, beginning on page 215. Census divisions represent all U.S. hospitals. Community hospitals are listed separately under United States. No estimates have been made for nonresponding hospitals. Definitions of facilities and services are listed in the Glossary, page 203.

CLASSIFICATION	HOSPITALS REPORTING	COMPUTER ASSISTED ORTHOPEDIC SURGERY (CAOS) No.	%	CRISIS PREVENTION No.	%	DIABETES PREVENTION PROGRAM No.	%	DENTAL SERVICES No.	%	EMPLOYMENT SUPPORT SERVICES No.	%	ENABLING SERVICES No.	%	ENROLLMENT ASSISTANCE SERVICES No.	%	EXTRACORPOREAL SHOCK WAVE LITHOTRIPTER (ESWL) No.	%	FERTILITY CLINIC No.	%	FITNESS CENTER No.	%	FREESTANDING OUTPATIENT CARE CENTER No.	%
UNITED STATES	4,097	1,004	24.5	1,148	28	1,724	42.1	786	19.2	977	23.8	1,429	34.9	2,557	62.4	1,254	30.6	202	4.9	1,123	27.4	1,420	34.7
COMMUNITY HOSPITALS	3,682	994	27	1,032	28	1,664	45.2	701	19	912	24.8	1,369	37.2	2,438	66.2	1,243	33.8	196	5.3	1,067	29	1,363	37
CENSUS DIVISION 1, NEW ENGLAND	148	48	32.4	66	44.6	85	57.4	31	20.9	61	41.2	84	56.8	128	86.5	75	50.7	23	15.5	43	29.1	80	54.1
Connecticut	24	15	62.5	20	83.3	11	45.8	11	45.8	16	66.7	18	75	22	91.7	16	66.7	7	29.2	14	58.3	17	70.8
Maine	29	1	3.4	6	20.7	21	72.4	3	10.3	4	13.8	13	44.8	22	75.9	12	41.4	1	3.4	7	24.1	14	48.3
Massachusetts	50	19	38	25	50	23	46	5	10	26	52	23	46	45	90	28	56	9	18	7	14	24	48
New Hampshire	26	7	26.9	12	46.2	19	73.1	7	26.9	8	30.8	17	65.4	24	92.3	9	34.6	5	19.2	9	34.6	15	57.7
Rhode Island	9	3	33.3	3	33.3	6	66.7	4	44.4	4	44.4	6	66.7	6	66.7	7	77.8	0	0	4	44.4	6	66.7
Vermont	10	3	30	0	0	5	50	1	10	3	30	7	70	9	90	3	30	1	10	2	20	4	40
CENSUS DIVISION 2, MIDDLE ATLANTIC	357	123	34.5	170	47.6	182	51	143	40.1	133	37.3	191	53.5	270	75.6	150	42	45	12.6	100	28	180	50.4
New Jersey	71	28	39.4	40	56.3	40	56.3	32	45.1	34	47.9	40	56.3	55	77.5	28	39.4	7	9.9	21	29.6	33	46.5
New York	122	56	45.9	72	59	77	63.1	61	50	55	45.1	70	57.4	107	87.7	69	56.6	25	20.5	39	32	74	60.7
Pennsylvania	164	39	23.8	58	35.4	65	39.6	50	30.5	44	26.8	81	49.4	108	65.9	53	32.3	13	7.9	40	24.4	73	44.5
CENSUS DIVISION 3, SOUTH ATLANTIC	541	167	30.9	161	29.8	246	45.5	118	21.8	140	25.9	240	44.4	373	68.9	206	38.1	20	3.7	169	31.2	232	42.9
Delaware	8	2	25	3	37.5	4	50	1	12.5	2	25	4	50	4	50	3	37.5	0	0	1	12.5	6	75
District of Columbia	9	4	44.4	5	55.6	6	66.7	5	55.6	6	66.7	6	66.7	7	77.8	4	44.4	0	0	4	44.4	6	66.7
Florida	154	58	37.7	35	22.7	63	40.9	26	16.9	48	31.2	62	40.3	102	66.2	69	44.8	3	1.9	42	27.3	59	38.3
Georgia	88	16	18.2	27	30.7	40	45.5	13	14.8	12	13.6	37	42	61	69.3	29	33	1	1.1	28	31.8	36	40.9
Maryland	40	19	47.5	27	67.5	30	75	18	45	23	57.5	32	80	38	95	32	80	4	10	13	32.5	22	55
North Carolina	68	21	30.9	23	33.8	37	54.4	21	30.9	13	19.1	35	51.5	50	73.5	9	13.2	2	2.9	23	33.8	34	50
South Carolina	78	17	21.8	14	17.9	6	7.7	12	15.4	7	9	17	21.8	38	48.7	21	26.9	3	3.8	22	28.2	21	26.9
Virginia	59	23	39	23	39	37	62.7	16	27.1	17	28.8	36	61	47	79.7	26	44.1	4	6.8	25	42.4	33	55.9
West Virginia	37	7	18.9	8	21.6	23	62.2	6	16.2	12	32.4	11	29.7	26	70.3	13	35.1	3	8.1	11	29.7	15	40.5
CENSUS DIVISION 4, EAST NORTH CENTRAL	621	159	25.6	221	35.6	319	51.4	104	16.7	168	27.1	267	43	400	64.4	213	34.3	25	4	218	35.1	274	44.1
Illinois	138	37	26.8	54	39.1	77	55.8	30	21.7	36	26.1	62	44.9	92	66.7	52	37.7	8	5.8	41	29.7	57	41.3
Indiana	108	25	23.1	25	23.1	55	50.9	18	16.7	28	25.9	40	37	82	75.9	37	34.3	1	0.9	37	34.3	39	36.1
Michigan	120	31	25.8	53	44.2	80	66.7	26	21.7	46	38.3	63	52.5	101	84.2	37	30.8	5	4.2	35	29.2	60	50
Ohio	108	41	38	46	42.6	71	65.7	30	27.8	43	39.8	59	54.6	79	73.1	44	40.7	7	6.5	49	45.4	59	54.6
Wisconsin	147	25	17	43	29.3	36	24.5	0	0	15	10.2	43	29.3	46	31.3	43	29.3	4	2.7	56	38.1	59	40.1
CENSUS DIVISION 5, EAST SOUTH CENTRAL	285	47	16.5	54	18.9	73	25.6	58	20.4	47	16.5	71	24.9	142	49.8	67	23.5	10	3.5	68	23.9	68	23.9
Alabama	52	13	25	7	13.5	17	32.7	4	7.7	14	26.9	12	23.1	31	59.6	14	26.9	2	3.8	15	28.8	17	32.7
Kentucky	72	11	15.3	15	20.8	25	34.7	11	15.3	14	19.4	24	33.3	49	68.1	20	27.8	3	4.2	10	13.9	19	26.4
Mississippi	96	6	6.3	10	10.4	16	16.7	26	27.1	7	7.3	8	8.3	26	27.1	13	13.5	1	1	24	25	14	14.6
Tennessee	65	17	26.2	22	33.8	15	23.1	17	26.2	12	18.5	27	41.5	36	55.4	20	30.8	4	6.2	19	29.2	18	27.7
CENSUS DIVISION 6, WEST NORTH CENTRAL	556	85	15.3	132	23.7	281	50.5	66	11.9	97	17.4	152	27.3	335	60.3	112	20.1	24	4.3	186	33.5	107	19.2
Iowa	122	22	18	27	22.1	79	64.8	10	8.2	25	20.5	37	30.3	97	79.5	17	13.9	1	0.8	41	33.6	16	13.1
Kansas	120	13	10.8	17	14.2	56	46.7	7	5.8	12	10	22	18.3	60	50	16	13.3	2	1.7	36	30	17	14.2
Minnesota	94	17	18.1	28	29.8	50	53.2	11	11.7	18	19.1	33	35.1	58	61.7	21	22.3	5	5.3	29	30.9	23	24.5
Missouri	130	16	12.3	38	29.2	47	36.2	27	20.8	19	14.6	43	33.1	75	57.7	40	30.8	12	9.2	44	33.8	34	26.2
Nebraska	39	12	30.8	13	33.3	22	56.4	5	12.8	13	33.3	11	28.2	29	74.4	10	25.6	2	5.1	18	46.2	8	20.5
North Dakota	12	3	25	4	33.3	8	66.7	3	25	4	33.3	3	25	5	41.7	4	33.3	1	8.3	3	25	4	33.3
South Dakota	39	2	5.1	5	12.8	19	48.7	3	7.7	6	15.4	3	7.7	11	28.2	4	10.3	1	2.6	15	38.5	5	12.8
CENSUS DIVISION 7, WEST SOUTH CENTRAL	842	153	18.2	116	13.8	207	24.6	114	13.5	130	15.4	146	17.3	379	45	180	21.4	14	1.7	171	20.3	183	21.7
Arkansas	98	16	16.3	17	17.3	31	31.6	13	13.3	23	23.5	23	23.5	49	50	14	14.3	2	2	36	22.4	18	18.4
Louisiana	79	17	21.5	22	27.8	27	34.2	20	25.3	17	21.5	24	30.4	47	59.5	18	22.8	1	1.3	16	20.3	26	32.9
Oklahoma	99	18	18.2	17	17.2	29	29.3	13	13.1	13	13.1	21	21.2	53	53.5	27	27.3	2	2	24	17.2	24	24.2
Texas	566	102	18	60	10.6	120	21.2	68	12	77	13.6	78	13.8	230	40.6	121	21.4	9	1.6	116	20.5	115	20.3
CENSUS DIVISION 8, MOUNTAIN	336	81	24.1	119	35.4	156	46.4	44	13.1	101	30.1	109	32.4	229	68.2	95	28.3	17	5.1	76	22.6	119	35.4
Arizona	70	26	37.1	23	32.9	27	38.6	5	7.1	22	31.4	34	48.6	48	68.6	30	42.9	5	7.1	19	27.1	24	34.3
Colorado	74	22	29.7	26	35.1	40	54.1	11	14.9	22	29.7	25	33.8	59	79.7	18	24.3	3	4.1	26	35.1	32	43.2
Idaho	26	10	38.5	8	30.8	12	46.2	4	15.4	5	19.2	7	26.9	21	80.8	6	23.1	1	3.8	5	19.2	14	53.8
Montana	45	4	8.9	10	22.2	25	55.6	3	6.7	7	15.6	8	17.8	23	51.1	8	17.8	2	4.4	11	24.4	15	33.3
Nevada	32	4	12.5	11	34.4	8	25	4	12.5	9	28.1	4	12.9	13	40.6	2	6.3	0	0	6	18.8	6	18.8
New Mexico	31	9	29	5	16.1	9	29	2	6.5	6	19.4	4	12.9	21	67.7	10	32.3	1	3.2	5	16.1	10	32.3
Utah	36	4	11.1	31	86.1	28	77.8	13	36.1	26	72.2	25	69.4	33	91.7	16	44.4	5	13.9	4	11.1	17	47.2
Wyoming	22	2	9.1	5	22.7	7	31.8	2	9.1	4	18.2	2	9.1	11	50	5	22.7	0	0	0	0	1	4.5
CENSUS DIVISION 9, PACIFIC	411	141	34.3	109	26.5	175	42.6	108	26.3	100	24.3	169	41.1	301	73.2	156	38	24	5.8	92	22.4	177	43.1
Alaska	9	2	22.2	3	33.3	4	44.4	1	11.1	4	44.4	4	44.4	7	77.8	3	33.3	0	0	1	11.1	3	33.3
California	268	98	36.6	67	25	113	42.2	91	34	77	28.7	108	40.3	192	71.6	106	39.6	20	7.5	53	19.8	123	45.9
Hawaii	15	4	26.7	3	20	7	46.7	4	26.7	3	20	11	73.3	11	73.3	4	26.7	0	0	3	20	7	46.7
Oregon	60	19	31.7	14	23.3	24	40	4	6.7	5	8.3	24	40	45	75	20	33.3	1	1.7	23	38.3	23	38.3
Washington	59	18	30.5	22	37.3	27	45.8	8	13.6	11	18.6	22	37.3	46	78	23	39	3	5.1	12	20.3	21	35.6

Note: The 2021 performance data do not reflect the full impact of the COVID-19 pandemic. Please refer to the discussion in the Introduction for more information.

Facilities and Services

Table 7 (Continued)

These data include only hospital-based facilities and services as reported by responding hospitals in Section C of the 2022 AHA Annual Survey, beginning on page 215. Census divisions represent all U.S. hospitals. Community hospitals are listed separately under United States. No estimates have been made for nonresponding hospitals. Definitions of facilities and services are listed in the Glossary, page 203.

CLASSIFICATION	HOSPITALS REPORTING	GENETIC TESTING/COUNSELING		GERIATRIC SERVICES		HEALTH FAIR		COMMUNITY HEALTH EDUCATION		HEALTH RESEARCH		HEALTH SCREENINGS		HEMODIALYSIS		HIV/AIDS SERVICES		HOME HEALTH SERVICES		HOSPICE	
		Number	Percent	Number	Percent	Number	Percent	Number	Percent	Number	Percent	Number	Percent	Number	Percent	Number	Percent	Number	Percent	Number	Percent
UNITED STATES	4,097	889	21.7	1,632	39.8	2,613	63.8	3,135	76.5	1,176	28.7	2,992	73	1,392	34	929	22.7	721	17.6	808	19.7
COMMUNITY HOSPITALS	3,682	875	23.8	1,539	41.8	2,535	68.8	3,025	82.2	1,112	30.2	2,888	78.4	1,347	36.6	885	24	688	18.7	770	20.9
CENSUS DIVISION 1, NEW ENGLAND	148	56	37.8	82	55.4	100	67.6	130	87.8	66	44.6	123	83.1	42	28.4	63	42.6	18	12.2	29	19.6
Connecticut	24	13	54.2	17	70.8	21	87.5	22	91.7	18	75	22	91.7	9	37.5	14	58.3	4	16.7	9	37.5
Maine	29	7	24.1	17	58.6	15	51.7	28	96.6	7	24.1	26	89.7	4	13.8	9	31	1	3.4	9	31
Massachusetts	50	18	36	23	46	32	64	39	78	25	50	36	72	21	42	25	50	6	12	7	14
New Hampshire	26	11	42.3	15	57.7	20	76.9	24	92.3	10	38.5	24	92.3	2	7.7	8	30.8	6	23.1	5	19.2
Rhode Island	9	4	44.4	7	77.8	7	77.8	7	77.8	4	44.4	7	77.8	5	55.6	5	55.6	1	11.1	2	22.2
Vermont	10	3	30	3	30	5	50	10	100	2	20	8	80	1	10	2	20	0	0	3	30
CENSUS DIVISION 2, MIDDLE ATLANTIC	357	149	41.7	187	52.4	255	71.4	279	78.2	175	49	284	79.6	178	49.9	139	38.9	62	17.4	103	28.9
New Jersey	71	40	56.3	44	62	51	71.8	58	81.7	48	67.6	55	77.5	47	66.2	36	50.7	9	12.7	27	38
New York	122	61	50	79	64.8	100	82	108	88.5	63	51.6	111	91	75	61.5	63	51.6	23	18.9	36	29.5
Pennsylvania	164	48	29.3	64	39	104	63.4	113	68.9	64	39	118	72	56	34.1	40	24.4	30	18.3	40	24.4
CENSUS DIVISION 3, SOUTH ATLANTIC	541	144	26.6	213	39.4	405	74.9	434	80.2	217	40.1	432	79.9	257	47.5	180	33.3	81	15	100	18.5
Delaware	8	3	37.5	3	37.5	5	62.5	5	62.5	3	37.5	5	62.5	4	50	4	50	3	37.5	1	12.5
District of Columbia	9	5	55.6	6	66.7	7	77.8	7	77.8	8	88.9	8	88.9	5	55.6	5	55.6	0	0	1	11.1
Florida	154	39	25.3	56	36.4	108	70.1	122	79.2	69	44.8	113	73.4	85	55.2	44	28.6	20	13	22	14.3
Georgia	88	21	23.9	28	31.8	64	72.7	72	81.8	30	34.1	77	87.5	37	42	30	34.1	10	11.4	22	25
Maryland	40	20	50	27	67.5	34	85	35	87.5	30	75	34	85	24	60	29	72.5	4	10	13	32.5
North Carolina	68	19	27.9	31	45.6	57	83.8	60	88.2	27	39.7	62	91.2	30	44.1	17	25	10	14.7	10	14.7
South Carolina	78	6	7.7	27	34.6	52	66.7	55	70.5	14	17.9	53	67.9	26	33.3	19	24.4	12	15.4	11	14.1
Virginia	59	23	39	23	39	49	83.1	49	83.1	30	50.8	50	84.7	36	61	24	40.7	16	27.1	19	32.2
West Virginia	37	8	21.6	12	32.4	29	78.4	29	78.4	6	16.2	30	81.1	10	27	8	21.6	6	16.2	1	2.7
CENSUS DIVISION 4, EAST NORTH CENTRAL	621	150	24.2	305	49.1	393	63.3	535	86.2	173	27.9	460	74.1	211	34	143	23	130	20.9	123	19.8
Illinois	138	37	26.8	64	46.4	108	78.3	122	88.4	43	31.2	125	90.6	54	39.1	37	26.8	27	19.6	26	18.8
Indiana	108	25	23.1	38	35.2	75	69.4	86	79.6	23	21.3	85	78.7	23	21.3	21	19.4	15	13.9	21	19.4
Michigan	120	29	24.2	63	52.5	80	66.7	104	86.7	45	37.5	106	88.3	45	37.5	41	34.2	38	31.7	32	26.7
Ohio	108	39	36.1	52	48.1	84	77.8	95	88	46	42.6	91	84.3	51	47.2	35	32.4	32	29.6	30	27.8
Wisconsin	147	20	13.6	88	59.9	46	31.3	128	87.1	16	10.9	53	36.1	38	25.9	9	6.1	18	12.2	14	9.5
CENSUS DIVISION 5, EAST SOUTH CENTRAL	285	44	15.4	68	23.9	178	62.5	192	67.4	61	21.4	195	68.4	79	27.7	47	16.5	32	11.2	36	12.6
Alabama	52	9	17.3	15	28.8	36	69.2	35	67.3	13	25	39	75	24	46.2	8	15.4	3	5.8	8	15.4
Kentucky	72	13	18.1	17	23.6	42	58.3	51	70.8	15	20.8	52	72.2	19	26.4	13	18.1	16	22.2	11	15.3
Mississippi	96	9	9.4	13	13.5	56	58.3	57	59.4	10	10.4	56	58.3	16	16.7	9	9.4	7	7.3	7	7.3
Tennessee	65	13	20	23	35.4	44	67.7	49	75.4	23	35.4	48	73.8	20	30.8	17	26.2	6	9.2	10	15.4
CENSUS DIVISION 6, WEST NORTH CENTRAL	556	83	14.9	235	42.3	373	67.1	451	81.1	104	18.7	455	81.8	117	21	91	16.4	153	27.5	135	24.3
Iowa	122	16	13.1	53	43.4	95	77.9	108	88.5	14	11.5	111	91	16	13.1	18	14.8	40	32.8	40	32.8
Kansas	120	19	15.8	45	37.5	68	56.7	83	69.2	14	11.7	91	75.8	13	10.8	14	11.7	23	19.2	16	13.3
Minnesota	94	12	12.8	44	46.8	67	71.3	81	86.2	20	21.3	78	83	15	16	13	13.8	33	35.1	28	29.8
Missouri	130	20	15.4	56	43.1	78	60	97	74.6	34	26.2	96	73.8	48	36.9	29	22.3	33	25.4	29	22.3
Nebraska	39	10	25.6	14	35.9	29	74.4	37	94.9	13	33.3	35	89.7	10	25.6	6	15.4	15	38.5	15	38.5
North Dakota	12	4	33.3	5	41.7	7	58.3	11	91.7	4	33.3	8	66.7	5	41.7	3	25	2	16.7	2	16.7
South Dakota	39	2	5.1	18	46.2	29	74.4	34	87.2	5	12.8	36	92.3	10	25.6	8	20.5	7	17.9	4	10.3
CENSUS DIVISION 7, WEST SOUTH CENTRAL	842	87	10.3	228	27.1	463	55	529	62.8	136	16.2	494	58.7	225	26.7	91	10.8	100	11.9	83	9.9
Arkansas	98	6	6.1	30	30.6	62	63.3	71	72.4	13	13.3	65	66.3	21	21.4	13	13.3	27	27.6	10	10.2
Louisiana	79	19	24.1	30	38	49	62	62	78.5	21	26.6	55	69.6	26	32.9	21	26.6	7	8.9	7	8.9
Oklahoma	99	8	8.1	25	25.3	47	47.5	62	62.6	19	19.2	63	63.6	21	21.2	7	7.1	14	14.1	10	10.1
Texas	566	54	9.5	143	25.3	305	53.9	334	59	83	14.7	311	54.9	157	27.7	50	8.8	52	9.2	56	9.9
CENSUS DIVISION 8, MOUNTAIN	336	75	22.3	135	40.2	204	60.7	263	78.3	83	24.7	258	76.8	108	32.1	65	19.3	56	16.7	96	28.6
Arizona	70	14	20	25	35.7	43	61.4	52	74.3	31	44.3	45	64.3	39	55.7	18	25.7	7	10	17	24.3
Colorado	74	23	31.1	30	40.5	45	60.8	64	86.5	22	29.7	69	93.2	20	27	21	28.4	13	17.6	20	27
Idaho	26	5	19.2	13	50	21	80.8	22	84.6	4	15.4	22	84.6	4	15.4	2	7.7	6	23.1	8	30.8
Montana	45	13	28.9	25	55.6	28	62.2	39	86.7	7	15.6	40	88.9	7	15.6	8	17.8	14	31.1	17	37.8
Nevada	32	2	6.3	9	28.1	11	34.4	13	40.6	5	15.6	13	40.6	6	18.8	7	21.9	3	9.4	4	12.5
New Mexico	31	2	6.5	10	32.3	21	67.7	22	71	3	9.7	21	67.7	8	25.8	3	9.7	7	22.6	8	25.8
Utah	36	12	33.3	12	33.3	25	69.4	33	91.7	10	27.8	33	91.7	19	52.8	4	11.1	2	5.6	19	52.8
Wyoming	22	4	18.2	11	50	10	45.5	18	81.8	0	0	15	68.2	5	22.7	2	9.1	4	18.2	3	13.6
CENSUS DIVISION 9, PACIFIC	411	101	24.6	179	43.6	242	58.9	322	78.3	161	39.2	291	70.8	175	42.6	110	26.8	89	21.7	103	25.1
Alaska	9	0	0	0	0	7	77.8	7	77.8	0	0	7	77.8	3	33.3	3	33.3	3	33.3	2	22.2
California	268	71	26.5	130	48.5	154	57.5	197	73.5	113	42.2	174	64.9	128	47.8	75	28	61	22.8	71	26.5
Hawaii	15	4	26.7	5	33.3	8	53.3	13	86.7	8	53.3	11	73.3	6	40	2	13.3	3	20	6	40
Oregon	60	9	15	20	33.3	39	65	54	90	14	23.3	53	88.3	16	26.7	14	23.3	13	21.7	13	21.7
Washington	59	17	28.8	24	40.7	34	57.6	51	86.4	26	44.1	46	78	22	37.3	16	27.1	9	15.3	11	18.6

Note: The 2021 performance data do not reflect the full impact of the COVID-19 pandemic. Please refer to the discussion in the Introduction for more information.

AHA Hospital Statistics © 2023 Health Forum LLC, an affiliate of the American Hospital Association

Table 7 (Continued)

These data include only hospital-based facilities and services as reported by responding hospitals in Section C of the 2022 AHA Annual Survey, beginning on page 215. Census divisions represent all U.S. hospitals. Community hospitals are listed separately under United States. No estimates have been made for nonresponding hospitals. Definitions of facilities and services are listed in the Glossary, page 203.

Facilities and Services

Classification	Hospitals Reporting	Hospital-Based Outpatient Care Center Services — Number	Percent	Immunization Program — Number	Percent	Indigent Care Clinic — Number	Percent	Linguistic/Translation Services — Number	Percent	Meal Delivery Services — Number	Percent	Mobile Health Services — Number	Percent	Neonatal Intermediate Care Units — Number	Percent	Neurological Services — Number	Percent	Nutrition Programs Center — Number	Percent	Obstetrics Inpatient Care Units — Number	Percent
UNITED STATES	4,097	3,007	73.4	1,999	48.8	645	15.7	2,273	55.5	285	7	531	13	618	15.1	2,060	50.3	3,033	74	2,114	51.6
COMMUNITY HOSPITALS	3,682	2,901	78.8	1,909	51.8	627	17	2,163	58.7	271	7.4	501	13.6	616	16.7	1,993	54.1	2,855	77.5	2,108	57.3
CENSUS DIVISION 1, NEW ENGLAND	148	125	84.5	103	69.6	29	19.6	104	70.3	5	3.4	31	20.9	22	14.9	103	69.6	135	91.2	89	60.1
Connecticut	24	19	79.2	19	79.2	10	41.7	21	87.5		0	7	29.2	2	8.3	20	83.3	23	95.8	20	83.3
Maine	29	26	89.7	22	75.9	2	6.9	13	44.8	1	3.4	4	13.8	2	6.9	14	48.3	21	72.4	21	72.4
Massachusetts	50	42	84	32	64	10	20	40	80	3	6	12	24	12	24	39	78	44	88	25	50
New Hampshire	26	24	92.3	18	69.2	4	15.4	16	61.5	1	3.8	6	23.1	5	19.2	17	65.4	25	96.2	13	50
Rhode Island	9	7	77.8	6	66.7	1	11.1	7	77.8		0	2	22.2		0	6	66.7	8	88.9	3	33.3
Vermont	10	7	70	6	60	2	20	7	70			0	0	1	10	7	70	8	80	7	70
CENSUS DIVISION 2, MIDDLE ATLANTIC	357	279	78.2	221	61.9	123	34.5	220	61.6	23	6.4	75	21	106	29.7	262	73.4	296	82.9	197	55.2
New Jersey	71	58	81.7	45	63.4	31	43.7	52	73.2	9	12.7	18	25.4	41	57.7	59	83.1	59	83.1	43	60.6
New York	122	107	87.7	85	69.7	61	50	93	76.2	7	5.7	39	32	45	36.9	94	77	110	90.2	83	68
Pennsylvania	164	114	69.5	91	55.5	31	18.9	75	45.7	7	4.3	18	11	20	12.2	109	66.5	127	77.4	71	43.3
CENSUS DIVISION 3, SOUTH ATLANTIC	541	412	76.2	237	43.8	103	19	329	60.8	20	3.7	100	18.5	120	22.2	359	66.4	443	81.9	304	56.2
Delaware	8	6	75	3	37.5	3	37.5	5	62.5	1	12.5	3	37.5	1	12.5	5	62.5	5	62.5	5	62.5
District of Columbia	9	7	77.8	7	77.8	3	33.3	8	88.9			6	66.7	2	22.2	8	88.9	9	100	5	55.6
Florida	154	111	72.1	54	35.1	23	14.9	83	53.9	5	3.2	20	13	20	13	121	78.6	127	82.5	74	48.1
Georgia	88	62	70.5	31	35.2	14	15.9	59	67	2	2.3	14	15.9	28	31.8	45	51.1	64	72.7	45	51.1
Maryland	40	36	90	27	67.5	19	47.5	37	92.5	2	5	16	40	6	15	35	87.5	39	97.5	29	72.5
North Carolina	68	60	88.2	33	48.5	16	23.5	44	64.7	3	4.4	15	22.1	25	36.8	45	66.2	58	85.3	53	77.9
South Carolina	78	50	64.1	23	29.5	8	10.3	33	42.3	2	2.6	9	11.5	26	33.3	41	52.6	58	74.4	38	48.7
Virginia	59	49	83.1	37	62.7	11	18.6	42	71.2	4	6.8	10	16.9	11	18.6	42	71.2	51	86.4	36	61
West Virginia	37	31	83.8	22	59.5	6	16.2	18	48.6	1	2.7	7	18.9	1	2.7	17	45.9	32	86.5	19	51.4
CENSUS DIVISION 4, EAST NORTH CENTRAL	621	510	82.1	310	49.9	112	18	337	54.3	75	12.1	89	14.3	79	12.7	313	50.4	496	79.9	363	58.5
Illinois	138	117	84.8	65	47.1	26	18.8	84	60.9	15	10.9	21	15.2	32	23.2	81	58.7	105	76.1	77	55.8
Indiana	108	80	74.1	54	50	15	13.9	59	54.6	20	18.5	16	14.8	16	14.8	50	46.3	85	78.7	69	63.9
Michigan	120	101	84.2	84	70	33	27.5	79	65.8	8	6.7	15	12.5	12	10	72	60	105	87.5	73	60.8
Ohio	108	87	80.6	57	52.8	22	20.4	67	62	9	8.3	25	23.1	19	17.6	75	69.4	90	83.3	58	53.7
Wisconsin	147	125	85	50	34	16	10.9	48	32.7	23	15.6	12	8.2	0	0	35	23.8	111	75.5	86	58.5
CENSUS DIVISION 5, EAST SOUTH CENTRAL	285	166	58.2	117	41.1	30	10.5	124	43.5	6	2.1	26	9.1	42	14.7	121	42.5	162	56.8	119	41.8
Alabama	52	29	55.8	18	34.6	4	7.7	29	55.8			4	7.7	9	7.7	32	61.5	23	44.2	23	44.2
Kentucky	72	48	66.7	29	40.3	8	11.1	34	47.2	4	5.6	7	9.7	9	12.5	31	43.1	48	66.7	32	44.4
Mississippi	96	46	47.9	40	41.7	10	10.4	36	37.5		0	6	6.3	21	21.9	22	22.9	31	32.3	33	34.4
Tennessee	65	43	66.2	30	46.2	8	12.3	25	38.5	2	3.1	9	13.8	8	12.3	36	55.4	54	83.1	31	47.7
CENSUS DIVISION 6, WEST NORTH CENTRAL	556	443	79.7	314	56.5	56	10.1	281	50.5	82	14.7	52	9.4	67	12.1	189	34	422	75.9	259	46.6
Iowa	122	106	86.9	77	63.1	15	12.3	69	56.6	23	18.9	11	9	9	7.4	31	25.4	105	86.1	52	42.6
Kansas	120	98	81.7	50	41.7	10	8.3	55	45.8	24	20	7	5.8	8	6.7	26	21.7	70	58.3	44	36.7
Minnesota	94	77	81.9	68	72.3	5	5.3	44	46.8	7	7.4	6	6.4	6	6.4	32	34	75	79.8	61	64.9
Missouri	130	88	67.7	61	46.9	17	13.1	71	54.6	16	12.3	11	8.5	35	26.9	69	53.1	102	78.5	59	45.4
Nebraska	39	28	71.8	24	61.5	3	7.7	24	61.5	6	15.4	9	23.1	5	12.8	20	51.3	32	82.1	21	53.8
North Dakota	12	11	91.7	7	58.3	2	16.7	5	41.7	1	8.3	2	16.7	3	25	6	50	11	91.7	7	58.3
South Dakota	39	35	89.7	27	69.2	4	10.3	13	33.3	5	12.8	6	15.4	1	2.6	5	12.8	27	69.2	15	38.5
CENSUS DIVISION 7, WEST SOUTH CENTRAL	842	517	61.4	296	35.2	81	9.6	359	42.6	33	3.9	64	7.6	72	8.6	316	37.5	498	59.1	309	36.7
Arkansas	98	63	64.3	26	26.5	8	8.2	44	44.9	7	7.1	7	7.1	9	9.2	26	26.5	52	53.1	35	35.7
Louisiana	79	54	68.4	40	50.6	14	17.7	40	50.6	3	3.8	9	11.4	7	8.9	35	44.3	50	63.3	32	40.5
Oklahoma	99	64	64.6	40	40.4	4	4	47	47.5	7	7.1	8	8.1	8	8.1	36	36.4	55	55.6	39	39.4
Texas	566	336	59.4	190	33.6	55	9.7	228	40.3	16	2.8	40	7.1	48	8.5	219	38.7	341	60.2	203	35.9
CENSUS DIVISION 8, MOUNTAIN	336	228	67.9	179	53.3	42	12.5	220	65.5	20	6	43	12.8	37	11	143	42.6	249	74.1	194	57.7
Arizona	70	45	64.3	28	40	8	11.4	48	68.6	7	10	14	11.4	11	15.7	37	52.9	56	80	32	45.7
Colorado	74	56	75.7	45	60.8	10	13.5	56	75.7	5	6.8	9	18.9	9	12.2	47	63.5	59	79.7	48	64.9
Idaho	26	20	84.6	20	76.9	8	30.8	22	84.6	1	3.8	7	26.9	0	0	9	34.6	23	88.5	18	69.2
Montana	45	37	82.2	31	68.9	5	11.1	18	40	5	11.1	2	15.6	2	4.4	10	22.2	29	64.4	24	53.3
Nevada	32	13	40.6	9	28.1	3	9.4	14	43.8	1	3.1	6	6.3	1	3.1	12	37.5	17	53.1	7	21.9
New Mexico	31	18	58.1	14	45.2	4	12.9	18	58.1	1	3.2	1	3.2	6	19.4	10	32.3	16	51.6	21	67.7
Utah	36	26	72.2	21	58.3	1	2.8	31	86.1		0	3	8.3	7	19.4	12	33.3	32	88.9	30	83.3
Wyoming	22	11	50	11	50	3	13.6	13	59.1		0	1	4.5	1	4.5	6	27.3	17	77.3	14	63.6
CENSUS DIVISION 9, PACIFIC	411	327	79.6	222	54	69	16.8	299	72.7	21	5.1	51	12.4	73	17.8	254	61.8	332	80.8	280	68.1
Alaska	9	8	88.9	8	88.9	1	11.1	5	55.6	2	22.2	0	0	0	0	2	22.2	7	77.8	7	77.8
California	268	207	77.2	142	53	53	19.8	200	74.6	14	5.2	34	12.7	41	15.3	179	66.8	212	79.1	178	66.4
Hawaii	15	12	80	5	46.7	1	6.7	12	80	2	13.3	1	6.7	3	20	10	66.7	11	73.3	8	53.3
Oregon	60	53	88.3	31	51.7	7	11.7	39	65		0	8	13.3	5	8.3	24	40	50	83.3	48	80
Washington	59	47	79.7	34	57.6	7	11.9	43	72.9	3	5.1	8	13.6	24	40.7	39	66.1	51	86.4	39	66.1

Note: The 2021 performance data do not reflect the full impact of the COVID-19 pandemic. Please refer to the discussion in the Introduction for more information.

Facilities and Services

Table 7 (Continued)

These data include only hospital-based facilities and services as reported by responding hospitals in Section C of the 2022 AHA Annual Survey, beginning on page 215. Census divisions represent all U.S. hospitals. Community hospitals are listed separately under United States. No estimates have been made for nonresponding hospitals. Definitions of facilities and services are listed in the Glossary, page 203.

CLASSIFICATION	HOSPITALS REPORTING	OCCUPATIONAL HEALTH SERVICES Number	Percent	ONCOLOGY SERVICES Number	Percent	ORTHOPEDIC SERVICES Number	Percent	OTHER SPECIAL CARE UNITS Number	Percent	OUTPATIENT SURGERY Number	Percent	PAIN MANAGEMENT PROGRAM Number	Percent	PALLIATIVE CARE PROGRAM Number	Percent	PALLIATIVE CARE INPATIENT UNIT Number	Percent	PATIENT CONTROLLED ANALGESIA (PCA) Number	Percent	PATIENT EDUCATION CENTER Number	Percent
UNITED STATES	4,097	2,689	66.6	2,100	51.3	2,785	68	793	19.4	3,182	77.7	2,174	53.1	1,695	41.4	402	9.8	2,764	67.5	2,161	52.7
COMMUNITY HOSPITALS	3,682	2,576	70	2,062	56	2,737	74.3	776	21.1	3,141	85.3	2,094	56.9	1,636	44.4	367	10	2,708	73.5	2,045	55.5
CENSUS DIVISION 1, NEW ENGLAND	148	117	79.1	92	62.2	114	77	26	17.6	118	79.7	103	69.6	86	58.1	26	17.6	118	79.7	96	64.9
Connecticut	24	18	75	19	79.2	20	83.3	5	20.8	20	83.3	17	70.8	20	83.3	7	29.2	20	83.3	18	75
Maine	29	24	82.8	17	58.6	23	79.3	8	27.6	24	82.8	21	72.4	18	62.1	2	6.9	24	82.8	15	51.7
Massachusetts	50	39	78	27	54	36	72	5	10	37	74	35	70	21	42	7	14	37	74	35	70
New Hampshire	26	22	84.6	17	65.4	21	80.8	7	26.9	22	84.6	17	65.4	16	61.5	8	30.8	21	80.8	20	76.9
Rhode Island	9	8	88.9	7	77.8	7	77.8	1	11.1	7	77.8	7	77.8	5	55.6	1	11.1	8	88.9	6	66.7
Vermont	10	6	60	5	50	7	70	0	0	8	80	6	60	6	60	1	10	8	80	2	20
CENSUS DIVISION 2, MIDDLE ATLANTIC	357	276	77.3	229	66.9	283	79.3	73	20.4	283	79.3	237	66.4	228	63.9	46	12.9	266	74.5	222	62.2
New Jersey	71	59	83.1	50	70.4	53	74.6	12	16.9	54	76.1	51	71.8	51	71.8	8	11.3	51	71.8	44	62
New York	122	105	86.1	94	77	108	88.5	28	23	105	86.1	91	74.6	91	74.6	26	21.3	99	81.1	82	67.2
Pennsylvania	164	112	68.3	95	57.9	122	74.4	33	20.1	124	75.6	95	57.9	86	52.4	12	7.3	116	70.7	96	58.5
CENSUS DIVISION 3, SOUTH ATLANTIC	541	423	78.2	329	60.8	426	78.7	145	26.8	437	80.8	310	57.3	279	51.6	58	10.7	412	76.2	337	62.3
Delaware	8	5	62.5	5	62.5	5	62.5	1	12.5	5	62.5	4	50	5	62.5	0	0	5	62.5	4	50
District of Columbia	9	8	88.9	7	77.8	7	77.8	4	44.4	6	66.7	6	66.7	6	66.7	1	11.1	5	55.6	8	88.9
Florida	154	121	78.6	97	63	126	81.8	53	34.4	126	81.8	94	61	81	52.6	15	9.7	123	79.9	89	57.8
Georgia	88	71	80.7	47	53.4	59	67	19	21.6	65	73.9	45	51.1	39	44.3	7	8	59	67	56	63.6
Maryland	40	40	100	34	85	36	90	8	20	37	92.5	34	85	36	90	9	22.5	38	95	31	77.5
North Carolina	68	57	83.8	50	73.5	60	88.2	13	19.1	63	92.6	47	69.1	36	52.9	7	10.3	58	85.3	51	75
South Carolina	78	47	60.3	30	38.5	57	73.1	25	32.1	54	69.2	28	35.9	27	34.6	1	1.3	53	67.9	36	46.2
Virginia	59	52	88.1	39	66.1	49	83.1	19	32.2	51	86.4	35	59.3	35	59.3	14	23.7	45	76.3	40	67.8
West Virginia	37	22	59.5	20	54.1	27	73	3	8.1	30	81.1	17	45.9	14	37.8	4	10.8	26	70.3	22	59.5
CENSUS DIVISION 4, EAST NORTH CENTRAL	621	415	66.8	391	63	443	71.3	190	30.6	531	85.5	383	61.7	250	40.3	62	10	430	69.2	421	67.8
Illinois	138	90	65.2	86	62.3	109	79	12	8.7	121	87.7	89	64.5	68	49.3	11	8	104	75.4	81	58.7
Indiana	108	70	64.8	61	56.5	80	74.1	16	14.8	92	85.2	53	49.1	35	32.4	13	12	86	79.6	55	50.9
Michigan	120	99	82.5	84	70	103	85.8	25	20.8	106	88.3	69	57.5	46	38.3	14	11.7	92	76.7	77	64.2
Ohio	108	79	73.1	77	71.3	90	83.3	30	27.8	89	82.4	80	74.1	54	50	14	13	84	77.8	70	64.8
Wisconsin	147	77	52.4	83	56.5	61	41.5	107	72.8	123	83.7	92	62.6	47	32	10	6.8	64	43.5	132	89.8
CENSUS DIVISION 5, EAST SOUTH CENTRAL	285	150	52.6	114	40	159	55.8	55	19.3	200	70.2	121	42.5	81	28.4	27	9.5	154	54	125	43.9
Alabama	52	34	65.4	32	61.5	33	63.5	10	19.2	37	71.2	18	34.6	18	34.6	9	17.3	36	69.2	25	48.1
Kentucky	72	39	54.2	49	68.1	49	68.1	10	13.9	56	77.8	36	50	25	34.7	9	12.5	44	61.1	36	50
Mississippi	96	30	31.3	28	29.2	28	29.2	15	15.6	57	59.4	27	28.1	16	16.7	7	7.3	31	32.3	31	32.3
Tennessee	65	47	72.3	49	75.4	49	75.4	20	30.8	50	76.9	31	47.7	22	33.8	2	3.1	43	66.2	33	50.8
CENSUS DIVISION 6, WEST NORTH CENTRAL	556	382	68.7	260	46.8	337	60.6	67	12.1	471	84.7	304	54.7	181	32.6	45	8.1	386	69.4	287	51.6
Iowa	122	89	73	62	50.8	81	66.4	6	4.9	112	91.8	79	64.8	33	27	4	3.3	96	78.7	59	48.4
Kansas	120	69	57.5	32	26.7	54	45	6	5	95	79.2	62	51.7	26	21.7	6	5	61	50.8	52	43.3
Minnesota	94	72	76.6	52	55.3	66	70.2	18	19.1	88	93.6	48	51.1	34	36.2	11	11.7	76	80.9	58	61.7
Missouri	130	90	69.2	74	56.9	89	68.5	29	22.3	100	76.9	64	49.2	50	38.5	11	8.5	97	74.6	81	62.3
Nebraska	39	31	79.5	25	64.1	29	74.4	4	10.3	34	87.2	21	53.8	21	53.8	3	7.7	29	74.4	18	46.2
North Dakota	12	7	58.3	4	33.3	6	50	2	16.7	11	91.7	8	66.7	6	50	3	25	6	50	5	41.7
South Dakota	39	24	61.5	11	28.2	12	30.8	2	5.1	31	79.5	15	38.5	11	28.2	7	17.9	21	53.8	14	35.9
CENSUS DIVISION 7, WEST SOUTH CENTRAL	842	416	49.4	247	29.3	447	53.1	105	12.5	517	61.4	314	37.3	195	23.2	42	5	451	53.6	314	37.3
Arkansas	98	43	43.9	31	31.6	46	46.9	10	10.2	65	66.3	29	29.6	17	17.3	4	4.1	52	53.1	29	29.6
Louisiana	79	41	51.9	36	45.6	42	53.2	8	10.1	52	65.8	29	36.7	27	34.2	3	3.8	44	55.7	41	51.9
Oklahoma	99	51	51.5	36	36.4	55	55.6	11	11.1	66	66.7	39	39.4	19	19.2	9	9.1	50	50.5	34	34.3
Texas	566	281	49.6	156	27.6	304	53.7	76	13.4	334	59	217	38.3	132	23.3	26	4.6	305	53.9	210	37.1
CENSUS DIVISION 8, MOUNTAIN	336	227	67.6	166	49.4	232	69	41	12.2	260	77.4	178	53	149	44.3	34	10.1	221	65.8	145	43.2
Arizona	70	49	70	36	51.4	48	68.6	12	17.1	51	72.9	36	51.4	33	47.1	12	17.1	47	67.1	34	48.6
Colorado	74	62	83.8	49	66.2	63	85.1	9	12.2	68	91.9	46	62.2	42	56.8	8	10.8	53	71.6	31	41.9
Idaho	26	22	84.6	11	42.3	19	73.1	1	3.8	23	88.5	15	57.7	8	30.8	2	7.7	18	69.2	12	46.2
Montana	45	22	48.9	19	42.2	24	53.3	3	6.7	31	68.9	24	53.3	19	42.2	6	13.3	25	55.6	18	40
Nevada	32	13	40.6	8	25	13	40.6	4	12.5	14	43.8	14	43.8	7	21.9	2	6.3	14	43.8	9	28.1
New Mexico	31	16	51.6	13	41.9	18	58.1	3	9.7	24	77.4	10	32.3	9	29	2	6.5	22	71	9	29
Utah	36	30	83.3	22	61.1	31	86.1	9	25	33	91.7	22	61.1	25	69.4	1	2.8	29	80.6	29	80.6
Wyoming	22	13	59.1	8	36.4	16	72.7	0	0	16	72.7	11	50	6	27.3	1	4.5	13	59.1	13	59.1
CENSUS DIVISION 9, PACIFIC	411	283	68.9	262	63.7	344	83.7	91	22.1	365	88.8	224	54.5	246	59.9	62	15.1	326	79.3	214	52.1
Alaska	9	8	88.9	3	33.3	5	55.6	2	22.2	6	66.7	4	44.4	3	33.3	1	11.1	6	66.7	6	66.7
California	268	180	67.2	168	62.7	229	85.4	56	20.9	237	88.4	147	54.9	173	64.6	45	16.8	211	78.7	140	52.2
Hawaii	15	12	80	12	80	12	80	5	33.3	11	73.3	7	46.7	9	60	1	6.7	11	73.3	7	46.7
Oregon	60	40	66.7	39	65	50	83.3	8	13.3	57	95	29	48.3	25	41.7	5	8.3	53	88.3	31	51.7
Washington	59	43	72.9	40	67.8	48	81.4	22	37.3	54	91.5	37	62.7	36	61	10	16.9	45	76.3	30	50.8

Note: The 2021 performance data do not reflect the full impact of the COVID-19 pandemic. Please refer to the discussion in the Introduction for more information.

Table 7 (Continued)

These data include only hospital-based facilities and services as reported by responding hospitals in Section C of the 2022 AHA Annual Survey, beginning on page 215. Census divisions represent all U.S. hospitals. Community hospitals are listed separately under United States. No estimates have been made for nonresponding hospitals. Definitions of facilities and services are listed in the Glossary, page 203.

CLASSIFICATION	HOSPITALS REPORTING	PATIENT REPRESENTATIVE SERVICES		PHYSICAL REHABILITATION INPATIENT CARE UNITS		PRIMARY CARE DEPARTMENT		ROBOTIC SURGERY		RURAL HEALTH CLINIC		SLEEP CENTER		SOCIAL WORK SERVICES		SPORTS MEDICINE		SUPPORT GROUPS	
		Number	Percent	Number	Percent	Number	Percent	Number	Percent	Number	Percent	Number	Percent	Number	Percent	Number	Percent	Number	Percent
UNITED STATES	4,097	2,925	71.4	1,170	28.6	1,815	44.3	1,728	42.2	1045	25.5	1,725	42.1	3,403	83.1	1,838	44.9	2,306	56.3
COMMUNITY HOSPITALS	3,682	2,757	74.9	1,132	30.7	1,743	47.3	1,710	46.4	1010	27.4	1,689	45.9	3,110	84.5	1,825	49.6	2,141	58.1
CENSUS DIVISION 1, NEW ENGLAND	148	130	87.8	33	22.3	97	65.5	65	43.9	26	17.6	78	52.7	135	91.2	93	62.8	117	79.1
Connecticut	24	23	95.8	7	29.2	16	66.7	19	79.2	0	0	16	66.7	23	95.8	17	70.8	23	95.8
Maine	29	25	86.2	5	17.2	25	86.2	6	20.7	13	44.8	12	41.4	27	93.1	16	55.2	21	72.4
Massachusetts	50	41	82	10	20	25	50	25	50	3	6	27	54	45	90	32	64	39	78
New Hampshire	26	24	92.3	6	23.1	19	73.1	8	30.8	7	26.9	14	53.8	24	92.3	18	69.2	18	76.9
Rhode Island	9	8	88.9	2	22.2	5	55.6	5	55.6	0	0	3	33.3	9	100	4	44.4	7	77.8
Vermont	10	9	90	3	30	7	70	2	20	3	30	6	60	7	70	6	60	7	70
CENSUS DIVISION 2, MIDDLE ATLANTIC	357	292	81.8	115	32.2	192	53.8	203	56.9	26	7.3	176	49.3	334	93.6	176	49.3	271	75.9
New Jersey	71	63	88.7	13	18.3	43	60.6	44	62	0	0	37	52.1	67	94.4	36	50.7	57	80.3
New York	122	111	91	38	31.1	92	75.4	76	62.3	17	13.9	60	49.2	118	96.7	68	55.7	97	79.5
Pennsylvania	164	118	72	64	39	57	34.8	83	50.6	9	5.5	79	48.2	149	90.9	72	43.9	117	71.3
CENSUS DIVISION 3, SOUTH ATLANTIC	541	415	76.7	171	31.6	199	36.8	301	55.6	87	16.1	244	45.1	456	84.3	274	50.6	355	65.6
Delaware	8	8	62.5	4	50	4	50	5	62.5	0	0	4	44.4	7	87.5	4	50	4	50
District of Columbia	9	8	88.9	3	33.3	6	66.7	6	66.7	0	0	4	44.4	9	100	5	55.6	7	77.8
Florida	154	120	77.9	45	29.2	44	28.6	100	64.9	20	13	55	35.7	124	80.5	75	48.7	98	63.6
Georgia	88	57	64.8	21	23.9	26	29.5	45	51.1	15	17	43	48.9	67	76.1	40	45.5	52	59.1
Maryland	40	39	97.5	7	17.5	21	52.5	29	72.5	4	10	18	45	40	100	22	55	34	85
North Carolina	68	57	83.8	21	30.9	27	39.7	38	55.9	10	14.7	37	54.4	62	91.2	42	61.8	50	73.5
South Carolina	78	48	61.5	46	59	20	25.6	29	37.2	17	21.8	26	33.3	59	75.6	32	41	44	56.4
Virginia	59	52	88.1	20	33.9	26	44.1	34	57.6	8	13.6	36	61	55	93.2	36	61	43	72.9
West Virginia	37	29	78.4	4	10.8	25	67.6	15	40.5	13	35.1	21	56.8	33	89.2	18	48.6	23	62.2
CENSUS DIVISION 4, EAST NORTH CENTRAL	621	499	80.4	204	32.9	321	51.7	276	44.4	152	24.5	341	54.9	548	88.2	370	59.6	386	62.2
Illinois	138	112	81.2	37	26.8	82	59.4	65	47.1	39	28.3	82	59.4	120	87	82	59.4	94	68.1
Indiana	108	81	75	31	28.7	47	43.5	44	40.7	22	20.4	66	61.1	85	78.7	50	46.3	73	67.6
Michigan	120	106	88.3	39	32.5	90	75	65	54.2	55	45.8	74	61.7	111	92.5	80	66.7	89	74.2
Ohio	108	89	82.4	37	34.3	57	52.8	63	58.3	12	11.1	71	65.7	99	91.7	77	71.3	82	75.9
Wisconsin	147	111	75.5	60	40.8	45	30.6	39	26.5	24	16.3	48	32.7	133	90.5	81	55.1	48	32.7
CENSUS DIVISION 5, EAST SOUTH CENTRAL	285	183	64.2	72	25.3	84	29.5	85	29.8	99	34.7	126	44.2	219	76.8	85	29.8	137	48.1
Alabama	52	34	65.4	11	21.2	15	28.8	24	46.2	11	21.2	27	51.9	36	69.2	18	34.6	30	57.7
Kentucky	72	51	70.8	11	15.3	28	38.9	22	30.6	31	43.1	43	59.7	50	69.4	25	34.7	38	52.8
Mississippi	96	54	56.3	34	35.4	23	24	16	16.7	48	50	24	25	76	79.2	16	16.7	30	31.3
Tennessee	65	44	67.7	16	24.6	18	27.7	23	35.4	9	13.8	32	49.2	57	87.7	26	40	39	60
CENSUS DIVISION 6, WEST NORTH CENTRAL	556	358	64.4	166	29.9	331	59.5	162	29.1	273	49.1	268	48.2	452	81.3	299	53.8	308	55.4
Iowa	122	74	60.7	24	19.7	77	63.1	36	29.5	68	55.7	64	52.5	102	83.6	68	55.7	68	70.5
Kansas	120	70	58.3	23	19.2	67	55.8	25	20.8	71	59.2	35	29.2	88	73.3	51	42.5	36	30
Minnesota	94	71	75.5	19	20.2	66	70.2	32	34	37	39.4	46	48.9	86	91.5	61	64.9	64	68.1
Missouri	130	95	73.1	83	63.8	58	44.6	45	34.6	50	38.5	77	59.2	110	84.6	67	51.5	69	53.1
Nebraska	39	26	66.7	8	20.5	23	61.5	15	38.5	23	59	24	61.5	33	84.6	29	74.4	26	66.7
North Dakota	12	7	58.3	3	25	8	66.7	4	33.3	3	25	6	50	7	58.3	7	58.3	8	66.7
South Dakota	39	15	38.5	6	15.4	31	79.5	5	12.8	21	53.8	16	41	26	66.7	16	41	19	48.7
CENSUS DIVISION 7, WEST SOUTH CENTRAL	842	490	58.2	220	26.1	244	29	275	32.7	211	25.1	239	28.4	611	72.6	232	27.6	312	37.1
Arkansas	98	54	55.1	30	30.6	33	33.7	27	27.6	32	32.7	45	45.9	70	71.4	24	24.5	32	32.7
Louisiana	79	56	70.9	28	35.4	43	54.4	31	39.2	20	25.3	29	36.7	65	82.3	25	31.6	41	51.9
Oklahoma	99	62	62.6	24	24.2	31	31.3	25	25.3	35	35.4	36	36.4	66	66.7	31	31.3	30	30.3
Texas	566	318	56.2	138	24.4	137	24.2	192	33.9	124	21.9	129	22.8	410	72.4	152	26.9	209	36.9
CENSUS DIVISION 8, MOUNTAIN	336	240	71.4	90	26.8	170	50.6	144	42.9	94	28	136	40.5	270	80.4	143	42.6	171	50.9
Arizona	70	51	72.9	20	28.6	20	28.6	36	51.4	8	11.4	18	25.7	55	78.6	24	34.3	39	55.7
Colorado	74	63	85.1	21	28.4	42	56.8	43	58.1	18	24.3	38	51.4	63	85.1	39	52.7	43	58.1
Idaho	26	20	76.9	6	23.1	23	88.5	10	38.5	19	73.1	15	57.7	24	92.3	15	57.7	13	50
Montana	45	30	66.7	7	15.6	34	75.6	14	31.1	26	57.8	22	48.9	34	75.6	17	37.8	21	46.7
Nevada	32	16	50	6	18.8	9	28.1	7	21.9	7	21.9	4	12.5	22	68.8	4	12.5	16	50
New Mexico	31	18	58.1	7	22.6	16	51.6	10	32.3	4	12.9	10	32.3	25	80.6	9	29	11	35.5
Utah	36	32	88.9	20	55.6	12	33.3	18	50	4	11.1	22	61.1	34	94.4	27	75	22	61.1
Wyoming	22	10	45.5	3	13.6	14	63.6	6	27.3	8	36.4	7	31.8	13	59.1	8	36.4	6	27.3
CENSUS DIVISION 9, PACIFIC	411	318	77.4	99	24.1	177	43.1	217	52.8	77	18.7	117	28.5	378	92	166	40.4	249	60.6
Alaska	9	7	77.8	2	22.2	7	77.8	3	33.3	7	77.8	4	44.4	7	77.8	3	33.3	3	33.3
California	268	203	75.7	69	25.7	92	34.3	150	56	35	13.1	49	18.3	246	91.8	95	35.4	152	56.7
Hawaii	15	10	66.7	2	13.3	6	40	8	53.3	4	26.7	3	20	14	93.3	9	60	12	80
Oregon	60	49	81.7	13	21.7	44	73.3	25	41.7	25	41.7	29	48.3	56	93.3	31	51.7	43	71.7
Washington	59	49	83.1	13	22	28	47.5	31	52.5	13	22	32	54.2	55	93.2	28	47.5	39	66.1

Note: The 2021 performance data do not reflect the full impact of the COVID-19 pandemic. Please refer to the discussion in the Introduction for more information.

AHA Hospital Statistics © 2023 Health Forum LLC, an affiliate of the American Hospital Association

Table 7 (Continued)

These data include only hospital-based facilities and services as reported by responding hospitals in Section C of the 2022 AHA Annual Survey, beginning on page 215. Census divisions represent all U.S. hospitals. Community hospitals are listed separately under United States. No estimates have been made for nonresponding hospitals. Definitions of facilities and services are listed in the Glossary, page 203.

CLASSIFICATION	HOSPITALS REPORTING	SWING BED SERVICES Number	Percent	TEEN OUTREACH SERVICES Number	Percent	TELEHEALTH Number	Percent	TOBACCO TREATMENT/ CESSATION PROGRAM Number	Percent	TRANSPORTATION TO HEALTH FACILITIES Number	Percent	URGENT CARE CENTER Number	Percent	VIOLENCE PREVENTION PROGRAM - COMMUNITY Number	Percent	VIOLENCE PREVENTION PROGRAM - WORKPLACE Number	Percent	VIRTUAL COLONOSCOPY Number	Percent	VOLUNTEER SERVICES DEPARTMENT Number	Percent	WOMEN'S HEALTH SERVICES Number	Percent	WOUND MANAGEMENT SERVICES Number	Percent
UNITED STATES	4,097	1,142	27.9	470	11.5	3,077	75.1	2,130	52	863	21.1	915	22.3	556	13.6	2,649	64.7	669	16.3	2,919	71.2	2,150	52.5	2,875	70.2
COMMUNITY HOSPITALS	3,682	1,122	30.5	444	12.1	2,815	76.5	1,961	53.3	753	20.5	886	24.1	520	14.1	2,461	66.8	660	17.9	2,786	75.7	2,097	57	2,772	75.3
CENSUS DIVISION 1, NEW ENGLAND	148	41	27.7	37	25	132	89.2	101	68.2	45	30.4	49	33.1	32	21.6	121	81.8	40	27	123	83.1	109	73.6	117	79.1
Connecticut	24	4	16.7	11	45.8	22	91.7	20	83.3	7	29.2	6	25	8	33.3	22	91.7	12	50	20	83.3	20	83.3	19	79.2
Maine	29	15	51.7	6	20.7	26	89.7	24	82.8	7	24.1	12	41.4	3	10.3	21	72.4	4	13.8	23	79.3	22	75.9	26	89.7
Massachusetts	50	4	8	14	28	44	88	26	52	17	34	16	32	16	32	42	84	15	30	42	84	32	64	35	70
New Hampshire	26	12	46.2	4	15.4	22	84.6	15	57.7	7	26.9	11	42.3	4	15.4	20	76.9	6	23.1	22	84.6	23	88.5	21	80.8
Rhode Island	9	1	11.1	1	11.1	8	88.9	6	66.7	5	55.6	0	0	1	11.1	7	77.8	1	11.1	7	77.8	6	66.7	8	88.9
Vermont	10	5	50	1	10	10	100	10	100	2	20	4	40	0	0	9	90	2	20	9	90	6	60	8	80
CENSUS DIVISION 2, MIDDLE ATLANTIC	357	42	11.8	84	23.5	310	86.8	240	67.2	102	28.6	80	22.4	97	27.2	289	81	101	28.3	294	82.4	223	62.5	271	75.9
New Jersey	71	5	7	23	32.4	66	93	45	63.4	36	50.7	13	18.3	24	33.8	64	90.1	23	32.4	56	78.9	45	63.4	56	78.9
New York	122	17	13.9	38	31.1	114	93.4	92	75.4	38	31.1	42	34.4	43	35.2	109	89.3	37	30.3	110	90.2	97	79.5	94	77
Pennsylvania	164	20	12.2	23	14	130	79.3	103	62.8	28	17.1	25	15.2	30	18.3	116	70.7	41	25	128	78	81	49.4	121	73.8
CENSUS DIVISION 3, SOUTH ATLANTIC	541	81	15	68	12.6	396	73.2	310	57.3	128	23.7	106	19.6	76	14	377	69.7	115	21.3	443	81.9	337	62.3	415	76.7
Delaware	8	0	0	2	25	5	62.5	5	62.5	1	12.5	4	50	1	12.5	8	100	1	12.5	6	75	5	55.6	8	100
District of Columbia	9	0	0	5	55.6	9	100	6	66.7	1	11.1	1	11.1	3	33.3	8	88.9	1	11.1	9	100	5	55.6	9	100
Florida	154	15	9.7	19	12.3	101	65.6	87	56.5	34	22.1	21	13.6	23	14.9	104	67.5	39	25.3	123	79.9	92	59.7	116	75.3
Georgia	88	24	27.3	5	5.7	70	79.5	48	54.5	20	22.7	23	26.1	3	3.4	64	72.7	12	13.6	67	76.1	48	54.5	62	70.5
Maryland	40	1	2.5	14	35	37	92.5	32	80	17	42.5	7	17.5	18	45	37	92.5	10	25	39	97.5	33	82.5	35	87.5
North Carolina	68	7	10.3	7	10.3	55	80.9	46	67.6	22	32.4	22	32.4	12	17.6	47	69.1	19	27.9	62	91.2	52	76.5	55	80.9
South Carolina	78	9	11.5	8	10.3	39	50	30	38.5	8	10.3	6	7.7	4	5.1	44	56.4	8	10.3	56	71.8	38	48.7	52	66.7
Virginia	59	8	13.6	5	8.5	52	88.1	31	52.5	14	23.7	11	18.6	7	11.9	44	74.6	16	27.1	52	88.1	40	67.8	54	91.5
West Virginia	37	17	45.9	3	8.1	28	75.7	25	67.6	11	29.7	11	29.7	5	13.5	21	56.8	8	21.6	29	78.4	24	64.9	24	64.9
CENSUS DIVISION 4, EAST NORTH CENTRAL	621	150	24.2	93	15	502	80.8	367	59.1	144	23.2	242	39	114	18.4	405	65.2	123	19.8	487	78.4	375	60.4	420	67.6
Illinois	138	42	30.4	23	16.7	117	84.8	72	52.2	44	31.9	52	37.7	28	20.3	110	79.7	31	22.5	115	83.3	80	58	99	71.7
Indiana	108	33	30.6	12	11.1	86	79.6	72	66.7	19	17.6	27	25	13	12	57	52.8	17	15.7	78	72.2	59	54.6	77	71.3
Michigan	120	28	23.3	22	18.3	109	90.8	85	70.8	33	27.5	49	40.8	23	19.2	98	81.7	23	19.2	105	87.5	85	70.8	91	75.8
Ohio	108	23	21.3	22	20.4	83	76.9	86	79.6	35	32.4	40	37	25	23.1	89	82.4	27	25	92	85.2	74	68.5	88	81.5
Wisconsin	147	24	16.3	14	9.5	107	72.8	52	35.4	13	8.8	74	50.3	25	17	51	34.7	25	17	97	66	77	52.4	65	44.2
CENSUS DIVISION 5, EAST SOUTH CENTRAL	285	109	38.2	22	7.7	182	63.9	123	43.2	41	14.4	34	11.9	22	7.7	145	50.9	36	12.6	183	64.2	115	40.4	169	59.3
Alabama	52	11	21.2	2	3.8	33	63.5	24	46.2	6	11.5	8	15.4	1	1.9	30	57.7	8	15.4	36	69.2	22	42.3	34	65.4
Kentucky	72	28	38.9	8	11.1	54	75	32	44.4	10	13.9	14	19.4	11	15.3	33	45.8	11	15.3	54	75	37	51.4	44	61.1
Mississippi	96	54	56.3	6	6.3	44	45.8	21	21.9	15	15.6	6	6.3	2	2.1	33	34.4	10	10.4	52	54.2	25	26	45	46.9
Tennessee	65	16	24.6	6	9.2	51	78.5	46	70.8	10	15.4	6	9.2	8	12.3	49	75.4	7	10.8	41	63.1	31	47.7	46	70.8
CENSUS DIVISION 6, WEST NORTH CENTRAL	556	330	59.4	51	9.2	437	78.6	282	50.7	131	23.6	141	25.4	64	11.5	332	59.7	73	13.1	373	67.1	247	44.4	408	73.4
Iowa	122	88	72.1	11	9	95	77.9	66	54.1	23	18.9	30	24.6	13	10.7	60	49.2	14	11.5	95	77.9	62	50.8	92	75.4
Kansas	120	82	68.3	3	2.5	80	66.7	43	35.8	24	20	30	25	5	4.2	58	48.3	17	14.2	61	50.8	43	35.8	84	70
Minnesota	94	52	55.3	15	16	84	89.4	68	72.3	18	19.1	36	38.3	11	11.7	80	85.1	11	11.7	75	79.8	49	52.1	72	76.6
Missouri	130	48	36.9	10	7.7	98	75.4	61	46.9	44	33.8	27	20.8	20	15.4	88	67.7	19	14.6	91	70	60	46.2	98	75.4
Nebraska	39	22	56.4	3	7.7	35	89.7	25	64.1	15	38.5	6	15.4	5	12.8	23	59	8	20.5	25	64.1	19	48.7	31	79.5
North Dakota	12	5	41.7	2	16.7	11	91.7	6	50	4	33.3	4	33.3	5	41.7	8	66.7	2	16.7	7	58.3	5	41.7	6	50
South Dakota	39	33	84.6	7	17.9	34	87.2	13	33.3	3	7.7	14	35.9	4	10.3	15	38.5	2	5.1	19	48.7	9	23.1	27	69.2
CENSUS DIVISION 7, WEST SOUTH CENTRAL	842	200	23.8	43	5.1	510	60.6	312	37.1	124	14.7	88	10.5	52	6.2	425	50.5	71	8.4	428	50.8	304	36.1	496	58.9
Arkansas	98	37	37.8	5	5.1	70	71.4	46	46.9	19	19.4	12	12.2	6	6.1	49	50	7	7.1	54	55.1	33	33.7	54	55.1
Louisiana	79	17	21.5	12	15.2	60	75.9	46	58.2	19	24.1	15	19	6	7.6	45	57	5	6.3	40	50.6	39	49.4	51	64.6
Oklahoma	99	35	35.4	4	4	71	71.7	49	49.5	22	22.2	14	14.1	4	4	61	61.6	3	3	61	61.6	43	43.4	56	56.6
Texas	566	111	19.6	22	3.9	309	54.6	171	30.2	64	11.3	47	8.3	36	6.4	270	47.7	56	9.9	273	48.2	189	33.4	337	59.5
CENSUS DIVISION 8, MOUNTAIN	336	119	35.4	28	8.3	262	78	175	52.1	59	17.6	75	22.3	51	15.2	212	63.1	44	13.1	241	71.7	185	55.1	247	73.5
Arizona	70	7	10	6	8.6	46	65.7	35	50	7	10	10	14.3	4	5.7	44	62.9	13	18.6	51	72.9	33	47.1	54	77.1
Colorado	74	25	33.8	5	6.8	60	81.1	43	58.1	12	16.2	15	20.3	9	12.2	48	64.9	9	12.2	62	83.8	52	70.3	63	85.1
Idaho	26	17	65.4	8	30.8	20	76.9	18	69.2	9	34.6	11	42.3	4	15.4	17	65.4	3	11.5	21	80.8	16	61.5	19	73.1
Montana	45	35	77.8	3	6.7	41	91.1	19	42.2	14	31.1	17	37.8	1	2.2	25	55.6	6	13.3	28	62.2	21	46.7	32	71.1
Nevada	32	5	15.6	0	0	22	68.8	12	37.5	6	18.8	6	18.8	4	12.5	22	68.8	3	9.4	16	50	9	28.1	17	53.1
New Mexico	31	9	29	1	3.2	21	67.7	13	41.9	5	16.1	8	25.8	3	9.7	13	41.9	2	6.5	21	67.7	17	54.8	19	61.3
Utah	36	9	25	4	11.1	34	94.4	27	75	1	2.8	3	8.3	24	66.7	27	75	4	11.1	27	75	27	75	30	83.3
Wyoming	22	12	54.5	1	4.5	18	81.8	8	36.4	5	22.7	5	22.7	2	9.1	16	72.7	4	18.2	15	68.2	10	45.5	13	59.1
CENSUS DIVISION 9, PACIFIC	411	70	17	44	10.7	346	84.2	220	53.5	89	21.7	100	24.3	48	11.7	343	83.5	66	16.1	347	84.4	255	62	332	80.8
Alaska	9	4	44.4	2	22.2	7	77.8	4	44.4	0	0	1	11.1	1	11.1	9	100			4	44.4	8	88.9	7	77.8
California	268	26	9.7	32	11.9	220	82.1	128	47.8	63	23.5	59	22	39	14.6	227	84.7	47	17.5	227	84.7	149	55.6	209	78
Hawaii	15	3	20	1	6.7	13	86.7	9	60	3	20	3	20	1	6.7	12	80	3	20	12	80	10	66.7	12	80
Oregon	60	26	43.3	7	11.7	53	88.3	45	75	15	25	22	36.7	1	1.7	47	78.3	11	18.3	55	91.7	45	75	56	93.3
Washington	59	11	18.6	2	3.4	53	89.8	34	57.6	8	13.6	14	23.7	6	10.2	48	81.4	5	8.5	49	83.1	43	72.9	48	81.4

Note: The 2021 performance data do not reflect the full impact of the COVID-19 pandemic. Please refer to the discussion in the Introduction for more information.

Table 7 (Continued)

These data include only hospital-based facilities and services as reported by responding hospitals in Section C of the 2022 AHA Annual Survey, beginning on page 215. Census divisions represent all U.S. hospitals. Community hospitals are listed separately under United States. No estimates have been made for nonresponding hospitals. Definitions of facilities and services are listed in the Glossary, page 203.

CLASSIFICATION	HOSPITALS REPORTING	GENERAL MEDICAL SURGICAL CARE UNITS – ADULT UNITS #	%	PEDIATRIC UNITS #	%	HOUSING – ASSISTED LIVING #	%	RETIREMENT HOUSING #	%	SUPPORTIVE HOUSING SERVICES #	%	INTENSIVE CARE – CARDIAC UNITS #	%	MEDICAL SURGICAL UNITS #	%	NEONATAL UNITS #	%	OTHER UNITS #	%	PEDIATRIC UNITS #	%	LONG-TERM CARE – ACUTE LONG-TERM CARE UNITS #	%	SKILLED NURSING CARE UNITS #	%	INTERMEDIATE NURSING CARE UNITS #	%	OTHER LONG-TERM CARE UNITS #	%
UNITED STATES	4,097	3,377	82.4	1,384	33.8	131	3.2	87	2.1	103	2.5	957	23.4	2,430	59.3	918	22.4	435	10.6	346	8.4	214	5.2	666	16.3	278	6.8	131	3.2
COMMUNITY HOSPITALS	3,682	3,316	90.1	1,374	37.3	113	3.1	84	2.3	68	1.8	951	25.8	2,387	64.8	916	24.9	425	11.5	344	9.3	158	4.3	614	16.7	263	7.1	102	2.8
CENSUS DIVISION 1, NEW ENGLAND	148	120	81.1	56	37.8	7	4.7	8	5.4	5	3.4	33	22.3	103	69.6	27	18.2	13	8.8	13	8.8	7	4.7	18	12.2	17	11.5	4	2.7
Connecticut	24	20	83.3	8	33.3	3	12.5	3	12.5	1	4.2	6	25	19	79.2	11	45.8	5	20.8	1	4.2	1	4.2	2	8.3	1	4.2	0	0
Maine	29	26	89.7	11	37.9	2	6.9	3	10.3	0	0	3	10.3	19	65.5	2	6.9	2	6.9	2	6.9	0	0	5	17.2	5	17.2	1	3.4
Massachusetts	50	36	72	23	46	1	2	1	2	3	6	16	32	32	64	10	20	2	4	6	12	2	3.4	4	8	4	8	2	4
New Hampshire	26	22	84.6	10	38.5	1	3.8	1	3.8	1	3.8	6	23.1	17	65.4	3	11.5	3	11.5	2	7.7	2	7.7	7	26.9	5	19.2	1	3.8
Rhode Island	9	9	77.8	1	11.1	0	0	0	0	0	0	1	11.1	7	77.8	1	11.1	1	11.1	1	11.1	1	11.1	0	0	2	22.2	2	22.2
Vermont	10	9	90	3	30	0	0	0	0	0	0	1	10	7	70	1	10	1	10	1	10	0	0	2	20	0	0	0	0
CENSUS DIVISION 2, MIDDLE ATLANTIC	357	290	81.2	139	38.9	6	1.7	3	0.8	17	4.8	127	35.6	260	72.8	106	29.7	46	12.9	42	11.8	16	4.5	58	16.2	13	3.6	7	2
New Jersey	71	57	80.3	32	45.1	2	2.8	2	2.8	4	5.6	25	35.2	55	77.5	21	29.6	9	12.7	12	16.9	4	5.6	4	5.6	3	4.2	3	4.2
New York	122	110	90.2	64	52.5	3	2.5	2	1.6	9	7.4	59	48.4	103	84.4	43	35.2	20	16.4	21	17.2	4	3.3	30	24.6	5	4.1	4	3.3
Pennsylvania	164	123	75	43	26.2	1	0.6	0	0	4	2.4	46	28	102	62.2	42	25.6	17	10.4	9	5.5	8	4.9	24	14.6	5	3	0	0
CENSUS DIVISION 3, SOUTH ATLANTIC	541	453	83.7	189	34.9	8	1.5	2	0.4	10	1.8	167	30.9	405	74.9	148	27.4	88	16.3	59	10.9	34	6.3	84	15.5	51	9.4	20	3.7
Delaware	8	5	62.5	4	50	1	12.5	0	0	0	0	4	44.4	5	62.5	3	37.5	1	12.5	1	12.5	1	12.5	0	0	1	12.5	0	0
District of Columbia	9	5	55.6	2	22.2	0	0	1	11.1	0	0	2	22.2	5	55.6	5	55.6	2	22.2	2	22.2	0	0	2	22.2	0	0	1	11.1
Florida	154	127	82.5	39	25.3	1	0.6	1	0.6	4	2.6	59	38.3	120	77.9	47	30.5	30	19.5	24	15.6	11	7.1	15	9.7	7	4.5	5	3.2
Georgia	88	76	86.4	19	21.6	3	3.4	2	2.3	2	2.3	20	22.7	57	64.8	22	25	13	15	2	2.3	4	4.5	21	23.9	6	6.8	5	5.7
Maryland	40	37	92.5	26	65	2	5	2	5	1	2.5	10	25	37	92.5	14	35	6	15	3	7.5	2	5	6	15	6	15	2	5
North Carolina	68	62	91.2	32	47.1	0	0	0	0	1	1.5	23	33.8	58	85.3	20	29.4	15	22.1	9	13.2	3	4.4	10	14.7	6	8.8	1	1.5
South Carolina	78	58	74.4	32	41	0	0	0	0	3	3.4	18	23.1	51	65.4	10	12.8	16	20.5	7	9	7	9	13	16.7	14	17.9	2	2.6
Virginia	59	51	86.4	19	32.2	1	1.7	1	1.7	0	0	22	37.3	48	81.4	21	35.6	7	11.9	8	13.6	3	5.1	9	15.3	4	6.8	1	1.7
West Virginia	37	32	86.5	16	43.2	0	0	0	0	0	0	12	32.4	24	64.9	6	16.2	4	10.8	3	8.1	3	8.1	8	21.6	4	10.8	1	2.7
CENSUS DIVISION 4, EAST NORTH CENTRAL	621	537	86.5	274	44.1	18	2.9	13	2.1	14	2.3	167	26.9	391	63	119	19.2	110	17.7	58	9.3	20	3.2	68	11	19	3.1	19	3.1
Illinois	138	121	87.7	68	49.3	3	2.2	3	2.2	3	2.2	35	25.4	95	68.8	27	19.6	10	7.2	13	9.4	3	2.2	4	2.9	4	2.9	5	3.6
Indiana	108	92	85.2	43	39.8	2	1.9	2	1.9	2	1.9	21	19.4	68	63	22	20.4	8	7.4	9	8.3	7	6.5	10	9.3	8	7.4	3	2.8
Michigan	120	109	90.8	40	33.3	3	2.5	3	2.5	3	2.5	21	17.5	85	70.8	20	16.7	18	15	11	9.2	7	5.8	21	17.5	3	2.5	6	5
Ohio	108	89	82.4	27	25	3	2.8	3	2.8	1	0.9	31	28.7	76	70.4	18	16.7	10	9.3	8	7.4	2	1.9	12	11.1	2	1.9	3	2.8
Wisconsin	147	126	85.7	96	65.3	7	4.8	4	2.7	4	2.7	54	36.7	67	45.6	32	21.8	64	43.5	17	11.6	5	3.4	12	8.2	1	0.7	2	1.4
CENSUS DIVISION 5, EAST SOUTH CENTRAL	285	232	81.4	97	34	5	1.8	3	1.1	3	1.1	69	24.2	151	53	51	17.9	33	11.6	19	6.7	16	5.6	47	16.5	13	4.6	11	3.9
Alabama	52	38	73.1	14	26.9	1	1.9	1	1.9	1	1.9	16	30.8	30	57.7	10	19.2	11	21.2	3	5.8	2	3.8	3	5.8	4	7.7	2	3.8
Kentucky	72	59	81.9	18	25	0	0	0	0	0	0	16	22.2	45	62.5	15	20.8	8	11.1	3	4.2	4	5.6	12	16.7	3	4.2	1	1.4
Mississippi	96	83	86.5	50	52.1	3	3.1	1	1	1	1	23	24	35	36.5	13	13.5	2	2.1	5	5.2	7	7.3	22	22.9	3	3	6	6.3
Tennessee	65	52	80	15	23.1	1	1.5	1	1.5	1	1.5	14	21.5	41	63.1	13	20	12	18.5	8	12.3	3	4.6	10	15.4	3	4.6	2	3.1
CENSUS DIVISION 6, WEST NORTH CENTRAL	556	502	90.3	232	41.7	43	7.7	45	8.1	21	3.8	90	16.2	236	42.4	73	13.1	33	5.9	36	6.5	25	4.5	214	38.5	93	16.7	38	6.8
Iowa	122	114	93.4	56	45.9	7	5.7	11	9	2	1.6	13	10.7	48	39.3	16	13.1	6	4.9	7	5.7	3	2.5	53	43.4	24	19.7	6	4.9
Kansas	120	110	91.7	35	29.2	6	5	12	10	3	2.5	8	6.7	38	31.7	11	9.2	2	1.7	4	3.3	5	4.2	48	40	32	26.7	10	8.3
Minnesota	94	90	95.7	33	35.1	13	13.8	13	13.8	9	9.6	15	16	39	41.5	10	10.6	4	4.3	9	9.6	3	3.2	36	38.3	5	5.3	8	8.5
Missouri	130	104	80	73	56.2	1	0.8	1	0.8	3	2.3	37	28.5	75	57.7	20	15.4	14	10.8	7	5.4	9	6.9	33	25.4	12	9.2	2	1.5
Nebraska	39	35	89.7	13	33.3	3	7.7	3	7.7	1	2.6	8	20.5	16	41	8	20.5	4	10.3	3	7.7	3	7.7	20	51.3	8	20.5	5	12.8
North Dakota	12	11	91.7	6	50	1	8.3	2	16.7	0	0	5	41.7	6	50	5	41.7	2	16.7	4	33.3	1	8.3	4	33.3	3	25	1	8.3
South Dakota	39	38	97.4	16	41	13	33.3	8	20.5	2	5.1	4	10.3	14	35.9	3	7.7	1	2.6	2	5.1	1	2.6	20	51.3	9	23.1	6	15.4
CENSUS DIVISION 7, WEST SOUTH CENTRAL	842	591	70.2	158	18.8	14	1.7	7	0.8	10	1.2	116	13.8	356	42.3	169	20.1	55	6.5	48	5.7	67	8	48	5.7	23	2.7	7	0.8
Arkansas	98	72	73.5	19	19.4	2	2	1	1	2	2	15	15.3	39	39.8	19	19.8	7	7.1	2	2	7	7.1	3	2.9	2	2	2	2
Louisiana	79	56	70.9	25	31.6	2	2.5	2	2.5	2	2.5	14	17.7	44	55.7	25	31.6	4	5.1	11	13.9	7	8.9	9	11.4	2	2.5	2	2.5
Oklahoma	99	80	80.8	27	27.3	1	1	1	1	3	3	13	13.1	42	42.4	12	12.1	7	7.1	7	7.1	3	3	14	14.1	10	10.1	2	2
Texas	566	383	67.7	87	15.4	9	1.6	5	0.9	3	0.5	70	12.4	231	40.8	122	21.6	37	6.5	32	5.7	50	8.8	15	2.7	9	1.6	1	0.2
CENSUS DIVISION 8, MOUNTAIN	336	285	84.8	107	31.8	20	6	10	2.9	11	3.3	57	17	199	59.2	77	22.9	20	6	27	8	19	5.6	58	17.3	31	9.2	18	5.4
Arizona	70	51	72.9	15	21.4	2	2.9	2	2.9	2	2.9	18	25.7	43	61.4	17	24.3	7	10	8	11.4	4	5.7	2	2.9	3	4.3	3	4.1
Colorado	74	70	94.6	20	27	6	8.1	3	4.1	3	4.1	13	17.6	53	71.6	25	33.8	5	6.8	5	6.8	1	1.4	8	10.8	7	9.5	3	4.1
Idaho	26	25	96.2	11	42.3	2	7.7	1	3.8	0	0	5	19.2	12	46.2	9	34.6	2	8.9	3	11.5	3	11.5	9	34.6	3	11.5	4	15.6
Montana	45	44	97.8	24	53.3	7	15.6	1	2.2	2	4.4	5	11.1	18	40.6	9	20	2	4.4	4	8.9	2	4.4	20	44.4	10	22.2	4	9.4
Nevada	32	16	50	5	15.6	1	3.1	0	0	1	3.1	3	9.4	24	74.2	4	12.5	3	9.4	2	6.3	6	18.8	4	12.5	6	18.8	0	0
New Mexico	31	27	87.1	11	35.5	0	0	0	0	0	0	5	16.1	16	52.8	4	12.9	3	9.7	3	9.7	1	3.2	1	3.2	3	9.7	1	3.2
Utah	36	33	91.7	12	33.3	0	0	0	0	1	2.8	8	22.2	23	63.6	9	25	3	8.3	3	8.3	1	2.8	8	22.2	1	2.8	1	2.8
Wyoming	22	19	86.4	9	40.9	2	9.1	0	0	2	9.1	0	0	14	63.6	0	0	0	0	1	5.6	0	0	6	27.3	2	9.1	2	9.1
CENSUS DIVISION 9, PACIFIC	411	367	89.3	132	32.1	10	2.4	3	0.7	12	2.9	131	31.9	329	80	148	36	37	9	44	10.7	12	2.9	71	17.3	18	4.4	7	1.7
Alaska	9	8	88.9	3	33.3	3	33.3	0	0	0	0	2	22.2	6	66.7	0	0	0	0	0	0	3	33.3	4	44.4	4	44.4	1	11.1
California	268	235	87.7	88	32.8	9	3.3	2	0.7	10	3.7	102	38.1	220	82.1	120	44.8	20	7.5	35	13.1	8	3	60	22.4	8	3	4	1.5
Hawaii	15	12	73.3	4	26.7	0	0	0	0	0	0	3	20	11	73.3	2	13.3	3	20	2	13.3	0	0	1	8.3	4	26.7	0	0
Oregon	60	59	98.3	21	35	2	3.3	1	1.7	1	1.7	10	16.7	49	81.7	11	18.3	6	10	4	6.7	5	8.3	1	1.7	4	6.7	4	6.7
Washington	59	54	91.5	16	27.1	2	3.4	0	0	1	1.7	14	23.7	43	72.9	14	23.7	8	13.6	3	5.1	1	1.7	10	8.3	2	3.4	2	3.4

Note: The 2021 performance data do not reflect the full impact of the COVID-19 pandemic. Please refer to the discussion in the Introduction for more information.

Table 7 (Continued)

These data include only hospital-based facilities and services as reported by responding hospitals in Section C of the 2022 AHA Annual Survey, beginning on page 215. Census divisions represent all U.S. hospitals. Community hospitals are listed separately under United States. No estimates have been made for nonresponding hospitals. Definitions of facilities and services are listed in the Glossary, page 203.

CARDIOLOGY AND CARDIAC SERVICES

CLASSIFICATION	HOSPITALS REPORTING	Adult Cardiology Services — Number	Percent	Pediatric Cardiology Services — Number	Percent	Adult Diagnostic Catheterization — Number	Percent	Pediatric Diagnostic Catheterization — Number	Percent	Adult Interventional Cardiac Catheterization — Number	Percent	Pediatric Interventional Cardiac Catheterization — Number	Percent	Adult Cardiac Surgery — Number	Percent	Pediatric Cardiac Surgery — Number	Percent	Adult Cardiac Electro-Physiology — Number	Percent	Pediatric Cardiac Electro-Physiology — Number	Percent	Cardiac Rehabilitation — Number	Percent
UNITED STATES	4,097	2,178	53.2	368	9	1,633	39.9	162	4	1,503	36.7	149	3.6	988	24.1	140	3.4	1,362	33.2	174	4.2	2,267	55.3
COMMUNITY HOSPITALS	3,682	2,139	58.1	367	10	1,609	43.7	162	4.4	1,478	40.1	149	4	969	26.3	140	3.8	1,339	36.4	174	4.7	2,238	60.8
CENSUS DIVISION 1, NEW ENGLAND	148	94	63.5	15	10.1	58	39.2	8	5.4	46	31.1	8	5.4	28	18.9	6	4.1	56	37.8	7	4.7	102	68.9
Connecticut	24	20	83.3	3	12.5	14	58.3	1	4.2	12	50	1	4.2	9	37.5	1	4.2	16	66.7	2	8.3	19	79.2
Maine	29	17	58.6	2	6.9	7	24.1	1	3.4	2	6.9	1	3.4	2	6.9	1	3.4	6	20.7	2	6.9	20	69
Massachusetts	50	32	64	6	12	21	42	3	6	19	38	3	6	11	22	2	4	19	38	1	2	30	60
New Hampshire	26	13	50	2	7.7	9	34.6	1	3.8	9	34.6	1	3.8	4	15.4	1	3.8	9	34.6	1	3.8	21	80.8
Rhode Island	9	7	77.8	1	11.1	6	66.7	1	11.1	3	33.3	1	11.1	1	11.1			5	55.6			5	55.6
Vermont	10	5	50	1	10	1	10	1	10	1	10	1	10	1	10	1	10	1	10	1	10	7	70
CENSUS DIVISION 2, MIDDLE ATLANTIC	357	251	70.3	56	15.7	186	52.1	16	4.5	171	47.9	14	3.9	90	25.2	13	3.6	153	42.9	20	5.6	201	56.3
New Jersey	71	52	73.2	14	19.7	45	63.4	1	1.4	40	56.3	1	1.4	16	22.5	1	1.4	26	36.6	2	2.8	44	62
New York	122	94	77	31	25.4	57	46.7	9	7.4	52	42.6	8	6.6	25	20.5	7	5.7	55	45.1	10	8.2	67	54.9
Pennsylvania	164	105	64	11	6.7	84	51.2	6	3.7	79	48.2	5	3	49	29.9	5	3	72	43.9	8	4.9	90	54.9
CENSUS DIVISION 3, SOUTH ATLANTIC	541	376	69.5	56	10.4	297	54.9	28	5.2	268	49.5	25	4.6	164	30.3	25	4.6	246	45.5	27	5	316	58.4
Delaware	8	5	62.5			5	62.5			5	62.5			4	50			3	37.5			6	75
District of Columbia	9	5	55.6	1	11.1	5	55.6	1	11.1	3	33.3	1	11.1	3	33.3	1	11.1	4	44.4	1	11.1	3	33.3
Florida	154	117	76	26	16.9	99	64.3	12	7.8	97	63	10	6.5	66	42.9	10	6.5	84	54.5	10	6.5	79	51.3
Georgia	88	52	59.1	1	1.1	43	48.9	1	1.1	39	44.3	1	1.1	18	20.5	1	1.1	37	42	1	1.1	43	48.9
Maryland	40	33	82.5	6	15	25	62.5	2	5	22	55	2	5	9	22.5	2	5	25	62.5	5	12.5	28	70
North Carolina	68	55	80.9	8	11.8	42	61.8	5	7.4	36	52.9	5	7.4	23	33.8	4	5.9	31	45.6	2	2.9	51	75
South Carolina	78	41	52.6	5	6.4	30	38.5	2	2.6	20	25.6	1	1.3	19	24.4	1	1.3	21	26.9	5	6.4	38	48.7
Virginia	59	46	78	7	11.9	34	57.6	4	6.8	33	55.9	4	6.8	16	27.1	5	8.5	32	54.2	2	3.4	44	74.6
West Virginia	37	22	59.5	2	5.4	14	37.8	1	2.7	13	35.1	1	2.7	6	16.2	1	2.7	9	24.3	1	2.7	24	64.9
CENSUS DIVISION 4, EAST NORTH CENTRAL	621	358	57.6	63	10.1	266	42.8	18	2.9	241	38.8	20	3.2	167	26.9	18	2.9	232	37.4	21	3.4	452	72.8
Illinois	138	100	72.5	24	17.4	73	52.9	7	5.1	70	50.7	7	5.1	49	35.5	7	5.1	65	47.1	8	5.8	105	76.1
Indiana	108	62	57.4	9	8.3	38	35.2	2	1.9	34	31.5	3	2.8	24	22.2	2	1.9	34	31.5	3	2.8	74	68.5
Michigan	120	77	64.2	18	15	52	43.3	3	2.5	44	36.7	3	2.5	32	26.7	3	2.5	52	43.3	3	2.5	88	73.3
Ohio	108	75	69.4	8	7.4	56	51.9	5	4.6	47	43.5	6	5.6	35	32.4	5	4.6	50	46.3	6	5.6	73	67.6
Wisconsin	147	44	29.9	4	2.7	47	32	1	0.7	46	31.3	1	0.7	27	18.4	1	0.7	31	21.1	1	0.7	112	76.2
CENSUS DIVISION 5, EAST SOUTH CENTRAL	285	135	47.4	18	6.3	96	33.7	10	3.5	80	28.1	7	2.5	56	19.6	9	3.2	71	24.9	13	4.6	136	47.7
Alabama	52	29	55.8	3	5.8	23	44.2	3	5.8	18	34.6	1	1.9	17	32.7	2	3.8	17	32.7	3	5.8	27	51.9
Kentucky	72	43	59.7	5	6.9	29	40.3	2	2.8	24	33.3	2	2.8	16	22.2	3	4.2	26	36.1	5	6.9	46	63.9
Mississippi	96	25	26	3	3.1	16	16.7	1	1	14	14.6	1	1	11	11.5	1	1	9	9.4	1	1	24	25
Tennessee	65	38	58.5	7	10.8	28	43.1	4	6.2	24	36.9	3	4.6	12	18.5	3	4.6	19	29.2	4	6.2	39	60
CENSUS DIVISION 6, WEST NORTH CENTRAL	556	219	39.4	38	6.8	138	24.8	16	2.9	133	23.9	15	2.7	81	14.6	13	2.3	117	21	19	3.4	411	73.9
Iowa	122	41	33.6	5	4.1	23	18.9	2	1.6	23	18.9	2	1.6	12	9.8	2	1.6	21	17.2	2	1.6	105	86.1
Kansas	120	31	25.8	5	4.2	21	17.5	1	0.8	22	18.3	1	0.8	14	11.7			14	11.7	2	1.7	64	53.3
Minnesota	94	42	44.7	7	7.4	16	17	2	2.1	16	17	2	2.1	12	12.8	2	2.1	16	17	3	3.2	82	87.2
Missouri	130	74	56.9	11	8.5	53	40.8	3	2.3	50	38.5	3	2.3	29	22.3	4	3.1	46	35.4	7	5.4	89	68.5
Nebraska	39	16	41	3	7.7	13	33.3	3	7.7	12	30.8	3	7.7	6	15.4	2	5.1	12	30.8	3	7.7	31	79.5
North Dakota	12	4	33.3	3	25	4	33.3	1	8.3	4	33.3	1	8.3	4	33.3	2	16.7	4	33.3	1	8.3	6	50
South Dakota	39	11	28.2	4	10.3	8	20.5	4	10.3	6	15.4	3	7.7	4	10.3	1	2.6	4	10.3	1	2.6	34	87.2
CENSUS DIVISION 7, WEST SOUTH CENTRAL	842	318	37.8	48	5.7	268	31.8	27	3.2	258	30.6	28	3.3	185	22	25	3	210	24.9	28	3.3	308	36.6
Arkansas	98	31	31.6	3	3.1	27	27.6	1	1	27	27.6	1	1	17	17.3	1	1	17	17.3	1	1	30	30.6
Louisiana	79	37	46.8	9	11.4	32	40.5	5	6.3	32	40.5	5	6.3	25	31.6	5	6.3	28	35.4	5	6.3	31	39.2
Oklahoma	99	44	44.4	4	4	30	30.3	2	2	29	29.3	2	2	13	13.1	2	2	21	21.2	5	5	35	35.4
Texas	566	206	36.4	32	5.7	179	31.6	19	3.4	170	30	20	3.5	130	23	17	3	144	25.4	17	3	212	37.5
CENSUS DIVISION 8, MOUNTAIN	336	161	47.9	24	7.1	120	35.7	13	3.9	121	36	10	3	74	22	10	3	96	28.6	12	3.6	155	46.1
Arizona	70	46	65.7	6	8.6	38	54.3	3	4.3	39	55.7	2	2.9	23	32.9	3	4.3	31	44.3	3	4.3	32	45.7
Colorado	74	48	64.9	5	6.8	39	52.7	2	2.7	39	52.7	2	2.7	21	28.4	2	2.7	31	41.9	3	4.1	41	55.4
Idaho	26	7	26.9	2	7.7	7	26.9	2	7.7	7	26.9	1	3.8	5	19.2	1	3.8	5	19.2	1	3.8	12	46.2
Montana	45	10	22.2	3	6.7	9	20	1	2.2	9	20	1	2.2	6	13.3			6	13.3	1	2.2	25	55.6
Nevada	32	9	28.1	2	6.3	7	21.9	1	3.1	7	21.9	1	3.1	7	21.9	1	3.1	7	21.9	2	6.3	7	21.9
New Mexico	31	16	51.6	4	12.9	8	25.8	3	9.7	8	25.8	2	6.5	5	16.1	2	6.5	7	22.6	2	6.5	10	32.3
Utah	36	18	50	1	2.8	9	25	1	2.8	9	25	1	2.8	6	16.7	1	2.8	7	19.4			13	36.1
Wyoming	22	7	31.8	1	4.5	3	13.6			3	13.6			1	4.5			2	9.1			15	68.2
CENSUS DIVISION 9, PACIFIC	411	266	64.7	50	12.2	204	49.6	26	6.3	185	45	22	5.4	143	34.8	21	5.1	181	44	27	6.6	186	45.3
Alaska	9	2	22.2			2	22.2			2	22.2											4	44.4
California	268	187	69.8	38	14.2	141	52.6	14	5.2	127	47.4	14	5.2	102	38.1	15	5.6	129	48.1	19	7.1	110	41
Hawaii	15	7	46.7	2	13.3	7	46.7	3	20	7	46.7	2	13.3	6	40	2	13.3	8	53.3	2	13.3	6	40
Oregon	60	31	51.7	6	10	23	38.3	5	8.3	21	35	2	3.3	15	25	2	3.3	20	33.3	3	5	34	56.7
Washington	59	39	66.1	4	6.8	31	52.5	4	6.8	28	47.5	4	6.8	20	33.9	2	3.4	24	40.7	3	5.1	32	54.2

Note: The 2021 performance data do not reflect the full impact of the COVID-19 pandemic. Please refer to the discussion in the Introduction for more information.

These data include only hospital-based facilities and services as reported by responding hospitals in Section C of the 2022 AHA Annual Survey, beginning on page 215. Census divisions represent all U.S. hospitals. Community hospitals are listed separately under United States. No estimates have been made for nonresponding hospitals. Definitions of facilities and services are listed in the Glossary, page 203.

Table 7 (Continued)

| | | EMERGENCY SERVICES | | | | | | | | ENDOSCOPIC SERVICES | | | | | | | | | |
| | HOSPITALS REPORTING | OFF-CAMPUS EMERGENCY DEPARTMENT | | ON-CAMPUS EMERGENCY DEPARTMENT | | PEDIATRIC EMERGENCY DEPARTMENT | | TRAUMA CENTER (CERTIFIED) | | ENDOSCOPIC ULTRASOUND | | ABLATION OF BARRETT'S ESOPHAGUS | | ESOPHAGEAL IMPEDANCE STUDY | | ENDOSCOPIC RETROGRADE CHOLANGIO-PANCREATOGRAPHY | | OPTICAL COLONOSCOPY | |
CLASSIFICATION		Number	Percent	Number	Percent	Number	Percent	Number	Percent	Number	Percent	Number	Percent	Number	Percent	Number	Percent	Number	Percent
UNITED STATES	4,097	328	8	3,327	81.2	894	21.8	1,670	40.8	1,583	38.6	1,174	28.7	1,135	27.7	1,719	42	2,747	67
COMMUNITY HOSPITALS	3,682	326	8.9	3,275	88.9	889	24.1	1,663	45.2	1,557	42.3	1,153	31.3	1,113	30.2	1,693	46	2,700	73.3
CENSUS DIVISION 1, NEW ENGLAND	148	9	6.1	120	81.1	35	23.6	44	29.7	69	46.6	58	39.2	56	37.8	74	50	110	74.3
Connecticut	24	5	20.8	20	83.3	8	33.3	10	41.7	16	66.7	15	62.5	14	58.3	19	79.2	19	79.2
Maine	29	3	10.3	26	89.7	4	13.8	6	20.7	10	34.5	6	20.7	7	24.1	8	27.6	23	79.3
Massachusetts	50	1	2	36	72	13	26	16	32	26	52	18	36	19	38	26	52	31	62
New Hampshire	26	0	0	22	84.6	9	34.6	10	38.5	11	42.3	12	46.2	11	42.3	13	50	22	84.6
Rhode Island	9	0	0	7	77.8	1	11.1	1	11.1	4	44.4	5	55.6	3	33.3	5	55.6	7	77.8
Vermont	10	0	0	9	90	0	0	1	10	2	20	2	20	2	20	3	30	8	80
CENSUS DIVISION 2, MIDDLE ATLANTIC	357	20	5.6	280	78.4	105	29.4	95	26.6	200	56	146	40.9	125	35	210	58.8	260	72.8
New Jersey	71	9	12.7	53	74.6	31	43.7	10	14.1	48	67.6	36	50.7	30	42.3	47	66.2	50	70.4
New York	122	8	6.6	105	86.1	51	41.8	43	35.2	76	62.3	62	50.8	49	40.2	81	66.4	99	81.1
Pennsylvania	164	3	1.8	122	74.4	23	14	42	25.6	76	46.3	48	29.3	46	28	82	50	111	67.7
CENSUS DIVISION 3, SOUTH ATLANTIC	541	80	14.8	447	82.6	129	23.8	143	26.4	269	49.7	205	37.9	209	38.6	318	58.8	414	76.5
Delaware	8	2	25	5	62.5	2	25	5	62.5	6	50	4	50	4	50	5	62.5	5	62.5
District of Columbia	9	1	11.1	6	66.7	1	11.1	4	44.4	6	66.7	3	33.3	5	55.6	6	66.7	6	66.7
Florida	154	35	22.7	126	81.8	46	29.9	29	18.8	87	56.5	65	42.2	64	41.6	109	70.8	122	79.2
Georgia	88	2	2.3	73	83	15	17	21	23.9	38	43.2	29	33	30	34.1	46	52.3	63	71.6
Maryland	40	1	2.5	37	92.5	18	45	10	25	22	55	18	45	17	42.5	30	75	33	82.5
North Carolina	68	10	14.7	62	91.2	12	17.6	18	26.5	38	55.9	27	39.7	28	41.2	41	60.3	62	91.2
South Carolina	78	9	11.5	54	69.2	6	7.7	17	21.8	27	34.6	19	24.4	18	23.1	30	38.5	45	57.7
Virginia	59	17	28.8	52	88.1	24	40.7	18	30.5	34	57.6	29	49.2	29	49.2	36	61	49	83.1
West Virginia	37	3	8.1	32	86.5	5	13.5	21	56.8	13	35.1	11	29.7	14	37.8	15	40.5	29	78.4
CENSUS DIVISION 4, EAST NORTH CENTRAL	621	57	9.2	531	85.5	141	22.7	293	47.2	246	39.6	196	31.6	184	29.6	263	42.4	417	67.1
Illinois	138	7	5.1	123	89.1	42	30.4	48	34.8	69	50	56	40.6	48	34.8	79	57.2	115	83.3
Indiana	108	9	8.3	89	82.4	18	16.7	19	17.6	38	35.2	33	30.6	28	25.9	43	39.8	78	72.2
Michigan	120	18	15	105	87.5	29	24.2	80	66.7	57	47.5	37	30.8	44	36.7	57	47.5	99	82.5
Ohio	108	23	21.3	89	82.4	28	25.9	37	34.3	46	42.6	37	34.3	43	39.8	50	46.3	75	69.4
Wisconsin	147	0	0	125	85	24	16.3	109	74.1	36	24.5	33	22.4	21	14.3	34	23.1	50	34
CENSUS DIVISION 5, EAST SOUTH CENTRAL	285	16	5.6	222	77.9	38	13.3	105	36.8	92	32.3	68	23.9	66	23.2	95	33.3	150	52.6
Alabama	52	7	13.5	39	75	8	15.4	23	44.2	23	44.2	13	25	12	23.1	23	44.2	33	63.5
Kentucky	72	4	5.6	60	83.3	8	11.1	14	19.4	22	30.6	24	33.3	23	31.9	33	45.8	43	59.7
Mississippi	96	2	2.1	72	75	7	7.3	62	64.6	20	20.8	12	12.5	11	11.5	14	14.6	34	35.4
Tennessee	65	3	4.6	51	78.5	15	23.1	6	9.2	27	41.5	19	29.2	20	30.8	25	38.5	40	61.5
CENSUS DIVISION 6, WEST NORTH CENTRAL	556	17	3.1	490	88.1	118	21.2	288	51.8	136	24.5	96	17.3	105	18.9	126	22.7	397	71.4
Iowa	122	1	0.8	114	93.4	19	15.6	93	76.2	24	19.7	16	13.1	16	13.1	18	14.8	96	78.7
Kansas	120	6	5	106	88.3	19	15.8	32	26.7	17	14.2	13	10.8	14	11.7	16	13.3	82	68.3
Minnesota	94	4	4.3	88	93.6	29	30.9	77	81.9	25	26.6	13	13.8	19	20.2	20	21.3	68	72.3
Missouri	130	3	2.3	96	73.8	25	19.2	29	22.3	43	33.1	32	24.6	33	25.4	52	40	86	66.2
Nebraska	39	2	5.1	36	92.3	15	38.5	20	51.3	16	41	13	33.3	14	35.9	11	28.2	30	76.9
North Dakota	12	0	0	11	91.7	2	16.7	9	75	5	41.7	3	25	2	16.7	4	33.3	10	83.3
South Dakota	39	1	2.6	39	100	9	23.1	28	71.8	6	15.4	6	15.4	7	17.9	5	12.8	25	64.1
CENSUS DIVISION 7, WEST SOUTH CENTRAL	842	83	9.9	597	70.9	123	14.6	354	42	222	26.4	154	18.3	142	16.9	251	29.8	443	52.6
Arkansas	98	4	4.1	74	75.5	6	6.1	47	48	21	21.4	11	11.2	15	15.3	19	19.4	63	64.3
Louisiana	79	9	11.4	54	68.4	15	19	12	15.2	31	39.2	17	21.5	16	20.3	30	38	46	58.2
Oklahoma	99	7	7.1	81	81.8	14	14.1	51	51.5	20	20.2	15	15.2	16	16.2	23	23.2	56	56.6
Texas	566	63	11.1	388	68.6	88	15.5	244	43.1	150	26.5	111	19.6	95	16.8	179	31.6	278	49.1
CENSUS DIVISION 8, MOUNTAIN	336	37	11	276	82.1	91	27.1	185	55.1	122	36.3	95	28.3	100	29.8	126	37.5	235	69.9
Arizona	70	7	10	48	68.6	19	27.1	28	40	33	47.1	27	38.6	27	38.6	35	50	46	65.7
Colorado	74	20	27	69	93.2	15	20.3	63	85.1	35	47.3	24	32.4	28	37.8	35	47.3	60	81.1
Idaho	26	2	7.7	25	96.2	8	30.8	17	65.4	12	46.2	7	26.9	7	26.9	8	30.8	21	80.8
Montana	45	2	4.4	44	97.8	13	28.9	29	64.4	9	20	7	15.6	9	20	9	20	26	57.8
Nevada	32	3	9.4	16	50	4	12.5	2	6.3	5	15.6	6	18.8	6	18.8	8	25	21	65.6
New Mexico	31	1	3.2	23	74.2	3	9.7	8	25.8	13	41.9	4	12.9	6	19.4	9	29	14	45.2
Utah	36	2	5.6	33	91.7	23	63.9	24	66.7	7	19.4	9	25	12	33.3	16	44.4	32	88.9
Wyoming	22	0	0	18	81.8	6	27.3	14	63.6	8	36.4	6	27.3	7	31.8	6	27.3	15	68.2
CENSUS DIVISION 9, PACIFIC	411	9	2.2	364	88.6	114	27.7	163	39.7	227	55.2	156	38	148	36	256	62.3	321	78.1
Alaska	9	0	0	8	88.9	2	22.2	4	44.4	3	33.3	2	22.2	2	22.2	2	22.2	6	66.7
California	268	1	0.4	229	85.4	86	32.1	70	26.1	159	59.3	107	39.9	103	38.4	190	70.9	204	76.1
Hawaii	15	0	0	13	86.7	4	26.7	7	46.7	7	46.7	4	26.7	5	33.3	10	66.7	8	53.3
Oregon	60	1	1.7	59	98.3	8	13.3	43	71.7	30	50	20	33.3	15	25	22	36.7	52	86.7
Washington	59	7	11.9	55	93.2	14	23.7	39	66.1	28	47.5	23	39	23	39	32	54.2	51	86.4

Note: The 2021 performance data do not reflect the full impact of the COVID-19 pandemic. Please refer to the discussion in the Introduction for more information.

AHA Hospital Statistics © 2023 Health Forum LLC, an affiliate of the American Hospital Association

Facilities and Services

Table 7 (Continued)

These data include only hospital-based facilities and services as reported by responding hospitals in Section C of the 2022 AHA Annual Survey, beginning on page 215. Census divisions represent all U.S. hospitals. Community hospitals are listed separately under United States. No estimates have been made for nonresponding hospitals. Definitions of facilities and services are listed in the Glossary, page 203.

CLASSIFICATION	HOSPITALS REPORTING Number	PHYSICAL REHABILITATION SERVICES — ASSISTIVE TECHNOLOGY CENTER Number	Percent	ELECTRODIAGNOSTIC SERVICES Number	Percent	PHYSICAL REHABILITATION OUTPATIENT SERVICES Number	Percent	PROSTHETIC ORTHOTIC SERVICES Number	Percent	ROBOT ASSISTED WALKING THERAPY Number	Percent	SIMULATED REHABILITATION ENVIRONMENT Number	Percent	PSYCHIATRIC SERVICES — PEDIATRIC CARE Number	Percent	CONSULTATION/ LIAISON SERVICES Number	Percent	EDUCATION SERVICES Number	Percent	EMERGENCY SERVICES Number	Percent
UNITED STATES	4,097	1,025	25	1,178	28.8	2,875	70.2	811	19.8	281	6.9	1,363	33.3	458	11.2	1,702	41.5	1,030	25.1	1,561	38.1
COMMUNITY HOSPITALS	3,682	970	26.3	1,141	31	2,801	76.1	759	20.6	267	7.3	1,324	36	299	8.1	1,481	40.2	817	22.2	1,423	38.6
CENSUS DIVISION 1, NEW ENGLAND	148	44	29.7	62	41.9	122	82.4	35	23.6	11	7.4	69	46.6	25	16.9	95	64.2	62	41.9	79	53.4
Connecticut	24	9	37.5	13	54.2	18	75	7	29.2	5	20.8	14	58.3	5	20.8	19	79.2	19	79.2	20	83.3
Maine	29	7	24.1	9	31	25	86.2	2	6.9	1	3.4	14	48.3	5	17.2	19	65.5	5	17.2	13	44.8
Massachusetts	50	11	22	20	40	39	78	10	20	2	4	17	34	9	18	37	74	22	44	23	46
New Hampshire	26	9	34.6	12	46.2	25	96.2	8	30.8	2	7.7	16	61.5	2	7.7	11	42.3	8	30.8	14	53.8
Rhode Island	9	5	55.6	4	44.4	6	66.7	5	55.6	0	0	4	44.4	2	22.2	5	55.6	5	55.6	5	55.6
Vermont	10	3	30	4	40	9	90	3	30	1	10	4	40	2	20	4	40	3	30	4	40
CENSUS DIVISION 2, MIDDLE ATLANTIC	357	113	31.7	175	49	262	73.4	113	31.7	38	10.6	174	48.7	48	13.4	241	67.5	156	43.7	204	57.1
New Jersey	71	35	49.3	41	57.7	56	78.9	33	46.5	9	12.7	36	50.7	11	15.5	54	76.1	47	66.2	51	71.8
New York	122	38	31.1	66	54.1	100	82	49	40.2	10	8.2	52	42.6	24	19.7	97	79.5	65	53.3	82	67.2
Pennsylvania	164	40	24.4	68	41.5	106	64.6	31	18.9	19	11.6	86	52.4	13	7.9	90	54.9	44	26.8	71	43.3
CENSUS DIVISION 3, SOUTH ATLANTIC	541	174	32.2	192	35.5	387	71.5	170	31.4	47	8.7	200	37	68	12.6	273	50.5	155	28.7	255	47.1
Delaware	8	2	25	2	25	6	75	3	37.5	1	12.5	5	62.5	1	12.5	3	37.5	3	25	2	25
District of Columbia	9	6	66.7	7	77.8	7	77.8	5	55.6	2	22.2	4	44.4	1	11.1	7	77.8	3	33.3	6	66.7
Florida	154	63	40.9	54	35.1	117	76	37	24	18	11.7	59	38.3	18	11.7	75	48.7	39	25.3	62	40.3
Georgia	88	16	18.2	22	25	64	72.7	19	21.6	4	4.5	20	22.7	5	5.7	42	47.7	20	22.7	33	37.5
Maryland	40	12	30	21	52.5	32	80	19	47.5	3	7.5	20	50	11	27.5	34	85	26	65	34	85
North Carolina	68	25	36.8	31	45.6	60	88.2	18	26.5	6	8.8	30	44.1	9	13.2	39	57.4	27	39.7	35	55.9
South Carolina	78	11	14.1	9	11.5	27	34.6	46	59	3	3.8	20	25.6	11	14.1	22	28.2	13	16.7	38	44.9
Virginia	59	34	57.6	33	55.9	51	86.4	19	32.2	9	15.3	35	59.3	10	16.9	36	61	20	33.9	38	64.4
West Virginia	37	5	13.5	13	35.1	23	62.2	4	10.8	1	2.7	7	18.9	2	5.4	15	40.5	5	13.5	7	18.9
CENSUS DIVISION 4, EAST NORTH CENTRAL	621	146	23.5	232	37.4	493	79.4	133	21.4	40	6.4	249	40.1	90	14.5	290	46.7	188	30.3	257	41.4
Illinois	138	34	24.6	64	46.4	110	79.7	33	23.9	6	4.3	58	42	23	16.7	68	49.3	48	34.8	63	45.7
Indiana	108	27	25	34	31.5	80	74.1	24	22.2	8	7.4	38	35.2	11	10.2	32	29.6	25	23.1	33	30.6
Michigan	120	31	25.8	54	45	103	85.8	16	13.3	8	6.7	54	45	12	10	73	60.8	50	41.7	60	50
Ohio	108	40	37	52	48.1	86	79.6	32	29.6	13	12	56	51.9	12	11.1	64	59.3	26	24.1	55	50.9
Wisconsin	147	14	9.5	28	19	114	77.6	28	19	5	3.4	43	29.3	32	21.8	53	36.1	39	26.5	46	31.3
CENSUS DIVISION 5, EAST SOUTH CENTRAL	285	52	18.2	64	22.5	178	62.5	44	15.4	12	4.2	71	24.9	29	10.2	70	24.6	62	21.8	76	26.7
Alabama	52	9	17.3	7	13.5	26	50	9	17.3	6	11.5	10	19.2	8	15.4	19	36.5	10	19.2	15	28.8
Kentucky	72	16	22.2	23	31.9	55	76.4	8	11.1	4	5.6	17	23.6	8	11.1	22	30.6	18	25	21	29.2
Mississippi	96	7	7.3	13	13.5	47	49	12	12.5	1	1	17	17.7	4	9.4	12	12.5	14	14.6	12	12.5
Tennessee	65	20	30.8	21	32.3	50	76.9	15	23.1	1	1.5	27	41.5	4	6.2	17	26.2	20	30.8	28	43.1
CENSUS DIVISION 6, WEST NORTH CENTRAL	556	120	21.6	128	23	447	80.4	102	18.3	23	4.1	180	32.4	64	11.5	170	30.6	123	22.1	184	33.1
Iowa	122	32	26.2	25	20.5	97	79.5	15	12.3	5	4.1	40	32.8	12	9.8	38	31.1	32	26.2	43	35.2
Kansas	120	17	14.2	20	16.7	101	84.2	13	10.8	4	5	22	18.3	4	3.3	18	15	9	7.5	26	21.7
Minnesota	94	32	34	19	20.2	79	84	20	21.3	4	4.3	43	45.7	9	9.6	44	46.8	29	30.9	40	42.6
Missouri	130	19	14.6	35	26.9	91	70	28	21.5	4	3.1	47	36.2	29	22.3	41	31.5	33	25.4	51	39.2
Nebraska	39	13	33.3	18	46.2	35	89.7	3	33.3	4	10.3	17	43.6	3	7.7	17	43.6	12	30.8	14	35.9
North Dakota	12	2	16.7	4	33.3	10	83.3	3	25	0	0	3	25	2	16.7	5	41.7	3	25	3	25
South Dakota	39	5	12.8	7	17.9	34	87.2	10	25.6	0	0	8	20.5	5	12.8	7	17.9	5	12.8	7	17.9
CENSUS DIVISION 7, WEST SOUTH CENTRAL	842	189	22.4	105	12.5	479	56.9	76	9	54	6.4	208	24.7	71	8.4	212	25.2	136	16.2	197	23.4
Arkansas	98	19	19.4	11	11.2	58	59.2	12	12.2	9	9.2	26	26.5	10	10.2	23	23.5	15	16.3	29	29.6
Louisiana	79	26	32.9	11	13.9	48	60.8	8	10.1	4	5.1	28	35.4	6	7.6	33	41.8	15	19	31	39.2
Oklahoma	99	29	29.3	15	15.2	66	66.7	11	11.1	5	5.1	20	20.2	8	8.1	35	35.4	18	18.2	29	29.3
Texas	566	115	20.3	68	12	307	54.2	45	8	36	6.4	134	23.7	47	8.3	121	21.4	87	15.4	108	19.1
CENSUS DIVISION 8, MOUNTAIN	336	80	23.8	85	25.3	227	67.6	48	14.3	28	8.3	92	27.4	32	9.5	145	43.2	57	17	144	42.9
Arizona	70	14	20	18	25.7	36	51.4	13	12.9	4	11.4	29	41.4	5	7.1	34	48.6	15	21.4	28	40
Colorado	74	24	32.4	29	39.2	57	77	13	17.6	4	5.4	29	39.2	5	6.8	26	35.1	12	16.2	36	48.6
Idaho	26	9	34.6	6	23.1	19	73.1	2	7.7	1	3.8	8	30.8	6	7.7	11	42.3	5	19.2	11	42.3
Montana	45	10	22.2	6	13.3	42	93.3	7	15.6	1	2.2	6	25	6	12.5	18	40	10	22.2	15	33.3
Nevada	32	5	15.6	4	12.9	14	43.8	5	15.6	4	12.5	8	25	4	12.5	10	34.4	6	18.8	9	28.1
New Mexico	31	6	19.4	4	12.9	20	64.5	2	6.5	1	3.2	6	19.4	3	9.7	10	32.3	3	9.7	9	29
Utah	36	10	27.8	12	33.3	26	72.2	7	19.4	9	25	8	22.2	4	9.7	28	77.8	3	8.3	30	83.3
Wyoming	22	2	9.1	3	13.6	13	59.1	3	13.6	0	0	4	18.2	3	13.6	7	31.8	3	13.6	6	27.3
CENSUS DIVISION 9, PACIFIC	411	107	26	135	32.8	280	68.1	90	21.9	28	6.8	120	29.2	31	7.5	206	50.1	91	22.1	165	40.1
Alaska	9	3	33.3	0	0	7	77.8	0	0	0	0	1	11.1	0	0	6	66.7	2	22.2	9	44.4
California	268	65	24.3	86	32.1	167	62.3	60	22.4	20	7.5	80	29.9	24	9	148	55.2	62	23.1	110	41
Hawaii	15	1	6.7	1	6.7	11	73.3	3	20	0	0	3	20	2	13.3	4	26.7	1	6.7	4	26.7
Oregon	60	19	31.7	20	33.3	48	80	8	13.3	2	3.3	11	18.3	2	3.3	21	35	8	13.3	19	31.7
Washington	59	19	32.2	24	40.7	47	79.7	19	32.2	6	10.2	25	42.4	3	5.1	27	45.8	18	30.5	27	45.8

Note: The 2021 performance data do not reflect the full impact of the COVID-19 pandemic. Please refer to the discussion in the Introduction for more information.

Table 7 (Continued)

These data include only hospital-based facilities and services as reported by responding hospitals in Section C of the 2022 AHA Annual Survey, beginning on page 215. Census divisions represent all U.S. hospitals. Community hospitals are listed separately under United States. No estimates have been made for nonresponding hospitals. Definitions of facilities and services are listed in the Glossary, page 203.

Facilities and Services

CLASSIFICATION	HOSPITALS REPORTING	Forensic Psychiatry No.	Forensic Psychiatry %	Geriatric No.	Geriatric %	Outpatient No.	Outpatient %	Partial Hosp. No.	Partial Hosp. %	Prenatal/Postpartum Psych No.	Prenatal/Postpartum Psych %	Psych Inpatient Care Units No.	Psych Inpatient Care Units %	Psych Intensive Outpatient No.	Psych Intensive Outpatient %	Residential Treatment No.	Residential Treatment %	Social & Community Psych No.	Social & Community Psych %	Suicide Prevention No.	Suicide Prevention %	CT Scanner No.	CT Scanner %	Diagnostic Radioisotope No.	Diagnostic Radioisotope %
UNITED STATES	4,097	166	4.1	736	18	1,230	30	522	12.7	497	12.1	1,321	32.2	641	15.6	190	4.6	484	11.8	1,268	30.9	3,406	83.1	2,343	57.2
COMMUNITY HOSPITALS	3,682	100	2.7	572	15.5	1,044	28.4	367	10	444	12.1	981	26.6	457	12.4	84	2.3	409	11.1	1,034	28.1	3,334	90.5	2,306	62.6
CENSUS DIVISION 1, NEW ENGLAND	148	12	8.1	34	23	82	55.4	38	25.7	31	20.9	74	50	45	30.4	12	8.1	35	23.6	71	48	121	81.8	102	68.9
Connecticut	24	5	20.8	9	37.5	19	79.2	12	50	8	33.3	21	87.5	18	75	6	25	13	54.2	21	87.5	20	83.3	20	83.3
Maine	29	0	0	4	13.8	17	58.6	4	13.8	2	6.9	8	27.6	5	17.2	0	0	4	13.8	6	20.7	26	89.7	24	82.8
Massachusetts	50	3	6	12	24	23	46	15	30	13	26	25	50	14	28	3	6	7	14	25	50	37	74	34	68
New Hampshire	26	1	3.8	6	23.1	12	46.2	2	7.7	4	15.4	9	34.6	5	19.2	1	3.8	6	23.1	8	30.8	22	84.6	12	46.2
Rhode Island	9	2	22.2	2	22.2	5	55.6	3	33.3	2	22.2	7	77.8	1	11.1	1	11.1	3	33.3	7	77.8	7	77.8	7	77.8
Vermont	10	1	10	1	10	6	60	2	20	2	20	4	40	2	20	1	10	2	20	4	40	9	90	7	70
CENSUS DIVISION 2, MIDDLE ATLANTIC	357	29	8.1	88	24.6	138	38.7	61	17.1	87	24.4	186	52.1	73	20.4	27	7.6	84	23.5	176	49.3	289	81	259	72.5
New Jersey	71	8	11.3	22	31	37	52.1	19	26.8	26	36.6	40	56.3	22	31	9	12.7	23	32.4	43	60.6	54	76.1	53	74.6
New York	122	17	13.9	35	28.7	72	59	24	19.7	34	27.9	78	63.9	36	29.5	8	6.6	44	36.1	63	51.6	109	89.3	93	76.2
Pennsylvania	164	4	2.4	31	18.9	29	17.7	18	11	27	16.5	68	41.5	15	9.1	10	6.1	17	10.4	70	42.7	126	76.8	113	68.9
CENSUS DIVISION 3, SOUTH ATLANTIC	541	23	4.3	111	20.5	154	28.5	85	15.7	68	12.6	205	37.9	88	16.3	25	4.6	74	13.7	177	32.7	462	85.4	378	69.9
Delaware	8	0	0	1	12.5	3	37.5	1	12.5	2	25	2	25	0	0	0	0	2	25	3	37.5	5	62.5	4	50
District of Columbia	7	1	11.1	2	22.2	4	55.6	3	33.3	3	33.3	7	77.8	1	11.1	1	11.1	2	22.2	5	55.6	6	66.7	5	55.6
Florida	154	5	3.2	31	20.1	32	20.8	21	13.6	11	7.1	46	29.9	19	12.3	7	4.5	14	9.1	52	33.8	135	87.7	117	76
Georgia	88	5	5.7	19	21.6	18	20.5	8	9.1	4	4.5	27	30.7	12	13.6	4	4.5	14	15.9	19	21.6	77	87.5	55	62.5
Maryland	40	0	0	10	25	28	70	18	45	14	35	27	67.5	19	47.5	3	7.5	17	42.5	25	62.5	36	90	32	80
North Carolina	68	4	5.9	12	17.6	19	27.9	10	14.7	9	13.2	31	45.6	9	13.2	1	1.5	4	5.9	20	29.4	63	92.6	45	66.2
South Carolina	78	1	1.3	18	23.1	12	15.4	8	10.3	3	3.8	25	32.1	8	10.3	0	0	4	5.1	16	20.5	56	71.8	46	59
Virginia	59	4	6.8	13	22	27	45.8	14	23.7	20	33.9	28	47.5	17	28.8	8	13.6	12	20.3	27	45.8	52	88.1	47	79.7
West Virginia	37	3	8.1	5	13.5	10	27	2	5.4	2	5.4	12	32.4	3	8.1	1	2.7	5	13.5	10	27	32	86.5	27	73
CENSUS DIVISION 4, EAST NORTH CENTRAL	621	21	3.4	129	20.8	227	36.6	87	14	83	13.4	210	33.8	100	16.1	27	4.3	81	13	188	30.3	543	87.4	410	66
Illinois	138	10	7.2	26	18.8	62	44.9	26	18.8	32	23.2	46	33.3	30	21.7	2	1.4	35	25.4	53	38.4	124	89.9	89	64.5
Indiana	108	2	1.9	15	13.9	31	28.7	11	10.2	12	11.1	30	27.8	19	17.6	7	6.5	11	10.2	22	20.4	92	85.2	63	58.3
Michigan	120	3	2.5	22	18.3	42	35	16	13.3	14	11.7	47	39.2	15	12.5	8	6.7	14	11.7	48	40	108	90	70	58.3
Ohio	108	4	3.7	24	22.2	39	36.1	25	23.1	16	14.8	47	43.5	28	25.9	7	6.5	14	13	42	38.9	92	85.2	75	69.4
Wisconsin	147	2	1.4	42	28.6	53	36.1	9	6.1	9	6.1	40	27.2	8	5.4	3	2	7	4.8	23	15.6	127	86.4	91	61.9
CENSUS DIVISION 5, EAST SOUTH CENTRAL	285	14	4.9	73	25.6	63	22.1	29	10.2	10	3.5	104	36.5	39	13.7	16	5.6	20	7	60	21.1	228	80	150	52.6
Alabama	52	1	1.9	15	28.8	9	17.3	4	7.7	2	3.8	23	44.2	6	11.5	6	11.5	3	5.8	15	28.8	40	76.9	31	59.6
Kentucky	72	1	1.4	11	15.3	18	25	7	9.7	5	6.9	23	31.9	8	11.1	1	1.4	8	11.1	20	27.8	59	81.9	42	58.3
Mississippi	96	1	1	32	33.3	29	30.2	15	15.6	0	0	38	39.6	20	20.8	9	9.4	4	4.2	9	9.4	77	80.2	40	41.7
Tennessee	65	11	16.9	15	23.1	7	10.8	3	4.6	3	4.6	20	30.8	5	7.7	0	0	5	7.7	16	24.6	52	80	37	56.9
CENSUS DIVISION 6, WEST NORTH CENTRAL	556	15	2.7	97	17.4	195	35.1	50	9	58	10.4	142	25.5	64	11.5	25	4.5	50	9	136	24.5	501	90.1	226	40.6
Iowa	122	3	2.5	16	13.1	47	38.5	6	5	8	6.6	29	23.8	15	12.3	3	2.5	11	9	23	18.9	113	92.6	38	31.1
Kansas	120	1	0.8	12	10	21	17.5	6	5	5	4.2	12	10	7	5.8	2	1.7	7	5.8	19	15.8	108	90	48	40
Minnesota	94	0	0	12	12.8	41	43.6	18	19.1	18	19.1	29	30.9	15	16	8	8.5	16	17	31	33	90	95.7	42	44.7
Missouri	130	7	5.4	47	36.2	48	36.9	12	9.2	16	12.3	55	42.3	19	14.6	9	6.9	8	6.2	37	28.5	105	80.8	65	50
Nebraska	39	1	2.6	4	10.3	24	61.5	3	7.7	4	10.3	10	25.6	5	12.8	2	5.1	3	7.7	16	41	37	94.9	16	41
North Dakota	12	1	8.3	2	16.7	5	41.7	2	16.7	3	25	4	33.3	1	8.3	0	0	1	8.3	3	25	10	83.3	7	58.3
South Dakota	39	2	5.1	4	10.3	9	23.1	2	5.1	4	10.3	3	7.7	2	5.1	1	2.6	4	10.3	7	17.9	38	97.4	10	25.6
CENSUS DIVISION 7, WEST SOUTH CENTRAL	842	22	2.6	130	15.4	163	19.4	86	10.2	58	6.9	210	24.9	127	15.1	27	3.2	59	7	184	21.9	606	72	343	40.7
Arkansas	98	2	2	23	23.5	25	25.5	9	9.2	9	9.2	38	38.8	22	22.4	7	7.1	13	13.3	28	28.6	74	75.5	39	39.8
Louisiana	79	4	5.1	16	20.3	29	36.7	9	11.4	11	13.9	36	45.6	19	24.1	3	3.8	13	16.5	25	31.6	57	72.2	43	54.4
Oklahoma	99	2	2	18	18.2	20	20.2	7	7.1	6	6.1	32	32.3	10	10.1	8	8.1	8	8.1	25	25.3	80	80.8	42	42.4
Texas	566	14	2.5	73	12.9	89	15.7	61	10.8	32	5.7	104	18.4	76	13.4	9	1.6	25	4.4	106	18.7	395	69.8	219	38.7
CENSUS DIVISION 8, MOUNTAIN	336	12	3.6	33	9.8	92	27.4	33	9.8	39	11.6	81	24.1	46	13.7	16	4.8	32	9.5	128	38.1	286	85.1	177	52.7
Arizona	70	2	2.9	7	10	18	25.7	7	10	5	7.1	18	25.7	13	18.6	2	2.9	3	4.3	21	30	50	71.4	45	64.3
Colorado	74	3	4.1	8	10.8	15	20.3	7	9.5	7	9.5	12	16.2	11	14.9	4	5.4	8	10.8	36	48.6	72	97.3	46	62.2
Idaho	26	1	3.8	1	3.8	10	38.5	1	3.8	1	3.8	7	26.9	0	0	1	3.8	5	19.2	10	38.5	25	96.2	14	53.8
Montana	45	1	2.2	4	8.9	18	40	5	11.1	10	22.2	7	15.6	5	11.1	3	6.7	4	8.9	13	28.9	42	93.3	15	33.3
Nevada	32	1	3.1	5	15.6	8	25	6	18.8	4	12.5	12	37.5	7	21.9	4	12.5	6	18.8	10	31.3	18	56.3	11	34.4
New Mexico	31	1	3.2	4	12.9	7	22.6	4	12.9	3	9.7	8	25.8	2	6.5	0	0	3	9.7	5	16.1	27	87.1	14	45.2
Utah	36	2	5.6	2	5.6	11	30.6	5	13.9	8	22.2	13	36.1	6	16.7	1	2.8	2	5.6	29	80.6	34	94.4	23	63.9
Wyoming	22	1	4.5	2	9.1	5	22.7	0	0	1	4.5	4	18.2	2	9.1	1	4.5	1	4.5	4	18.2	18	81.8	9	40.9
CENSUS DIVISION 9, PACIFIC	411	18	4.4	41	10	116	28.2	53	12.9	63	15.3	109	26.5	59	14.4	15	3.6	49	11.9	148	36	370	90	298	72.5
Alaska	18	0	0	0	0	6	33.3	2	11.1	2	11.1	4	22.2	2	11.1	2	11.1	2	11.1	2	11.1	18	100	8	44.4
California	268	13	4.9	33	12.3	72	26.9	39	14.6	46	17.2	72	26.9	43	16	10	3.7	37	13.8	97	36.2	237	88.4	198	73.9
Hawaii	15	1	6.7	0	0	3	20	2	13.3	2	13.3	5	33.3	2	13.3	0	0	0	0	4	26.7	12	80	11	73.3
Oregon	60	1	1.7	4	6.7	14	23.3	6	10	5	8.3	14	23.3	5	8.3	3	5	3	5	15	25	57	95	41	68.3
Washington	59	3	5.1	4	6.8	24	40.7	5	8.5	8	13.6	16	27.1	7	11.9	0	0	6	10.2	29	49.2	55	93.2	44	74.6

Note: The 2021 performance data do not reflect the full impact of the COVID-19 pandemic. Please refer to the discussion in the Introduction for more information.

AHA Hospital Statistics © 2023 Health Forum LLC, an affiliate of the American Hospital Association

Facilities and Services

Table 7 (Continued)

These data include only hospital-based facilities and services as reported by responding hospitals in Section C of the 2022 AHA Annual Survey; beginning on page 215. Census divisions represent all U.S. hospitals. Community hospitals are listed separately under United States. No estimates have been made for nonresponding hospitals. Definitions of facilities and services are listed in the Glossary; page 203.

RADIOLOGY, DIAGNOSTIC

Classification	Hospitals Reporting	EBCT No.	EBCT %	FFDM No.	FFDM %	MRI No.	MRI %	Intraop. No.	Intraop. %	Magneto. No.	Magneto. %	Multi-Slice <64 No.	Multi-Slice <64 %	Multi-Slice 64+ No.	Multi-Slice 64+ %	PET No.	PET %	PET/CT No.	PET/CT %	SPECT No.	SPECT %
UNITED STATES	4,097	335	8.2	2,469	60.3	2,808	68.5	244	6	118	2.9	1,904	46.5	2,593	63.3	773	18.9	979	23.9	1,562	38.1
COMMUNITY HOSPITALS	3,682	328	8.9	2,447	66.5	2,758	74.9	238	6.5	115	3.1	1,872	50.8	2,552	69.3	749	20.3	954	25.9	1,538	41.8
CENSUS DIVISION 1, NEW ENGLAND	148	11	7.4	112	75.7	101	68.2	11	7.4	4	2.7	75	50.7	104	70.3	35	23.6	44	29.7	71	48
Connecticut	24	2	8.3	20	83.3	19	79.2	5	20.8	0	0	17	70.8	20	83.3	15	62.5	16	66.7	16	66.7
Maine	29	1	3.4	23	79.3	21	72.4	0	0	0	0	9	31	22	75.9	5	17.2	8	27.6	10	34.5
Massachusetts	50	6	12	34	68	31	62	4	8	3	6	26	52	33	66	10	20	13	26	21	42
New Hampshire	26	1	3.8	22	84.6	16	61.5	2	7.7	1	3.8	13	50	18	69.2	2	7.7	3	11.5	13	50
Rhode Island	9	0	0	5	55.6	7	77.8	0	0	0	0	5	55.6	5	55.6	2	22.2	2	22.2	5	55.6
Vermont	10	0	0	8	80	7	70	0	0	0	0	5	50	6	60	1	10	2	20	6	60
CENSUS DIVISION 2, MIDDLE ATLANTIC	357	43	12	241	67.5	267	74.8	35	9.8	13	3.6	189	52.9	254	71.1	98	27.5	125	35	186	52.1
New Jersey	71	12	16.9	46	64.8	51	71.8	7	9.9	3	4.2	37	52.1	46	64.8	29	40.8	32	45.1	35	49.3
New York	122	17	13.9	93	76.2	98	80.3	16	13.1	4	3.3	72	59	100	82	32	26.2	44	36.1	66	54.1
Pennsylvania	164	14	8.5	102	62.2	118	72	12	7.3	6	3.7	80	48.8	108	65.9	37	22.6	49	29.9	85	51.8
CENSUS DIVISION 3, SOUTH ATLANTIC	541	52	9.6	382	70.6	418	77.3	33	6.1	17	3.1	312	57.7	388	71.7	132	24.4	171	31.6	269	49.7
Delaware	8	1	12.5	5	62.5	6	75	1	12.5	0	0	5	62.5	5	62.5	4	50	4	50	5	62.5
District of Columbia	9	0	0	5	55.6	6	66.7	2	22.2	0	0	2	22.2	4	44.4	0	0	5	55.6	5	55.6
Florida	154	28	18.2	104	67.5	122	79.2	16	10.4	9	5.8	97	63	113	73.4	46	29.9	51	33.1	81	52.6
Georgia	88	6	6.8	64	72.7	67	76.1	4	4.5	4	4.5	47	53.4	60	68.2	23	26.1	31	35.2	28	31.8
Maryland	40	3	7.5	33	82.5	33	82.5	2	5	1	2.5	25	62.5	34	85	14	35	14	35	29	72.5
North Carolina	68	5	7.4	53	77.9	60	88.2	3	4.4	1	1.5	48	70.6	55	80.9	15	22.1	23	33.8	43	63.2
South Carolina	78	2	2.6	51	65.4	52	66.7	1	1.3	1	1.3	36	46.2	46	59	4	5.1	15	19.2	23	29.5
Virginia	59	5	8.5	46	78	50	84.7	4	6.8	1	1.7	30	50.8	46	78	16	27.1	18	30.5	37	62.7
West Virginia	37	2	5.4	29	78.4	23	62.2	0	0	0	0	19	51.4	23	62.2	10	27	10	27	18	48.6
CENSUS DIVISION 4, EAST NORTH CENTRAL	621	46	7.4	418	67.3	475	76.5	43	6.9	28	4.5	283	45.6	412	66.3	153	24.6	177	28.5	305	49.1
Illinois	138	8	5.8	109	79	105	76.1	11	8	3	2.2	78	56.5	107	77.5	34	24.6	47	34.1	62	44.9
Indiana	108	9	8.3	77	71.3	87	80.6	6	5.6	4	3.7	56	51.9	70	64.8	27	25	27	25	41	38
Michigan	120	8	6.7	101	84.2	89	74.2	6	5	5	4.2	54	45	99	82.5	23	19.2	32	26.7	62	51.7
Ohio	108	10	9.3	77	71.3	86	79.6	14	13	9	8.3	66	61.1	78	72.2	35	32.4	40	37	66	61.1
Wisconsin	147	11	7.5	54	36.7	108	73.5	6	4.1	7	4.8	29	19.7	58	39.5	34	23.1	31	21.1	74	50.3
CENSUS DIVISION 5, EAST SOUTH CENTRAL	285	30	10.5	154	54	176	61.8	16	5.6	5	1.8	116	40.7	159	55.8	55	19.3	58	20.4	102	35.8
Alabama	52	5	9.6	30	57.7	37	71.2	2	3.8	2	3.8	23	44.2	32	61.5	15	28.8	16	30.8	20	38.5
Kentucky	72	6	8.3	45	62.5	52	72.2	3	4.2	2	2.8	27	37.5	49	68.1	15	20.8	17	23.6	30	41.7
Mississippi	96	7	7.3	33	34.4	40	41.7	7	7.3	0	0	36	37.5	35	36.5	13	13.5	10	10.4	28	29.2
Tennessee	65	12	18.5	46	70.8	47	72.3	4	6.2	1	1.5	30	46.2	43	66.2	12	18.5	15	23.1	24	36.9
CENSUS DIVISION 6, WEST NORTH CENTRAL	556	27	4.9	361	64.9	344	61.9	19	3.4	14	2.5	208	37.4	345	62.1	75	13.5	107	19.2	158	28.4
Iowa	122	3	2.5	105	86.1	72	59	2	1.6	1	0.8	53	43.4	76	62.3	17	13.9	24	19.7	32	26.2
Kansas	120	7	5.8	53	44.2	59	49.2	3	2.5	1	0.8	46	38.3	57	47.5	9	7.5	13	10.8	22	18.3
Minnesota	94	4	4.3	67	71.3	61	64.9	5	5.3	4	4.3	29	30.9	71	75.5	17	18.1	16	17	33	35.1
Missouri	130	7	5.4	82	63.1	99	76.2	4	3.1	3	2.3	41	31.5	84	64.6	22	16.9	41	31.5	47	36.2
Nebraska	39	4	10.3	29	74.4	28	71.8	2	5.1	2	5.1	18	46.2	29	74.4	7	17.9	7	17.9	11	28.2
North Dakota	12	1	8.3	7	58.3	6	50	2	16.7	0	0	6	50	6	50	2	16.7	2	16.7	5	41.7
South Dakota	39	1	2.6	18	46.2	19	48.7	1	2.6	0	0	15	38.5	22	56.4	1	2.6	4	10.3	8	20.5
CENSUS DIVISION 7, WEST SOUTH CENTRAL	842	47	5.6	356	42.3	457	54.3	37	4.4	14	1.7	353	41.9	387	46	76	9	100	11.9	187	22.2
Arkansas	98	7	7.1	50	51	58	59.2	3	3.1	0	0	39	39.8	50	51	10	10.2	10	10.2	19	19.4
Louisiana	79	6	7.6	49	62	48	60.8	7	8.9	1	1.3	34	43	41	51.9	19	24.1	20	25.3	21	26.6
Oklahoma	99	6	6.1	53	53.5	61	61.6	0	0	0	0	46	46.5	57	57.6	9	9.1	16	16.2	26	26.3
Texas	566	28	4.9	204	36	290	51.2	27	4.8	13	2.3	234	41.3	239	42.2	38	6.7	54	9.5	121	21.4
CENSUS DIVISION 8, MOUNTAIN	336	30	8.9	185	55.1	238	70.8	24	7.1	9	2.7	132	39.3	236	70.2	48	14.3	73	21.7	104	31
Arizona	70	7	10	23	32.9	46	65.7	8	11.4	3	4.3	32	45.7	43	61.4	10	14.3	14	20	23	32.9
Colorado	74	9	12.2	52	70.3	63	85.1	6	8.1	3	4.1	39	52.7	62	83.8	16	21.6	23	31.1	27	36.5
Idaho	26	3	11.5	16	61.5	20	76.9	2	7.7	1	3.8	11	42.3	21	80.8	4	15.4	5	19.2	11	42.3
Montana	45	1	2.2	24	53.3	28	62.2	2	4.4	0	0	14	31.1	23	51.1	4	8.9	6	13.3	9	20
Nevada	32	2	6.3	9	28.1	13	40.6	0	0	0	0	9	28.1	11	34.4	3	9.4	4	12.5	5	15.6
New Mexico	31	4	12.9	19	61.3	20	64.5	2	6.5	0	0	16	51.6	19	61.3	3	9.7	7	22.6	8	25.8
Utah	36	2	5.6	30	83.3	33	91.7	3	8.3	2	5.6	7	19.4	31	86.1	7	19.4	10	27.8	17	47.2
Wyoming	22	2	9.1	12	54.5	15	68.2	1	4.5	0	0	4	18.2	16	72.7	1	4.5	4	18.2	4	18.2
CENSUS DIVISION 9, PACIFIC	411	49	11.9	260	63.3	332	80.8	26	6.3	14	3.4	236	57.4	308	74.9	101	24.6	124	30.2	180	43.8
Alaska	9	0	0	5	55.6	6	66.7	0	0	0	0	6	66.7	6	66.7	0	0	0	0	2	22.2
California	268	31	11.6	165	61.6	213	79.5	21	7.8	14	5.2	153	57.1	198	73.9	71	26.5	88	32.8	121	45.1
Hawaii	15	0	0	11	73.3	11	73.3	0	0	0	0	3	20	11	73.3	0	0	2	13.3	4	26.7
Oregon	60	5	8.3	45	75	52	86.7	4	6.7	0	0	33	55	43	71.7	15	25	15	25	29	48.3
Washington	59	13	22	34	57.6	50	84.7	1	1.7	0	0	41	69.5	50	84.7	15	25.4	19	32.2	24	40.7

Note: The 2021 performance data do not reflect the full impact of the COVID-19 pandemic. Please refer to the discussion in the Introduction for more information.

Table 7 (Continued)

These data include only hospital-based facilities and services as reported by responding hospitals in Section C of the 2022 AHA Annual Survey, beginning on page 215. Census divisions represent all U.S. hospitals. Community hospitals are listed separately under United States. No estimates have been made for nonresponding hospitals. Definitions of facilities and services are listed in the Glossary, page 203.

Facilities and Services

CLASSIFICATION	HOSPITALS REPORTING	ULTRASOUND Number	ULTRASOUND Percent	BASIC INTERVENTIONAL RADIOLOGY Number	BASIC INTERVENTIONAL RADIOLOGY Percent	IGRT Number	IGRT Percent	IMRT Number	IMRT Percent	PROTON BEAM THERAPY Number	PROTON BEAM THERAPY Percent	SHAPED BEAM RADIATION SYSTEM Number	SHAPED BEAM RADIATION SYSTEM Percent	STEREOTACTIC RADIOSURGERY Number	STEREOTACTIC RADIOSURGERY Percent	MED. ASSISTED TREATMENT OTHER SUBSTANCE Number	MED. ASSISTED TREATMENT OTHER SUBSTANCE Percent	MED. ASSISTED TREATMENT OPIOID Number	MED. ASSISTED TREATMENT OPIOID Percent
UNITED STATES	4,097	3,321	81.1	1,902	46.4	1,088	26.6	1,086	26.5	124	3	893	21.8	917	22.4	646	15.8	789	19.3
COMMUNITY HOSPITALS	3,682	3,244	88.1	1,869	50.8	1,070	29.1	1,073	29.1	119	3.2	882	24	908	24.7	535	14.5	664	18
CENSUS DIVISION 1, NEW ENGLAND	148	128	86.5	79	53.4	49	33.1	51	34.5	8	5.4	45	30.4	47	31.8	66	44.6	85	57.4
Connecticut	24	20	83.3	20	83.3	18	75	18	75	0	0	14	58.3	15	62.5	16	66.7	16	66.7
Maine	29	26	89.7	11	37.9	11	13.8	5	17.2	0	0	4	13.8	4	13.8	10	34.5	20	69
Massachusetts	50	42	84	28	56	17	34	17	34	5	10	16	32	19	38	23	46	27	54
New Hampshire	26	23	88.5	11	42.3	6	23.1	6	23.1	1	3.8	6	23.1	6	23.1	12	46.2	15	57.7
Rhode Island	9	8	88.9	6	66.7	1	11.1	2	22.2	2	22.2	2	22.2	1	11.1	3	33.3	2	22.2
Vermont	10	9	90	3	30	3	30	3	30	0	0	3	30	2	20	2	20	5	50
CENSUS DIVISION 2, MIDDLE ATLANTIC	357	289	81	235	65.8	156	43.7	159	44.5	14	3.9	138	38.7	127	35.6	97	27.2	121	33.9
New Jersey	71	52	73.2	47	66.2	34	47.9	33	46.5	1	1.4	32	45.1	31	43.7	19	26.8	19	26.8
New York	122	111	91	87	71.3	54	44.3	56	45.9	7	5.7	46	37.7	48	39.3	45	36.9	63	51.6
Pennsylvania	164	126	76.8	101	61.6	68	41.5	70	42.7	6	3.7	60	36.6	48	29.3	33	20.1	39	23.8
CENSUS DIVISION 3, SOUTH ATLANTIC	541	465	86	285	52.7	196	36.2	194	35.9	19	3.5	162	29.9	153	28.3	80	14.8	91	16.8
Delaware	8	6	75	6	75	4	50	4	50	0	0	4	50	3	37.5	1	12.5	2	25
District of Columbia	9	7	77.8	6	66.7	5	55.6	4	44.4	2	22.2	5	55.6	3	33.3	3	33.3	3	33.3
Florida	154	132	85.7	91	59.1	50	32.5	45	29.2	2	4.5	39	25.3	43	27.9	18	11.7	20	13
Georgia	88	77	87.5	47	53.4	28	31.8	29	33	1	1.1	24	27.3	26	29.5	9	10.2	9	10.2
Maryland	40	37	92.5	34	85	19	47.5	19	47.5	5	5	13	32.5	19	47.5	15	37.5	20	50
North Carolina	68	64	94.1	43	63.2	38	55.9	39	57.4	5	7.4	34	50	20	29.4	11	16.2	12	17.6
South Carolina	78	57	73.1	12	15.4	15	19.2	16	20.5	0	0	13	16.7	11	14.1	3	3.8	2	2.6
Virginia	59	53	89.8	33	55.9	27	45.8	28	47.5	2	3.4	22	37.3	20	33.9	13	22	14	23.7
West Virginia	37	32	86.5	15	40.5	10	27	10	27	0	0	8	21.6	8	21.6	7	18.9	9	24.3
CENSUS DIVISION 4, EAST NORTH CENTRAL	621	537	86.5	311	50.1	192	30.9	199	32	22	3.5	158	25.4	156	25.1	111	17.9	134	21.6
Illinois	138	124	89.9	81	58.7	49	35.5	52	37.7	5	3.6	40	29	44	31.9	25	18.1	34	24.6
Indiana	108	92	85.2	49	45.4	36	33.3	39	36.1	6	5.6	28	25.9	28	22.2	22	20.4	25	23.1
Michigan	120	111	92.5	67	55.8	40	33.3	44	36.7	4	3.3	37	30.8	35	29.2	29	24.2	35	29.2
Ohio	108	95	88	65	60.2	38	35.2	35	32.4	5	4.6	25	23.1	34	31.5	19	17.6	21	19.4
Wisconsin	147	115	78.2	49	33.3	29	19.7	29	19.7	2	1.4	28	19	19	12.9	16	10.9	19	12.9
CENSUS DIVISION 5, EAST SOUTH CENTRAL	285	227	79.6	100	35.1	70	24.6	67	23.5	6	2.1	49	17.2	61	21.4	21	7.4	22	7.7
Alabama	52	39	75	24	46.2	14	26.9	13	25	0	0	8	15.4	12	23.1	2	3.8	2	3.8
Kentucky	72	59	81.9	26	36.1	19	26.4	18	25	2	2.8	13	18.1	17	23.6	8	11.1	10	13.9
Mississippi	96	75	78.1	16	16.7	13	13.5	11	11.5	2	2.1	10	10.4	12	12.5	6	6.3	5	5.2
Tennessee	65	54	83.1	34	52.3	24	36.9	25	38.5	2	3.1	18	27.7	20	30.8	5	7.7	5	7.7
CENSUS DIVISION 6, WEST NORTH CENTRAL	556	447	80.4	176	31.7	111	20	109	19.6	8	1.4	90	16.2	80	14.4	71	12.8	85	15.3
Iowa	122	110	90.2	37	30.3	16	15.6	19	15.6	1	0.8	18	14.8	13	10.7	16	10.7	16	13.1
Kansas	120	89	74.2	33	27.5	16	13.3	14	11.7	1	0.8	13	10.8	12	10	5	4.2	7	5.8
Minnesota	94	78	83	27	28.7	19	20.2	19	20.2	1	1.1	13	13.8	12	12.8	22	23.4	27	28.7
Missouri	130	99	76.2	52	40	35	26.9	36	27.7	2	1.5	30	23.1	28	21.5	19	14.6	20	15.4
Nebraska	39	35	89.7	18	46.2	13	33.3	11	28.2	0	0	10	25.6	10	25.6	5	12.8	7	17.9
North Dakota	12	8	66.7	3	25	2	16.7	2	16.7	1	8.3	2	16.7	2	16.7	2	16.7	3	25
South Dakota	39	28	71.8	6	15.4	7	17.9	8	20.5	0	0	4	10.3	3	7.7	5	12.8	4	12.8
CENSUS DIVISION 7, WEST SOUTH CENTRAL	842	577	68.5	293	34.8	96	11.4	100	11.9	14	1.7	80	9.5	98	11.6	66	7.8	76	9
Arkansas	98	77	78.6	31	31.6	10	10.2	10	10.2	0	0	7	7.1	12	12.2	11	11.2	15	15.3
Louisiana	79	58	73.4	37	46.8	16	20.3	17	21.5	2	2.5	16	20.3	17	21.5	11	19	17	21.5
Oklahoma	99	76	76.8	37	37.4	20	20.2	19	19.2	1	1	14	14.1	12	12.1	13	9.1	16	16.2
Texas	566	366	64.7	188	33.2	50	8.8	54	9.5	11	1.9	43	7.6	57	10.1	31	5.5	28	4.9
CENSUS DIVISION 8, MOUNTAIN	336	276	82.1	147	43.8	82	24.4	79	23.5	16	4.8	62	18.5	72	21.4	45	13.4	67	19.9
Arizona	70	50	71.4	34	48.6	15	21.4	15	21.4	4	5.7	12	17.1	17	24.3	3	4.3	8	11.4
Colorado	74	70	94.6	43	58.1	24	32.4	22	29.7	4	5.4	19	25.7	16	21.6	11	14.9	19	25.7
Idaho	26	24	92.3	10	38.5	4	15.4	6	23.1	1	3.8	3	11.5	5	19.2	8	30.8	7	26.9
Montana	45	39	86.7	17	37.8	10	22.2	11	24.4	3	6.7	8	17.8	12	26.7	6	13.3	9	20
Nevada	32	18	56.3	10	31.3	2	6.3	1	3.1	0	0	1	3.1	3	6.3	4	12.5	5	15.6
New Mexico	31	24	77.4	11	35.5	8	25.8	7	22.6	1	3.2	4	12.9	3	9.7	6	19.4	6	19.4
Utah	36	34	94.4	15	41.7	12	33.3	12	33.3	1	2.8	11	30.6	12	33.3	5	13.9	6	16.7
Wyoming	22	17	77.3	7	31.8	7	31.8	5	22.7	0	0	4	18.2	5	22.7	2	9.1	4	18.2
CENSUS DIVISION 9, PACIFIC	411	375	91.2	276	67.2	136	33.1	128	31.1	17	4.1	109	26.5	123	29.9	89	21.7	108	26.3
Alaska	9	9	100	5	55.6	1	11.1	1	11.1	0	0	1	11.1	1	0	2	55.6	3	33.3
California	268	241	89.9	184	68.7	92	34.3	85	31.7	12	4.5	73	27.2	87	32.5	63	23.5	80	29.9
Hawaii	15	13	86.7	10	66.7	3	20	3	20	0	0	2	13.3	1	6.7	2	13.3	2	13.3
Oregon	60	58	96.7	38	63.3	16	26.7	15	25	2	3.3	14	23.3	11	18.3	6	10	8	13.3
Washington	59	54	91.5	39	66.1	24	40.7	24	40.7	3	5.1	19	32.2	24	40.7	13	22	15	25.4

Note: The 2021 performance data do not reflect the full impact of the COVID-19 pandemic. Please refer to the discussion in the Introduction for more information.

Table 7 (Continued)

These data include only hospital-based facilities and services as reported by responding hospitals in Section C of the 2022 AHA Annual Survey, beginning on page 215. Census divisions represent all U.S. hospitals. Community hospitals are listed separately under United States. No estimates have been made for nonresponding hospitals. Definitions of facilities and services are listed in the Glossary, page 203.

CLASSIFICATION	HOSPITALS REPORTING	SUBSTANCE USE DISORDER INPATIENT CARE UNITS Number	Percent	SUBSTANCE USE DISORDER PEDIATRIC SERVICES Number	Percent	SUBSTANCE USE DISORDER OUTPATIENT SERVICES Number	Percent	SUBSTANCE USE DISORDER PARTIAL HOSPITALIZATION SERVICES Number	Percent	BONE MARROW Number	Percent	HEART Number	Percent	KIDNEY Number	Percent	LIVER Number	Percent	LUNG Number	Percent	TISSUE Number	Percent	OTHER Number	Percent
UNITED STATES	4,097	401	9.8	105	2.6	666	16.3	311	7.6	191	4.7	142	3.5	215	5.2	140	3.4	82	2	473	11.5	223	5.4
COMMUNITY HOSPITALS	3,682	267	7.3	68	1.8	529	14.4	212	5.8	190	5.2	139	3.8	211	5.7	137	3.7	80	2.2	469	12.7	221	6
CENSUS DIVISION 1, NEW ENGLAND	148	17	11.5	7	4.7	63	42.6	29	19.6	11	7.4	8	5.4	17	11.5	10	6.8	4	2.7	23	15.5	11	7.4
Connecticut	24	3	12.5	1	4.2	15	62.5	10	41.7	1	4.2	4	16.7	4	16.7	4	16.7	1	4.2	7	29.2	2	8.3
Maine	29	2	6.9	1	3.4	15	51.7	2	6.9	0	0	0	0	0	0	0	0	0	0	1	3.4	0	0
Massachusetts	50	7	14	2	4	17	34	9	18	8	16	4	8	9	18	6	12	3	6	10	20	7	14
New Hampshire	26	2	7.7	2	7.7	11	42.3	3	11.5	1	3.8	0	0	1	3.8	0	0	0	0	1	3.8	1	3.8
Rhode Island	9	1	11.1	1	11.1	2	22.2	3	33.3	0	0	0	0	1	11.1	0	0	0	0	2	22.2	0	0
Vermont	10	2	20	0	0	3	30	2	20	1	10	0	0	1	10	0	0	0	0	2	20	1	10
CENSUS DIVISION 2, MIDDLE ATLANTIC	357	58	16.2	11	3.1	90	25.2	28	7.8	26	7.3	16	4.5	31	8.7	19	5.3	12	3.4	96	26.9	39	10.9
New Jersey	71	6	8.5	3	4.2	20	28.2	8	11.3	3	4.2	2	2.8	4	5.6	2	2.8	1	1.4	25	35.2	6	8.5
New York	122	28	23	5	4.1	53	43.4	16	13.1	12	9.8	6	4.9	10	8.2	6	4.9	5	4.1	40	32.8	15	12.3
Pennsylvania	164	24	14.6	3	1.8	17	10.4	4	2.4	11	6.7	8	4.9	17	10.4	11	6.7	6	3.7	31	18.9	18	11
CENSUS DIVISION 3, SOUTH ATLANTIC	541	58	10.7	14	2.6	80	14.8	41	7.6	39	7.2	26	4.8	33	6.1	20	3.7	14	2.6	86	15.9	38	7
Delaware	8	0	0	0	0	2	25	0	0	1	12.5	0	0	1	12.5	0	0	0	0	4	44.4	0	0
District of Columbia	9	0	0	0	0	2	22.2	0	0	3	33.3	2	22.2	3	33.3	2	22.2	0	0	0	0	3	33.3
Florida	154	15	9.7	3	1.9	13	8.4	11	7.1	14	9.1	9	5.8	10	6.5	7	4.5	6	3.9	32	20.8	7	4.5
Georgia	88	4	4.5	1	1.1	4	9.1	4	4.5	3	3.4	2	2.3	4	3.4	2	2.3	1	1.1	11	12.5	3	3.4
Maryland	40	7	17.5	2	5	16	40	5	12.5	4	5	2	5	4	5	2	5	2	5	9	22.5	5	12.5
North Carolina	68	7	10.3	2	2.9	10	14.7	5	4.4	6	8.8	5	5.9	5	5.9	3	4.4	2	2.9	8	11.8	10	14.7
South Carolina	78	13	16.7	2	2.6	5	6.4	4	5.1	4	5.1	1	1.3	1	1.3	1	1.3	1	1.3	6	7.7	4	5.1
Virginia	59	11	18.6	2	3.4	17	28.8	10	16.9	4	6.8	5	8.5	7	11.9	3	5.1	2	3.4	14	23.7	4	6.8
West Virginia	37	1	2.7	2	5.4	7	18.9	4	10.8	2	5.4	1	2.7	2	5.4	0	0	0	0	2	5.4	2	5.4
CENSUS DIVISION 4, EAST NORTH CENTRAL	621	81	13	16	2.6	130	20.9	60	9.7	28	4.5	23	3.7	30	4.8	18	2.9	17	2.7	71	11.4	31	5.1
Illinois	138	14	10.1	6	4.3	26	18.8	18	13	9	6.5	9	4.3	9	6.5	6	4.3	3	2.2	15	10.9	8	5.7
Indiana	108	10	9.3	8	7.4	24	20.4	11	10.2	1	0.9	3	2.8	3	2.8	1	0.9	1	0.9	7	6.5	4	3.7
Michigan	120	15	12.5	1	0.8	24	20	7	5.8	4	3.3	3	2.5	6	5	3	2.5	3	2.5	19	15.8	8	7.4
Ohio	108	10	9.3	0	0.9	22	20.4	16	14.8	8	7.4	6	5.6	8	7.4	6	5.6	5	4.6	20	18.5	8	4.1
Wisconsin	147	32	21.8	0	0	36	24.5	8	5.4	6	4.1	2	3.4	4	2.7	2	1.4	5	3.4	10	6.8	5	4.1
CENSUS DIVISION 5, EAST SOUTH CENTRAL	285	21	7.4	8	2.8	22	7.7	15	5.3	12	4.2	11	3.9	13	4.6	9	3.2	10	3.4	26	9.1	14	4.9
Alabama	52	2	3.8	2	1.4	4	7.7	1	1.9	2	3.8	3	3.8	3	5.8	3	3.8	1	1.9	1	1.9	3	5.8
Kentucky	72	4	5.6	2	5.2	11	15.3	6	8.3	3	5.6	3	4.2	3	4.2	2	2.8	2	2.8	8	11.1	3	4.2
Mississippi	96	13	13.5	5	3.1	5	5.2	6	6.3	1	1	1	1	1	1	0	0	3	3.1	4	4.2	3	3.2
Tennessee	65	2	3.1	1	2.6	6	3.1	3	3.1	6	9.2	5	7.7	6	9.2	4	4.6	2	3.1	13	20	6	9.2
CENSUS DIVISION 6, WEST NORTH CENTRAL	556	60	10.8	11	2	87	15.6	34	6.1	15	2.7	13	2.3	21	3.8	13	2.4	8	1.4	38	6.8	27	4.9
Iowa	122	8	6.6	1	0.8	21	17.2	7	5.7	1	0.8	1	0.8	1	0.8	1	0.8	2	1.6	2	1.6	3	2.5
Kansas	120	2	1.7	1	0.8	6	5	2	1.7	1	1.6	1	1.6	1	0.8	2	1.6	0	0	4	3.3	3	2.5
Minnesota	94	13	13.8	4	4.3	22	23.4	9	9.6	6	3.2	5	3.2	8	4.3	3	3.2	3	3.2	7	7.4	3	3.2
Missouri	130	31	23.8	4	3.1	20	15.4	8	6.2	6	4.6	5	3.8	8	6.2	7	5.4	2	1.5	16	12.3	12	9.2
Nebraska	39	4	10.3	0	2.6	9	23.1	3	7.7	2	5.1	2	5.1	2	2.6	2	5.1	1	2.6	5	12.8	5	5.1
North Dakota	12	1	8.3	0	0	3	25	0	0	1	8.3	0	0	0	16.7	0	0	0	0	2	16.7	2	16.7
South Dakota	39	1	2.6	1	2.6	6	15.4	4	10.3	1	2.6	0	0	3	5.1	0	2.6	0	0	2	5.1	2	5.1
CENSUS DIVISION 7, WEST SOUTH CENTRAL	842	47	5.6	16	1.9	76	9	49	5.8	21	2.5	18	2.1	31	3.7	20	2.4	9	1.1	40	4.8	26	3.1
Arkansas	98	8	8.2	2	1.9	9	9.2	7	7.1	4	5.1	2	1.3	2	5.1	1	1	0	0	4	4.1	1	1
Louisiana	79	8	10.1	3	3.8	12	15.2	3	3.8	4	5.1	1	1.3	4	5.1	2	2.5	1	1.3	4	5.1	5	6.3
Oklahoma	99	5	5.1	2	3.8	10	10.1	6	6.1	1	6.7	1	1	2	6.7	2	6.7	1	1	5	5.3	2	1
Texas	566	26	4.6	10	1.8	45	8	33	5.8	13	2.3	14	2.5	22	3.9	13	2.3	7	1.2	30	5.3	18	3.2
CENSUS DIVISION 8, MOUNTAIN	336	32	9.5	11	3.3	57	17	25	7.4	14	4.2	9	2.7	14	4.2	13	3.9	4	1.2	43	12.8	8	2.4
Arizona	70	7	10	3	4.1	14	20	5	7.1	3	4.3	2	2.7	5	7.1	5	7.1	2	2.9	8	11.4	3	4.3
Colorado	74	7	9.5	3	4.1	12	16.2	6	8.1	3	4.1	2	2.7	4	5.4	2	2.7	1	1.4	8	10.8	2	2.7
Idaho	26	3	11.5	1	3.8	6	23.1	6	11.5	1	3.8	0	0	0	0	0	0	0	0	2	7.7	0	0
Montana	45	3	6.7	1	2.1	7	15.6	4	8.1	1	2.2	0	0	0	0	0	0	0	0	2	4.4	0	0
Nevada	32	5	15.6	2	3.1	5	15.6	4	12.5	1	3.2	0	0	0	0	0	0	1	3.2	1	3.1	0	0
New Mexico	31	3	9.7	1	6.5	5	16.1	3	9.7	1	3.2	0	0	3	6.5	3	6.5	0	0	0	0	1	3.2
Utah	36	3	8.3	2	4.5	6	16.7	0	0	3	8.3	3	8.3	3	8.3	3	8.3	1	2.8	21	58.3	2	5.6
Wyoming	22	1	4.5	1	4.5	2	9.1	1	4.5	0	0	0	0	0	0	0	0	0	0	1	4.5	0	0
CENSUS DIVISION 9, PACIFIC	411	27	6.6	11	2.7	61	14.8	30	7.3	25	6.1	18	4.4	25	6.1	16	3.9	9	2.2	50	12.2	29	7.1
Alaska	9	2	22.2	0	0	2	44.4	2	22.2	0	0	0	0	0	0	0	0	0	0	0	0	0	0
California	268	18	6.7	10	3.7	43	16	24	9	18	6.7	14	5.2	18	6.7	12	4.5	8	2.8	37	13.8	21	7.8
Hawaii	15	1	6.7	0	0	2	6.7	1	6.7	1	6.7	0	0	1	6.7	0	6.7	0	0	2	13.3	0	0
Oregon	60	2	3.3	0	0	6	10	1	1.7	2	3.3	2	3.3	2	3.3	2	1.7	0	0	5	8.3	3	5
Washington	59	4	6.8	7	1.7	7	11.9	2	3.4	4	6.8	2	3.4	4	6.8	2	3.4	1	1.7	6	10.2	5	8.5

Note: The 2021 performance data do not reflect the full impact of the COVID-19 pandemic. Please refer to the discussion in the Introduction for more information.

Table 8

Table		Page
8	**Utilization and Personnel in Community Hospitals By Metropolitan Area for 2022**	171
	U.S. Census Division 1	172
	U.S. Census Division 2	174
	U.S. Census Division 3	176
	U.S. Census Division 4	182
	U.S. Census Division 5	186
	U.S. Census Division 6	188
	U.S. Census Division 7	192
	U.S. Census Division 8	194
	U.S. Census Division 9	198

Core-Based Statistical Areas

A core-based statistical area is a U.S. geographic area defined by the Office of Management and Budget (OMB) that consists of one or more counties (or equivalents) anchored by an urban center of at least 10,000 people plus adjacent counties that are socioeconomically tied to the urban center by commuting. Areas defined on the basis of these standards applied to Census 2000 data were announced by OMB in June 2003.

When a CBSA encompasses two or more central cities, up to three cities may be specified in the CBSA title. They will be listed in order of population size. When a single central city exists, the CBSA is named for that particular city. A CBSA may extend beyond a single state.

A CBSA containing a single core with a population of 2.5 million or more may be subdivided to form smaller groupings of counties referred to as Metropolitan Divisions. Where they exist, Metropolitan Divisions are shown in this table rather than the entire CBSA.

Note: The 2021 performance data do not reflect the full impact of the COVID-19 pandemic. Please refer to the discussion in the Introduction for more information.

TABLE 8

U.S. CENSUS DIVISION 1, NEW ENGLAND

U.S. Community Hospitals
(Nonfederal, short-term general and other special hospitals)

2022 Utilization and Personnel

CLASSIFICATION	Hospitals	Beds	Admissions	Inpatient Days	Adjusted Inpatient Days	Average Daily Census	Adjusted Average Daily Census	Average Stay (days)	Surgical Operations	NEWBORNS	
										Bassinets	Births
UNITED STATES	5,129	784,112	31,555,807	188,912,326	427,815,753	517,547	1,172,213	6	27,415,410	52,767	3,510,787
Nonmetropolitan	1,810	101,773	2,674,924	18,315,169	70,605,601	50,170	193,475	6.8	3,612,917	8,171	329,480
Metropolitan	3,319	682,339	28,880,883	170,597,157	357,210,152	467,377	978,738	5.9	23,802,493	44,596	3,181,307
CENSUS DIVISION 1, NEW ENGLAND	191	33,234	1,461,305	9,195,363	24,051,275	25,190	65,898	6.3	1,293,610	2,222	141,485
Nonmetropolitan	56	3,441	117,255	818,398	3,389,404	2,242	9,288	7	183,876	309	12,226
Metropolitan	135	29,793	1,344,050	8,376,965	20,661,871	22,948	56,610	6.2	1,109,734	1,913	129,259
Connecticut	31	7,473	361,956	2,262,500	5,133,633	6,198	14,065	6.3	279,036	452	35,009
Nonmetropolitan	3	199	10,934	52,535	142,814	144	391	4.8	8,135	21	1,274
Metropolitan	28	7,274	351,022	2,209,965	4,990,819	6,054	13,674	6.3	270,901	431	33,735
Bridgeport-Stamford-Danbury	6	1,657	88,404	491,887	1,197,504	1,348	3,281	5.6	65,524	119	12,194
Hartford-West Hartford-East Hartford	10	2,478	118,695	752,736	1,620,210	2,061	4,439	6.3	95,947	136	10,215
New Haven	5	1,844	85,413	612,607	1,277,985	1,678	3,501	7.2	64,321	64	6,192
Norwich-New London-Willimantic	3	501	26,851	142,156	421,043	390	1,154	5.3	20,149	54	2,158
Waterbury-Shelton	4	794	31,659	210,579	474,077	577	1,299	6.7	24,960	58	2,976
Maine	34	3,510	109,409	941,674	2,690,912	2,579	7,374	8.6	147,906	241	11,395
Nonmetropolitan	21	1,108	28,781	259,929	1,141,988	713	3,129	9	50,669	117	3,460
Metropolitan	13	2,402	80,628	681,745	1,548,924	1,866	4,245	8.5	97,237	124	7,935
Bangor	4	497	21,019	144,157	366,644	394	1,005	6.9	21,792	28	1,598
Lewiston-Auburn	2	540	13,325	168,445	361,803	462	992	12.6	13,754	25	1,004
Portland-South Portland	7	1,365	46,284	369,143	820,477	1,010	2,248	8	61,691	71	5,333
Massachusetts	73	15,959	730,753	4,427,563	11,344,897	12,131	31,084	6.1	575,869	1,049	65,855
Nonmetropolitan	3	186	5,750	34,985	213,841	96	586	6.1	6,082	28	672
Metropolitan	70	15,773	725,003	4,392,578	11,131,056	12,035	30,498	6.1	569,787	1,021	65,183
Amherst Town-Northampton	1	140	5,756	30,877	118,433	85	324	5.4	4,508	11	601
Barnstable Town	3	388	21,424	112,526	304,907	308	836	5.3	13,853	10	986
Boston	25	6,750	308,527	1,992,869	4,955,443	5,461	13,577	6.5	273,321	311	27,979
Cambridge-Newton-Framingham	18	3,891	180,590	1,010,386	2,580,095	2,768	7,068	5.6	117,610	399	16,713
Pittsfield	2	296	12,197	63,061	241,809	173	663	5.2	12,772	24	748
Providence-Warwick	4	1,055	47,983	271,350	687,277	743	1,883	5.7	34,770	63	4,409
Springfield	7	1,531	68,380	412,821	1,042,537	1,130	2,857	6	47,143	73	5,589
Worcester	10	1,722	80,146	498,688	1,200,555	1,367	3,290	6.2	65,810	130	8,158
New Hampshire	28	2,856	115,320	696,657	2,382,099	1,907	6,526	6	146,853	252	12,978
Nonmetropolitan	17	1,221	47,989	301,466	1,224,489	824	3,356	6.3	82,910	73	4,285
Metropolitan	11	1,635	67,331	395,191	1,157,610	1,083	3,170	5.9	63,943	179	8,693
Manchester-Nashua	5	901	37,999	218,516	632,287	599	1,732	5.8	31,906	110	5,120
Rockingham County-Strafford County	6	734	29,332	176,675	525,323	484	1,438	6	32,037	69	3,573
Rhode Island	11	2,124	97,630	546,235	1,363,914	1,496	3,737	5.6	83,796	117	11,106
Metropolitan	11	2,124	97,630	546,235	1,363,914	1,496	3,737	5.6	83,796	117	11,106
Providence-Warwick	11	2,124	97,630	546,235	1,363,914	1,496	3,737	5.6	83,796	117	11,106
Vermont	14	1,312	46,237	320,734	1,135,820	879	3,112	6.9	60,150	111	5,142
Nonmetropolitan	12	727	23,801	169,483	666,272	465	1,826	7.1	36,080	70	2,535
Metropolitan	2	585	22,436	151,251	469,548	414	1,286	6.7	24,070	41	2,607
Burlington-South Burlington	2	614	22,383	138,121	419,991	379	1,151	6.2	22,019	44	2,446

Note: The 2021 performance data do not reflect the full impact of the COVID-19 pandemic. Please refer to the discussion in the Introduction for more information.

TABLE 8

U.S. CENSUS DIVISION 1, NEW ENGLAND

U.S. Community Hospitals
(Nonfederal, short-term general and other special hospitals)

2022 Utilization and Personnel

OUTPATIENT VISITS		FULL-TIME EQUIVALENT PERSONNEL					FULL-TIME EQUIV. TRAINEES		
Emergency	Total	Physicians and Dentists	Registered Nurses	Licensed Practical Nurses	Other Salaried Personnel	Total Personnel	Medical and Dental Residents	Other Trainees	Total Trainees
136,969,033	799,667,133	156,181	1,595,765	81,078	3,559,675	5,392,699	127,277	15,852	143,129
21,104,862	138,249,897	18,747	154,066	20,198	443,074	636,085	3,269	858	4,127
115,864,171	661,417,236	137,434	1,441,699	60,880	3,116,601	4,756,614	124,008	14,994	139,002
6,975,161	53,890,095	15,224	82,785	2,654	222,094	322,757	9,767	2,923	12,690
881,533	9,278,054	2,077	7,736	412	25,320	35,545	528	184	712
6,093,628	44,612,041	13,147	75,049	2,242	196,774	287,212	9,239	2,739	11,978
1,610,068	10,215,927	1,376	18,221	446	40,621	60,664	2,294	156	2,450
88,791	478,152	49	507	18	1,264	1,838	4	5	9
1,521,277	9,737,775	1,327	17,714	428	39,357	58,826	2,290	151	2,441
368,346	2,450,106	310	3,732	53	8,703	12,798	466	15	481
529,709	3,228,825	629	6,225	170	14,213	21,237	202	122	324
286,063	2,345,375	98	5,665	81	9,668	15,512	1,518	3	1,521
187,690	942,719	85	962	1	2,499	3,547	1	8	9
149,469	770,750	205	1,130	123	4,274	5,732	103	3	106
698,707	7,974,080	1,890	7,073	175	20,740	29,878	387	52	439
275,418	3,379,162	502	1,865	53	6,750	9,170	4	6	10
423,289	4,594,918	1,388	5,208	122	13,990	20,708	383	46	429
70,014	1,163,474	516	1,283	17	3,484	5,300	34	6	40
141,338	768,609	67	873	38	1,914	2,892	35	5	40
211,937	2,662,835	805	3,052	67	8,592	12,516	314	35	349
3,225,024	23,744,721	8,508	42,412	1,385	115,675	167,980	5,324	2,333	7,657
53,000	282,565	109	369	16	939	1,433	5	0	5
3,172,024	23,462,156	8,399	42,043	1,369	114,736	166,547	5,319	2,333	7,652
36,557	281,880	109	334	14	1,117	1,574	0	6	6
105,574	757,831	136	614	15	1,885	2,650	0	3	3
1,012,788	10,605,756	6,397	21,609	438	64,571	93,015	4,086	2,118	6,204
927,009	5,817,714	486	8,863	438	20,991	30,778	414	36	450
72,687	485,615	80	744	96	2,789	3,709	75	0	75
338,527	1,505,484	73	1,848	44	4,502	6,467	21	1	22
297,189	1,662,455	605	3,218	80	8,382	12,285	350	113	463
381,693	2,345,421	513	4,813	244	10,499	16,069	373	56	429
651,205	6,269,301	1,623	6,918	318	21,397	30,256	529	170	699
244,857	3,468,231	1,084	3,366	160	10,855	15,465	508	160	668
406,348	2,801,070	539	3,552	158	10,542	14,791	21	10	31
158,830	1,504,813	353	1,819	63	5,374	7,609	0	8	8
247,518	1,296,257	186	1,733	95	5,168	7,182	21	2	23
482,421	2,422,189	425	4,703	104	12,700	17,932	864	159	1,023
482,421	2,422,189	425	4,703	104	12,700	17,932	864	159	1,023
482,421	2,422,189	425	4,703	104	12,700	17,932	864	159	1,023
307,736	3,263,877	1,402	3,458	226	10,961	16,047	369	53	422
219,467	1,669,944	333	1,629	165	5,512	7,639	7	13	20
88,269	1,593,933	1,069	1,829	61	5,449	8,408	362	40	402
70,796	1,340,817	1,000	1,875	72	5,339	8,286	353	44	397

Note: The 2021 performance data do not reflect the full impact of the COVID-19 pandemic. Please refer to the discussion in the Introduction for more information.

TABLE 8 U.S. CENSUS DIVISION 2, MIDDLE ATLANTIC

U.S. Community Hospitals
(Nonfederal, short-term general and other special hospitals)

2022 Utilization and Personnel

CLASSIFICATION	Hospitals	Beds	Admissions	Inpatient Days	Adjusted Inpatient Days	Average Daily Census	Adjusted Average Daily Census	Average Stay (days)	Surgical Operations	NEWBORNS Bassinets	Births
UNITED STATES	5,129	784,112	31,555,807	188,912,326	427,815,753	517,547	1,172,213	6	27,415,410	52,767	3,510,787
Nonmetropolitan	1,810	101,773	2,674,924	18,315,169	70,605,601	50,170	193,475	6.8	3,612,917	8,171	329,480
Metropolitan	3,319	682,339	28,880,883	170,597,157	357,210,152	467,377	978,738	5.9	23,802,493	44,596	3,181,307
CENSUS DIVISION 2, MIDDLE ATLANTIC	424	106,265	4,314,139	27,976,453	57,765,843	76,654	158,334	6.5	3,785,182	5,869	425,696
Nonmetropolitan	77	8,264	237,992	1,853,557	6,092,229	5,077	16,690	7.8	327,600	431	21,081
Metropolitan	347	98,001	4,076,147	26,122,896	51,673,614	71,577	141,644	6.4	3,457,582	5,438	404,615
New Jersey	79	21,837	874,171	5,336,288	9,661,193	14,622	26,473	6.1	567,460	1,407	99,960
Metropolitan	79	21,837	874,171	5,336,288	9,661,193	14,622	26,473	6.1	567,460	1,407	99,960
Allentown-Bethlehem-Easton	2	187	7,172	36,041	90,655	99	249	5	6,096	0	0
Atlantic City-Hammonton	4	957	37,388	204,482	456,724	560	1,252	5.5	17,823	74	3,014
Camden	11	2,809	125,426	689,566	1,232,381	1,890	3,376	5.5	84,290	182	12,003
Lakewood-New Brunswick	20	5,340	240,532	1,370,908	2,307,738	3,756	6,323	5.7	137,402	376	29,082
New York-Jersey City-White Plains	16	5,745	190,029	1,320,250	2,359,780	3,619	6,464	6.9	128,888	340	23,713
Newark	18	5,299	212,008	1,361,245	2,476,747	3,728	6,789	6.4	131,678	325	25,202
Trenton-Princeton	4	692	30,611	181,238	388,673	497	1,065	5.9	31,165	36	3,763
Vineland	2	384	16,349	101,561	207,273	279	568	6.2	14,836	24	1,651
Wilmington	2	424	14,656	70,997	141,222	194	387	4.8	15,282	50	1,532
New York	160	49,726	2,030,070	14,038,591	28,635,499	38,465	78,449	6.9	1,924,824	2,921	200,809
Nonmetropolitan	35	3,843	87,859	899,176	2,995,936	2,465	8,205	10.2	122,394	208	8,313
Metropolitan	125	45,883	1,942,211	13,139,415	25,639,563	36,000	70,244	6.8	1,802,430	2,713	192,496
Albany-Schenectady-Troy	8	2,459	102,063	624,247	1,452,124	1,710	3,979	6.1	75,931	81	8,089
Binghamton	2	618	25,903	164,749	435,982	451	1,195	6.4	27,493	52	2,116
Buffalo-Cheektowaga	9	3,789	118,322	1,124,521	2,148,092	3,079	5,886	9.5	128,283	227	11,271
Elmira	1	266	10,639	50,203	107,129	138	294	4.7	6,483	20	945
Glens Falls	1	243	11,644	58,596	154,832	161	424	5	9,211	22	1,120
Ithaca	1	159	5,903	30,113	73,767	83	202	5.1	6,359	21	815
Kingston	3	280	8,913	54,153	148,651	149	407	6.1	7,502	20	760
Kiryas Joel-Poughkeepsie-Newburgh	6	1,177	58,587	309,263	611,477	848	1,675	5.3	38,632	68	6,785
Nassau County-Suffolk County	18	7,366	355,875	2,215,479	4,006,007	6,071	10,975	6.2	294,320	395	34,591
New York-Jersey City-White Plains	53	23,788	1,018,676	6,860,495	12,146,439	18,796	33,276	6.7	1,016,735	1,430	106,814
Rochester	10	3,060	113,137	957,612	2,621,791	2,623	7,183	8.5	107,313	174	10,115
Syracuse	6	1,812	77,904	491,693	1,135,648	1,347	3,111	6.3	54,390	123	5,392
Utica-Rome	4	656	25,153	147,023	392,198	403	1,074	5.8	15,897	48	1,860
Watertown-Fort Drum	3	210	9,492	51,268	205,426	141	563	5.4	13,881	32	1,823
Pennsylvania	185	34,702	1,409,898	8,601,574	19,469,151	23,567	53,412	6.1	1,292,898	1,541	124,927
Nonmetropolitan	42	4,421	150,133	954,381	3,096,293	2,612	8,485	6.4	205,206	223	12,768
Metropolitan	143	30,281	1,259,765	7,647,193	16,372,858	20,955	44,927	6.1	1,087,692	1,318	112,159
Allentown-Bethlehem-Easton	9	2,338	109,584	629,688	1,327,704	1,726	3,697	5.7	82,039	93	8,894
Altoona	4	496	19,784	121,145	318,138	332	872	6.1	19,050	28	1,579
Chambersburg	2	331	15,007	69,951	191,467	191	524	4.7	10,312	25	1,680
Erie	6	1,045	34,966	230,345	487,875	632	1,337	6.6	33,656	58	3,401
Gettysburg	1	76	4,916	21,884	89,711	60	246	4.5	4,497	12	347
Harrisburg-Carlisle	9	2,237	78,766	533,278	1,134,831	1,461	3,122	6.8	84,014	71	7,681
Johnstown	3	574	14,930	92,754	188,781	254	517	6.2	13,242	14	1,427
Lancaster	4	866	40,133	219,102	526,916	600	1,443	5.5	41,423	74	5,347
Lebanon	1	163	7,489	38,959	110,307	107	302	5.2	5,503	19	647
Montgomery County-Bucks County-Chester County	19	3,709	173,180	878,015	1,710,332	2,407	4,685	5.1	111,782	239	20,602
Philadelphia	23	7,150	308,789	1,972,537	3,742,915	5,403	10,254	6.4	253,801	237	22,084
Pittsburgh	38	7,179	284,954	1,824,628	4,109,748	4,999	11,260	6.4	284,567	283	24,613
Reading	5	1,031	44,364	279,987	610,995	768	1,673	6.3	19,890	56	3,688
Scranton-Wilkes-Barre	8	1,431	53,621	301,642	724,626	827	1,985	5.6	59,816	51	3,683
State College	2	294	11,106	60,345	129,576	165	355	5.4	10,734	5	1,309
Williamsport	3	413	12,404	108,086	410,244	296	1,124	8.7	14,666	15	1,063
York-Hanover	6	948	45,772	264,847	558,692	727	1,531	5.8	38,700	38	4,114

Note: The 2021 performance data do not reflect the full impact of the COVID-19 pandemic. Please refer to the discussion in the Introduction for more information.

174 AHA Hospital Statistics © 2024 Health Forum LLC, an affiliate of the American Hospital Association

TABLE 8

U.S. CENSUS DIVISION 2, MIDDLE ATLANTIC

U.S. Community Hospitals
(Nonfederal, short-term general and other special hospitals)

2022 Utilization and Personnel

OUTPATIENT VISITS		FULL-TIME EQUIVALENT PERSONNEL					FULL-TIME EQUIV. TRAINEES		
Emergency	Total	Physicians and Dentists	Registered Nurses	Licensed Practical Nurses	Other Salaried Personnel	Total Personnel	Medical and Dental Residents	Other Trainees	Total Trainees
136,969,033	799,667,133	156,181	1,595,765	81,078	3,559,675	5,392,699	127,277	15,852	143,129
21,104,862	138,249,897	18,747	154,066	20,198	443,074	636,085	3,269	858	4,127
115,864,171	661,417,236	137,434	1,441,699	60,880	3,116,601	4,756,614	124,008	14,994	139,002
17,442,118	119,589,789	32,285	228,295	9,131	555,174	824,885	34,303	1,284	35,587
1,899,064	12,652,677	1,683	12,339	1,436	36,449	51,907	836	47	883
15,543,054	106,937,112	30,602	215,956	7,695	518,725	772,978	33,467	1,237	34,704
3,375,540	16,084,922	4,244	40,873	974	88,336	134,427	3,972	85	4,057
3,375,540	16,084,922	4,244	40,873	974	88,336	134,427	3,972	85	4,057
40,440	171,569	12	294	8	728	1,042	1	1	2
153,316	571,424	293	1,506	70	3,486	5,355	82	6	88
457,292	1,527,615	1,085	4,823	156	12,795	18,859	682	9	691
897,696	3,105,385	359	11,553	156	20,326	32,394	1,097	7	1,104
658,741	5,375,461	1,044	9,213	226	20,426	30,909	797	31	828
862,561	4,189,541	1,334	10,600	217	23,418	35,569	1,036	18	1,054
138,981	510,045	106	1,523	52	3,349	5,030	38	8	46
91,264	412,231	1	677	54	2,260	2,992	174	1	175
75,249	221,651	10	684	35	1,548	2,277	65	4	69
8,233,170	61,622,951	17,786	114,609	4,923	302,227	439,545	19,842	683	20,525
826,207	5,629,393	492	5,356	607	15,174	21,629	112	19	131
7,406,963	55,993,558	17,294	109,253	4,316	287,053	417,916	19,730	664	20,394
352,397	2,619,653	757	4,789	286	11,903	17,735	432	43	475
244,281	2,597,220	222	1,854	162	4,502	6,740	136	14	150
504,580	2,429,236	478	6,605	343	13,485	20,911	294	78	372
73,739	381,899	80	956	39	2,215	3,290	36	5	41
42,856	664,019	62	439	26	1,317	1,844	0	0	0
54,342	290,202	37	412	23	987	1,459	11	2	13
24,370	134,270	43	460	27	1,143	1,673	12	4	16
224,521	885,944	38	2,196	36	4,810	7,080	125	4	129
1,148,999	5,293,829	4,974	20,649	442	57,912	83,977	3,839	67	3,906
3,854,817	28,179,995	8,704	59,772	1,614	157,995	228,085	13,075	396	13,471
402,178	8,188,764	1,519	6,222	875	17,617	26,233	916	28	944
308,303	2,741,240	202	3,339	243	8,344	12,128	782	18	800
111,147	1,113,973	115	1,031	109	3,138	4,393	60	2	62
60,433	473,314	63	529	91	1,685	2,368	12	3	15
5,833,408	41,881,916	10,255	72,813	3,234	164,611	250,913	10,489	516	11,005
1,072,857	7,023,284	1,191	6,983	829	21,275	30,278	724	28	752
4,760,551	34,858,632	9,064	65,830	2,405	143,336	220,635	9,765	488	10,253
407,098	2,578,287	1,188	5,567	197	12,728	19,680	612	41	653
64,951	518,022	73	751	52	1,556	2,432	2	22	24
71,935	448,268	0	384	11	1,242	1,637	0	0	0
129,571	492,583	25	1,732	100	3,207	5,064	96	4	100
30,513	298,578	0	200	4	495	699	0	3	3
271,013	2,755,997	1,199	5,151	448	10,862	17,660	930	10	940
36,625	535,275	1	508	42	1,685	2,236	85	4	89
161,872	2,110,286	199	1,719	78	5,626	7,622	88	20	108
45,133	279,474	0	203	8	556	767	20	0	20
562,377	3,301,905	648	7,294	170	14,759	22,871	439	13	452
1,092,314	8,441,773	3,545	21,627	410	43,277	68,859	5,084	234	5,318
1,248,464	7,953,216	1,617	13,816	379	30,173	45,985	1,874	83	1,957
148,929	1,383,596	50	1,708	61	4,759	6,578	225	6	231
218,543	1,423,394	398	2,034	213	4,860	7,505	117	0	117
62,093	340,879	37	482	24	1,111	1,654	16	2	18
62,846	462,763	18	611	96	1,819	2,544	0	0	0
146,274	1,534,336	66	2,043	112	4,621	6,842	177	46	223

CBSAs

Note: The 2021 performance data do not reflect the full impact of the COVID-19 pandemic. Please refer to the discussion in the Introduction for more information.

AHA Hospital Statistics © 2024 Health Forum LLC, an affiliate of the American Hospital Association **175**

TABLE 8 U.S. CENSUS DIVISION 3, SOUTH ATLANTIC

U.S. Community Hospitals
(Nonfederal, short-term general and other special hospitals)

2022 Utilization and Personnel

CLASSIFICATION	Hospitals	Beds	Admissions	Inpatient Days	Adjusted Inpatient Days	Average Daily Census	Adjusted Average Daily Census	Average Stay (days)	Surgical Operations	NEWBORNS	
										Bassinets	Births
UNITED STATES	5,129	784,112	31,555,807	188,912,326	427,815,753	517,547	1,172,213	6	27,415,410	52,767	3,510,787
Nonmetropolitan	1,810	101,773	2,674,924	18,315,169	70,605,601	50,170	193,475	6.8	3,612,917	8,171	329,480
Metropolitan	3,319	682,339	28,880,883	170,597,157	357,210,152	467,377	978,738	5.9	23,802,493	44,596	3,181,307
CENSUS DIVISION 3, SOUTH ATLANTIC	748	154,452	6,660,227	39,353,416	83,653,861	107,815	229,196	5.9	5,370,811	9,754	691,234
Nonmetropolitan	187	15,280	474,618	3,200,522	10,047,705	8,768	27,535	6.7	542,605	1,112	50,869
Metropolitan	561	139,172	6,185,609	36,152,894	73,606,156	99,047	201,661	5.8	4,828,206	8,642	640,365
Delaware	8	2,338	102,143	697,248	1,393,040	1,909	3,817	6.8	85,094	157	10,906
Nonmetropolitan	2	254	14,096	72,897	215,093	199	590	5.2	19,217	25	1,515
Metropolitan	6	2,084	88,047	624,351	1,177,947	1,710	3,227	7.1	65,877	132	9,391
Dover	2	463	19,607	135,120	308,762	370	846	6.9	16,376	36	2,396
Wilmington	4	1,621	68,440	489,231	869,185	1,340	2,381	7.1	49,501	96	6,995
District of Columbia	10	3,363	108,392	875,234	1,539,127	2,397	4,217	8.1	90,029	168	12,216
Metropolitan	10	3,363	108,392	875,234	1,539,127	2,397	4,217	8.1	90,029	168	12,216
Washington	10	3,363	108,392	875,234	1,539,127	2,397	4,217	8.1	90,029	168	12,216
Florida	213	55,144	2,545,316	13,725,366	26,211,128	37,606	71,809	5.4	1,599,060	2,649	212,163
Nonmetropolitan	17	705	24,399	109,526	414,114	301	1,134	4.5	27,418	25	1,343
Metropolitan	196	54,439	2,520,917	13,615,840	25,797,014	37,305	70,675	5.4	1,571,642	2,624	210,820
Cape Coral-Fort Myers	4	1,887	84,407	456,446	911,571	1,250	2,498	5.4	56,199	161	6,721
Crestview-Fort Walton Beach-Destin	5	568	26,675	120,033	253,701	329	694	4.5	24,373	51	3,402
Deltona-Daytona Beach-Ormond Beach	7	1,663	77,699	415,562	856,786	1,139	2,348	5.3	43,318	61	4,275
Fort Lauderdale-Pompano Beach-Sunrise	15	4,772	198,109	1,167,474	2,113,431	3,201	5,790	5.9	108,838	220	19,264
Gainesville	4	1,647	80,221	493,361	807,953	1,351	2,214	6.2	63,432	40	6,560
Homosassa Springs	2	332	16,694	69,596	124,949	191	342	4.2	11,249	20	1,696
Jacksonville	14	4,376	199,438	1,124,951	2,198,948	3,083	6,023	5.6	169,324	264	19,467
Lakeland-Winter Haven	5	1,656	75,881	398,474	854,060	1,091	2,340	5.3	40,767	87	6,400
Miami-Miami Beach-Kendall	23	7,175	286,659	1,712,844	3,354,157	4,692	9,190	6	177,837	364	22,594
Naples-Marco Island	3	919	39,431	200,929	373,580	550	1,024	5.1	24,404	38	3,606
North Port-Sarasota-Bradenton	9	2,224	99,230	527,345	919,350	1,444	2,519	5.3	56,154	80	6,582
Ocala	4	746	36,929	189,230	349,855	519	958	5.1	18,600	30	1,967
Orlando-Kissimmee-Sanford	16	6,691	360,058	1,918,410	3,367,171	5,255	9,224	5.3	246,657	283	32,529
Palm Bay-Melbourne-Titusville	9	1,598	68,744	361,552	624,981	990	1,711	5.3	40,801	70	5,946
Panama City-Panama City Beach	5	541	25,425	143,475	357,046	392	978	5.6	14,849	25	899
Pensacola-Ferry Pass-Brent	8	1,411	67,707	367,525	842,110	1,007	2,308	5.4	49,508	72	7,328
Port St. Lucie	4	1,079	61,228	277,387	528,075	761	1,446	4.5	30,165	64	4,713
Punta Gorda	3	681	25,347	131,242	227,311	359	622	5.2	18,802	22	1,298
Sebastian-Vero Beach-West Vero Corridor	3	448	21,985	108,311	229,382	297	629	4.9	11,132	22	753
Sebring	2	284	15,049	73,205	153,773	201	422	4.9	11,259	29	1,492
St. Petersburg-Clearwater-Largo	13	3,264	135,421	724,880	1,319,338	1,986	3,616	5.4	74,002	89	10,296
Tallahassee	4	798	43,485	221,816	449,446	608	1,231	5.1	25,584	62	3,541
Tampa	20	6,011	293,560	1,504,673	2,965,413	4,123	8,123	5.1	151,381	246	23,194
West Palm Beach-Boca Raton-Delray Beach	13	3,628	181,148	896,225	1,602,623	2,456	4,392	4.9	101,432	224	16,297
Wildwood-The Villages	1	40	387	10,894	12,004	30	33	28.1	1,575	0	0
Georgia	141	24,625	956,736	6,471,991	14,605,933	17,729	40,020	6.8	752,500	1,724	117,996
Nonmetropolitan	55	5,236	126,660	1,161,137	3,542,673	3,181	9,708	9.2	138,904	303	16,631
Metropolitan	86	19,389	830,076	5,310,854	11,063,260	14,548	30,312	6.4	613,596	1,421	101,365
Albany	2	426	17,721	122,475	304,162	335	833	6.9	11,902	29	1,940
Athens-Clarke County	3	597	27,596	151,090	308,919	414	847	5.5	32,285	54	3,425
Atlanta-Sandy Springs-Roswell	38	8,779	391,623	2,476,906	4,926,222	6,786	13,497	6.3	256,402	682	53,177
Augusta-Richmond County	7	1,441	59,737	393,377	804,077	1,076	2,202	6.6	63,051	106	5,559
Brunswick-St. Simons	1	564	13,336	141,087	305,406	387	837	10.6	9,326	8	1,166
Chattanooga	1	35	494	1,332	17,820	4	49	2.7	60	0	0
Columbus	4	974	29,686	174,456	338,427	478	928	5.9	27,869	76	3,239
Dalton	2	242	9,039	43,163	109,908	118	301	4.8	6,692	40	1,535
Gainesville	1	937	38,409	288,452	553,547	790	1,517	7.5	27,471	52	4,927
Hinesville	1	100	3,335	36,589	95,199	100	261	11	2,215	4	447
Macon-Bibb County	5	1,044	43,630	298,749	500,162	820	1,371	6.8	26,021	50	3,509
Marietta	6	1,641	85,649	504,635	1,032,608	1,382	2,829	5.9	58,728	145	11,717
Rome	2	584	27,579	149,347	324,388	409	889	5.4	17,159	30	2,261
Savannah	7	1,345	52,958	378,295	1,065,226	1,036	2,919	7.1	49,046	81	4,918
Valdosta	3	379	14,621	79,106	190,434	217	521	5.4	12,552	30	1,591
Warner Robins	3	301	14,663	71,795	186,755	196	511	4.9	12,817	34	1,954

Note: The 2021 performance data do not reflect the full impact of the COVID-19 pandemic. Please refer to the discussion in the Introduction for more information.

176 AHA Hospital Statistics © 2024 Health Forum LLC, an affiliate of the American Hospital Association

TABLE 8 — U.S. CENSUS DIVISION 3, SOUTH ATLANTIC

U.S. Community Hospitals
(Nonfederal, short-term general and other special hospitals)

2022 Utilization and Personnel

OUTPATIENT VISITS		FULL-TIME EQUIVALENT PERSONNEL					FULL-TIME EQUIV. TRAINEES		
Emergency	Total	Physicians and Dentists	Registered Nurses	Licensed Practical Nurses	Other Salaried Personnel	Total Personnel	Medical and Dental Residents	Other Trainees	Total Trainees
136,969,033	799,667,133	156,181	1,595,765	81,078	3,559,675	5,392,699	127,277	15,852	143,129
21,104,862	138,249,897	18,747	154,066	20,198	443,074	636,085	3,269	858	4,127
115,864,171	661,417,236	137,434	1,441,699	60,880	3,116,601	4,756,614	124,008	14,994	139,002
27,712,049	123,650,884	20,788	303,302	14,720	653,921	992,731	20,901	2,626	23,527
3,297,850	15,199,681	2,064	22,664	3,035	62,473	90,236	372	114	486
24,414,199	108,451,203	18,724	280,638	11,685	591,448	902,495	20,529	2,512	23,041
433,317	2,405,013	955	5,731	212	14,003	20,901	471	28	499
86,092	868,824	143	947	60	2,450	3,600	4	0	4
347,225	1,536,189	812	4,784	152	11,553	17,301	467	28	495
98,309	638,030	125	690	44	3,189	4,048	66	24	90
248,916	898,159	687	4,094	108	8,364	13,253	401	4	405
361,541	2,943,676	1,670	6,921	143	16,232	24,966	1,293	22	1,315
361,541	2,943,676	1,670	6,921	143	16,232	24,966	1,293	22	1,315
361,541	2,943,676	1,670	6,921	143	16,232	24,966	1,293	22	1,315
9,944,409	32,469,671	4,440	103,088	4,154	208,827	320,509	6,636	808	7,444
240,432	724,627	71	1,163	177	3,021	4,432	11	2	13
9,703,977	31,745,044	4,369	101,925	3,977	205,806	316,077	6,625	806	7,431
275,471	577,828	257	3,747	178	9,042	13,224	800	51	851
141,479	410,130	12	890	55	1,441	2,398	8	2	10
323,439	1,583,728	229	2,586	147	6,583	9,545	93	19	112
815,132	3,031,354	531	8,354	242	14,155	23,282	433	41	474
236,069	1,330,554	22	3,777	77	6,458	10,334	1,011	14	1,025
111,981	273,135	17	645	41	1,110	1,813	19	2	21
859,977	2,854,603	216	8,838	321	16,422	25,797	498	42	540
330,350	642,500	29	2,431	34	5,376	7,870	9	1	10
1,212,764	4,400,066	827	15,307	489	29,976	46,599	1,965	159	2,124
238,579	685,149	157	1,669	71	2,903	4,800	35	0	35
309,726	1,091,160	269	3,795	271	7,978	12,313	110	11	121
84,044	275,650	50	1,217	77	2,275	3,619	45	3	48
1,484,788	3,470,622	102	12,027	496	28,612	41,237	988	85	1,073
342,747	984,841	29	2,320	77	3,909	6,335	34	2	36
122,146	377,131	19	664	55	1,230	1,968	14	2	16
342,042	1,721,709	17	2,988	103	4,390	7,498	12	59	71
212,404	367,373	232	1,886	122	4,643	6,883	25	1	26
88,967	219,574	23	915	60	1,545	2,543	24	2	26
63,232	139,099	144	712	24	2,115	2,995	10	0	10
77,642	203,144	34	469	60	1,258	1,821	26	2	28
488,428	1,470,857	280	5,634	206	9,964	16,084	145	4	149
152,351	1,074,660	174	2,419	186	4,946	7,725	105	6	111
846,258	3,184,203	601	12,649	313	27,858	41,421	114	214	328
543,961	1,362,402	98	5,935	258	11,490	17,781	102	84	186
0	13,572	0	51	14	127	192	0	0	0
4,084,147	21,188,510	2,559	43,983	2,836	98,587	147,965	2,158	932	3,090
802,764	3,359,756	484	5,816	1,036	16,730	24,066	88	47	135
3,281,383	17,828,754	2,075	38,167	1,800	81,857	123,899	2,070	885	2,955
63,017	1,197,650	4	690	44	1,679	2,417	33	86	119
117,389	537,331	19	1,489	77	2,713	4,298	100	8	108
1,578,885	8,836,310	1,084	19,095	641	40,945	61,765	903	453	1,356
257,622	1,396,578	80	2,821	146	5,515	8,562	59	75	134
46,132	735,592	109	301	78	1,436	1,924	0	0	0
19,454	34,337	0	31	4	74	109	0	0	0
84,876	480,377	100	1,271	69	2,439	3,879	90	9	99
47,622	235,105	34	399	20	944	1,397	13	2	15
147,030	494,696	88	2,110	77	3,402	5,677	199	53	252
10,675	55,105	13	118	12	305	448	3	0	3
144,791	605,929	16	1,819	163	3,811	5,809	135	39	174
380,151	1,458,805	90	3,812	136	8,003	12,041	262	131	393
116,145	393,693	55	919	81	2,721	3,776	32	2	34
144,954	684,653	224	2,073	130	4,895	7,322	173	19	192
50,007	323,349	154	596	35	1,588	2,373	49	6	55
72,633	359,244	5	623	87	1,387	2,102	19	2	21

Table continues

Note: The 2021 performance data do not reflect the full impact of the COVID-19 pandemic. Please refer to the discussion in the Introduction for more information.

AHA Hospital Statistics © 2024 Health Forum LLC, an affiliate of the American Hospital Association **177**

TABLE 8

U.S. CENSUS DIVISION 3, SOUTH ATLANTIC CONTINUED

U.S. Community Hospitals
(Nonfederal, short-term general and other special hospitals)

2022 Utilization and Personnel

CLASSIFICATION	Hospitals	Beds	Admissions	Inpatient Days	Adjusted Inpatient Days	Average Daily Census	Adjusted Average Daily Census	Average Stay (days)	Surgical Operations	NEWBORNS Bassinets	NEWBORNS Births
Maryland	47	11,169	482,892	2,956,970	5,281,093	8,099	14,472	6.1	420,331	952	63,451
Nonmetropolitan	5	584	22,633	135,620	343,540	372	941	6	24,527	50	1,915
Metropolitan	42	10,585	460,259	2,821,350	4,937,553	7,727	13,531	6.1	395,804	902	61,536
Baltimore-Columbia-Towson	23	7,017	290,386	1,888,208	3,222,853	5,171	8,832	6.5	276,414	472	32,933
Frederick-Gaithersburg-Bethesda	8	1,852	86,097	496,681	835,187	1,361	2,288	5.8	50,248	256	19,803
Hagerstown-Martinsburg	1	327	13,964	68,643	129,784	188	356	4.9	8,108	41	1,834
Lexington Park	2	176	12,138	48,838	116,742	134	319	4	12,026	17	1,815
Salisbury	2	330	16,158	82,448	153,892	226	422	5.1	18,802	28	2,045
Washington	5	764	35,345	204,726	404,399	560	1,109	5.8	25,668	76	2,693
Wilmington	1	119	6,171	31,806	74,696	87	205	5.2	4,538	12	413
North Carolina	111	22,106	976,423	5,933,571	14,363,340	16,252	39,354	6.1	865,322	1,556	117,144
Nonmetropolitan	43	3,616	146,667	795,518	2,525,447	2,176	6,922	5.4	158,284	376	17,644
Metropolitan	68	18,490	829,756	5,138,053	11,837,893	14,076	32,432	6.2	707,038	1,180	99,500
Asheville	5	1,142	54,046	321,370	703,909	881	1,928	5.9	46,591	51	3,836
Burlington	1	189	10,170	48,798	113,411	134	311	4.8	6,665	20	1,152
Charlotte-Concord-Gastonia	19	4,633	227,555	1,335,539	2,888,236	3,659	7,911	5.9	174,084	375	28,092
Durham-Chapel Hill	7	2,424	96,385	740,896	1,715,584	2,030	4,700	7.7	103,586	69	10,965
Fayetteville	2	679	33,364	191,949	388,655	526	1,064	5.8	14,125	48	4,667
Goldsboro	1	233	9,208	46,836	119,859	128	328	5.1	8,951	16	1,200
Greensboro-High Point	6	1,610	63,813	400,522	967,251	1,098	2,650	6.3	43,269	106	8,423
Greenville	1	974	39,228	265,469	509,442	727	1,396	6.8	20,169	47	3,341
Hickory-Lenoir-Morganton	4	798	29,896	170,918	456,603	467	1,252	5.7	28,125	59	3,297
Jacksonville	1	149	5,411	29,177	111,650	80	306	5.4	6,246	23	982
Pinehurst-Southern Pines	1	362	21,339	106,598	212,432	292	582	5	9,656	14	1,570
Raleigh-Cary	5	2,024	99,696	588,790	1,565,802	1,613	4,291	5.9	112,632	177	16,300
Rocky Mount	3	368	14,579	86,520	198,087	237	543	5.9	10,917	34	1,786
Wilmington	4	833	40,379	256,103	648,515	702	1,777	6.3	45,458	40	5,140
Winston-Salem	8	2,072	84,687	548,568	1,238,457	1,502	3,393	6.5	76,564	101	8,749
South Carolina	70	11,798	507,295	2,954,162	6,570,618	8,097	17,999	5.8	551,269	787	51,788
Nonmetropolitan	15	1,394	43,886	276,594	743,644	759	2,037	6.3	48,508	118	3,144
Metropolitan	55	10,404	463,409	2,677,568	5,826,974	7,338	15,962	5.8	502,761	669	48,644
Augusta-Richmond County	2	324	12,418	58,640	108,657	161	298	4.7	9,346	18	1,160
Charleston-North Charleston	8	2,021	96,289	552,274	1,201,815	1,513	3,293	5.7	118,703	116	10,837
Charlotte-Concord-Gastonia	4	629	19,956	142,101	380,112	389	1,041	7.1	15,739	23	1,653
Columbia	9	1,886	83,880	502,831	985,008	1,379	2,698	6	82,819	167	9,581
Florence	5	1,072	38,503	255,198	535,985	699	1,468	6.6	48,772	55	3,232
Greenville-Anderson-Greer	13	2,103	104,468	564,237	1,345,227	1,546	3,684	5.4	120,322	126	11,832
Hilton Head Island-Bluffton-Port Royal	4	373	18,277	76,659	160,531	211	439	4.2	23,606	46	1,981
Myrtle Beach-Conway-North Myrtle Beach	5	952	49,081	257,132	512,464	704	1,404	5.2	52,747	61	3,635
Spartanburg	4	822	32,322	227,460	479,437	624	1,314	7	22,167	33	3,653
Sumter	1	222	8,215	41,036	117,738	112	323	5	8,540	24	1,080
Virginia	94	17,476	758,915	4,275,325	9,699,711	11,715	26,577	5.6	724,201	1,401	88,129
Nonmetropolitan	26	1,945	54,623	348,001	1,042,882	954	2,858	6.4	63,320	126	5,431
Metropolitan	68	15,531	704,292	3,927,324	8,656,829	10,761	23,719	5.6	660,881	1,275	82,698
Arlington-Alexandria-Reston	20	4,526	193,468	1,028,842	2,358,584	2,819	6,461	5.3	145,094	499	34,766
Blacksburg-Christiansburg-Radford	4	258	14,368	68,176	201,719	187	552	4.7	17,394	32	1,616
Charlottesville	3	849	34,183	242,083	610,078	663	1,672	7.1	154,728	41	3,361
Harrisonburg	1	214	19,235	48,775	153,120	134	420	2.5	12,996	16	1,807
Kingsport-Bristol	2	141	6,985	27,301	67,870	74	186	3.9	7,037	16	778
Lynchburg	2	615	27,631	158,937	350,601	435	961	5.8	19,960	39	2,636
Richmond	15	3,698	160,820	915,444	1,780,266	2,508	4,878	5.7	103,259	254	13,812
Roanoke	3	1,105	56,286	350,604	628,373	960	1,722	6.2	45,921	67	4,626
Staunton-Stuarts Draft	1	215	9,440	44,937	169,904	123	465	4.8	11,720	21	901
Virginia Beach-Chesapeake-Norfolk	16	3,369	159,218	918,258	2,072,430	2,518	5,679	5.8	127,823	253	15,935
Winchester	1	541	22,658	123,967	263,884	340	723	5.5	14,949	37	2,460

Note: The 2021 performance data do not reflect the full impact of the COVID-19 pandemic. Please refer to the discussion in the Introduction for more information.

CBSAs

178 AHA Hospital Statistics © 2024 Health Forum LLC, an affiliate of the American Hospital Association

TABLE 8

U.S. CENSUS DIVISION 3, SOUTH ATLANTIC CONTINUED

U.S. Community Hospitals
(Nonfederal, short-term general and other special hospitals)

2022 Utilization and Personnel

OUTPATIENT VISITS		FULL-TIME EQUIVALENT PERSONNEL					FULL-TIME EQUIV. TRAINEES		
Emergency	Total	Physicians and Dentists	Registered Nurses	Licensed Practical Nurses	Other Salaried Personnel	Total Personnel	Medical and Dental Residents	Other Trainees	Total Trainees
1,920,902	7,330,840	2,255	24,550	563	54,890	82,258	2,602	322	2,924
111,041	841,201	103	1,097	94	3,128	4,422	13	5	18
1,809,861	6,489,639	2,152	23,453	469	51,762	77,836	2,589	317	2,906
1,039,427	4,224,546	1,693	16,129	336	35,763	53,921	2,558	287	2,845
352,741	991,077	95.	3,854	25	7,311	11,285	0	6	6
58,458	172,502	10	543	21	1,386	1,960	18	0	18
73,533	207,158	75	556	4	1,278	1,913	0	15	15
75,213	432,499	99	855	38	2,293	3,285	0	0	0
175,273	336,070	151	1,283	36	2,946	4,416	13	9	22
35,216	125,787	29	233	9	785	1,056	0	0	0
4,215,823	20,724,076	3,868	51,290	2,259	113,328	170,745	3,961	235	4,196
973,923	4,119,902	477	6,528	650	17,595	25,250	166	51	217
3,241,900	16,604,174	3,391	44,762	1,609	95,733	145,495	3,795	184	3,979
149,033	1,393,428	367	2,234	88	5,512	8,201	241	26	267
49,576	272,216	3	259	14	788	1,064	0	0	0
1,005,773	3,344,947	234	11,661	368	20,608	32,871	85	20	105
232,225	2,576,008	135	8,715	106	14,459	23,415	1,717	56	1,773
131,575	534,389	246	1,149	115	3,539	5,049	194	1	195
59,342	155,892	0	356	21	1,064	1,441	0	0	0
271,134	1,321,240	485	2,939	277	8,816	12,517	82	0	82
25,695	192,504	262	1,728	51	3,784	5,825	259	26	285
159,087	1,024,985	247	1,368	72	3,590	5,277	30	0	30
46,579	108,239	2	277	15	628	922	0	0	0
31,344	173,698	79	1,121	39	2,332	3,571	73	4	77
499,547	2,672,221	647	6,348	86	11,796	18,877	216	38	254
77,957	453,388	23	554	43	1,783	2,403	3	0	3
175,390	668,270	185	1,577	121	5,513	7,396	101	0	101
327,643	1,712,749	476	4,476	193	11,521	16,666	794	13	807
2,273,244	10,281,319	1,354	21,696	1,173	46,644	70,867	420	7	427
364,548	1,616,011	256	2,088	224	5,634	8,202	1	0	1
1,908,696	8,665,308	1,098	19,608	949	41,010	62,665	419	7	426
49,540	112,669	15	319	21	737	1,092	0	0	0
353,846	1,924,794	162	4,104	162	10,344	14,772	29	5	34
98,276	257,987	53	769	88	1,951	2,861	0	0	0
319,336	1,338,483	45	3,610	126	7,086	10,867	0	0	0
123,014	497,309	162	1,759	103	3,623	5,647	46	0	46
417,985	2,627,222	394	4,474	179	8,531	13,578	41	0	41
101,991	378,537	20	610	25	1,293	1,948	27	2	29
247,010	906,843	90	1,811	204	2,832	4,937	210	0	210
145,256	441,181	156	1,851	30	4,029	6,066	66	0	66
52,442	180,283	1	301	11	584	897	0	0	0
3,501,737	18,721,090	2,590	35,207	2,049	71,657	111,503	2,623	213	2,836
381,691	1,703,167	207	2,946	280	7,235	10,668	53	8	61
3,120,046	17,017,923	2,383	32,261	1,769	64,422	100,835	2,570	205	2,775
966,251	3,165,589	1,065	9,659	385	15,034	26,143	293	50	343
87,141	562,797	8	725	161	1,617	2,511	2	3	5
116,228	2,372,929	7	2,449	95	5,300	7,851	754	25	779
61,046	310,362	0	451	21	787	1,259	0	1	1
44,022	235,099	42	489	30	1,193	1,754	13	2	15
116,178	415,123	10	1,237	116	3,230	4,593	26	2	28
491,161	2,626,284	179	6,498	336	14,401	21,414	970	62	1,032
310,280	2,248,448	661	2,903	216	6,106	9,886	374	17	391
58,351	882,787	117	371	77	1,593	2,158	0	2	2
797,600	3,753,539	270	6,591	310	13,564	20,735	138	39	177
71,788	444,966	24	888	22	1,597	2,531	0	2	2

Table continues

Note: The 2021 performance data do not reflect the full impact of the COVID-19 pandemic. Please refer to the discussion in the Introduction for more information.

TABLE 8 U.S. CENSUS DIVISION 3, SOUTH ATLANTIC CONTINUED

U.S. Community Hospitals
(Nonfederal, short-term general and other special hospitals)

2022 Utilization and Personnel

CLASSIFICATION	Hospitals	Beds	Admissions	Inpatient Days	Adjusted Inpatient Days	Average Daily Census	Adjusted Average Daily Census	Average Stay (days)	Surgical Operations	NEWBORNS	
										Bassinets	Births
West Virginia	54	6,433	222,115	1,463,549	3,989,871	4,011	10,931	6.6	283,005	360	17,441
Nonmetropolitan	24	1,546	41,654	301,229	1,220,312	826	3,345	7.2	62,427	89	3,246
Metropolitan	30	4,887	180,461	1,162,320	2,769,559	3,185	7,586	6.4	220,578	271	14,195
Arlington-Alexandria-Reston	1	25	1,276	4,669	30,550	13	84	3.7	3,003	4	173
Beckley	4	480	16,245	101,336	246,003	278	673	6.2	19,295	29	653
Charleston	6	1,201	41,658	248,280	582,774	680	1,596	6	62,441	68	3,587
Hagerstown-Martinsburg	2	231	9,216	58,191	191,551	159	525	6.3	13,975	21	983
Huntington-Ashland	4	832	30,188	230,147	494,145	631	1,353	7.6	33,245	55	2,709
Morgantown	5	1,046	44,060	274,110	529,459	751	1,451	6.2	52,758	9	3,204
Parkersburg-Vienna	2	323	16,524	74,130	178,389	203	488	4.5	11,764	22	1,149
Weirton-Steubenville	2	216	6,455	46,015	127,471	126	350	7.1	5,131	21	543
Wheeling	3	489	14,371	112,610	307,442	309	842	7.8	18,842	42	1,194
Winchester	1	44	468	12,832	81,775	35	224	27.4	124	0	0

Note: The 2021 performance data do not reflect the full impact of the COVID-19 pandemic. Please refer to the discussion in the Introduction for more information.

Table 8

U.S. CENSUS DIVISION 3, SOUTH ATLANTIC CONTINUED

U.S. Community Hospitals
(Nonfederal, short-term general and other special hospitals)

2022 Utilization and Personnel

OUTPATIENT VISITS		FULL-TIME EQUIVALENT PERSONNEL					FULL-TIME EQUIV. TRAINEES		
Emergency	Total	Physicians and Dentists	Registered Nurses	Licensed Practical Nurses	Other Salaried Personnel	Total Personnel	Medical and Dental Residents	Other Trainees	Total Trainees
976,929	7,586,689	1,097	10,836	1,331	29,753	43,017	737	59	796
337,359	1,966,193	323	2,079	514	6,680	9,596	36	1	37
639,570	5,620,496	774	8,757	817	23,073	33,421	701	58	759
19,623	116,491	0	80	0	177	257	0	1	1
64,279	215,210	37	512	76	1,246	1,871	4	0	4
169,523	1,270,453	220	2,229	189	6,083	8,721	189	0	189
52,040	337,062	2	352	11	870	1,235	0	1	1
88,374	927,281	147	1,659	223	4,012	6,041	0	0	0
107,185	1,526,300	78	2,486	128	5,725	8,417	463	44	507
37,182	45,684	71	464	73	1,549	2,157	18	11	29
38,044	500,463	48	303	24	911	1,286	0	0	0
53,507	627,219	166	647	87	2,377	3,277	27	1	28
9,813	54,333	5	25	6	123	159	0	0	0

Note: The 2021 performance data do not reflect the full impact of the COVID-19 pandemic. Please refer to the discussion in the Introduction for more information.

TABLE 8 — U.S. CENSUS DIVISION 4, EAST NORTH CENTRAL

U.S. Community Hospitals
(Nonfederal, short-term general and other special hospitals)

2022 Utilization and Personnel

CLASSIFICATION	Hospitals	Beds	Admissions	Inpatient Days	Adjusted Inpatient Days	Average Daily Census	Adjusted Average Daily Census	Average Stay (days)	Surgical Operations	NEWBORNS Bassinets	NEWBORNS Births
UNITED STATES	5,129	784,112	31,555,807	188,912,326	427,815,753	517,547	1,172,213	6	27,415,410	52,767	3,510,787
Nonmetropolitan	1,810	101,773	2,674,924	18,315,169	70,605,601	50,170	193,475	6.8	3,612,917	8,171	329,480
Metropolitan	3,319	682,339	28,880,883	170,597,157	357,210,152	467,377	978,738	5.9	23,802,493	44,596	3,181,307
CENSUS DIVISION 4, EAST NORTH CENTRAL	771	116,292	4,662,619	26,231,354	68,813,979	71,861	188,575	5.6	4,485,536	8,798	469,439
Nonmetropolitan	266	14,863	454,198	2,518,736	12,875,982	6,904	35,288	5.5	710,092	1,514	53,797
Metropolitan	505	101,429	4,208,421	23,712,618	55,937,997	64,957	153,287	5.6	3,775,444	7,284	415,642
Illinois	181	30,671	1,195,512	6,788,731	16,505,119	18,599	45,246	5.7	1,027,309	2,244	122,734
Nonmetropolitan	61	3,459	102,684	540,554	2,084,031	1,481	5,709	5.3	136,601	261	9,899
Metropolitan	120	27,212	1,092,828	6,248,177	14,421,088	17,118	39,537	5.7	890,708	1,983	112,835
Bloomington	2	328	14,753	71,471	160,858	196	441	4.8	11,664	52	2,084
Champaign-Urbana	4	717	30,175	164,251	482,755	450	1,323	5.4	22,178	49	3,314
Chicago-Naperville-Schaumburg	64	18,479	748,850	4,380,155	9,589,622	12,001	26,271	5.8	554,330	1,319	76,028
Davenport-Moline-Rock Island	6	522	14,526	79,152	287,107	217	815	5.4	15,288	40	1,330
Decatur	2	425	12,233	68,746	221,621	189	607	5.6	18,645	38	1,191
Elgin	7	1,098	39,527	199,382	525,755	545	1,441	5	28,673	80	4,690
Kankakee	2	482	14,379	71,487	240,222	196	658	5	15,962	35	1,190
Lake County	5	877	43,246	197,088	497,818	540	1,363	4.6	38,853	110	4,495
Paducah	1	25	367	1,596	16,168	4	44	4.3	292	0	0
Peoria	6	1,162	44,303	282,460	700,356	775	1,918	6.4	64,502	57	3,698
Rockford	4	820	36,298	209,665	435,157	574	1,192	5.8	35,329	69	5,454
Springfield	2	935	39,874	245,503	483,306	673	1,325	6.2	35,494	37	3,439
St. Louis	15	1,342	54,297	277,221	780,343	758	2,139	5.1	49,498	97	5,922
Indiana	130	18,043	707,815	4,028,917	9,867,703	11,029	27,041	5.7	624,272	1,563	76,846
Nonmetropolitan	41	2,433	68,784	419,206	1,539,177	1,146	4,222	6.1	93,319	269	10,230
Metropolitan	89	15,610	639,031	3,609,711	8,328,526	9,883	22,819	5.6	530,953	1,294	66,616
Bloomington	2	254	12,270	64,541	166,135	177	455	5.3	8,952	24	1,720
Cincinnati	1	61	3,535	12,849	28,505	35	78	3.6	2,544	10	319
Columbus	1	245	9,963	42,743	105,981	117	290	4.3	10,725	20	1,125
Elkhart-Goshen	2	333	16,093	73,327	155,614	200	427	4.6	14,625	54	2,091
Evansville	6	1,187	54,129	360,884	842,485	989	2,309	6.7	44,901	62	4,335
Fort Wayne	9	1,791	79,921	424,542	937,235	1,163	2,568	5.3	86,290	156	7,249
Indianapolis-Carmel-Greenwood	31	5,565	228,369	1,328,917	3,131,010	3,638	8,578	5.8	180,710	490	28,233
Kokomo	2	225	9,550	39,424	123,468	108	338	4.1	8,703	31	1,005
Lafayette-West Lafayette	4	460	22,372	108,908	294,087	298	806	4.9	17,113	50	2,599
Lake County-Porter County-Jasper County	13	3,050	99,220	607,788	1,236,835	1,664	3,388	6.1	77,586	224	7,086
Louisville-Jefferson County	6	545	24,302	111,031	317,501	303	871	4.6	24,137	48	2,176
Michigan City-La Porte	2	255	11,956	54,355	127,188	149	348	4.5	11,111	30	1,307
Muncie	2	369	15,924	97,508	208,118	267	571	6.1	5,885	20	1,202
South Bend-Mishawaka	3	711	31,167	166,862	313,011	457	857	5.4	22,391	40	3,650
Terre Haute	5	559	20,260	116,032	341,353	318	935	5.7	15,280	35	2,519
Michigan	140	24,569	1,004,007	5,736,102	16,498,642	15,722	45,202	5.7	926,394	1,612	96,729
Nonmetropolitan	51	2,713	76,710	486,327	4,573,893	1,337	12,534	6.3	146,396	250	8,682
Metropolitan	89	21,856	927,297	5,249,775	11,924,749	14,385	32,668	5.7	779,998	1,362	88,047
Ann Arbor	5	1,752	87,124	510,968	1,273,943	1,400	3,490	5.9	87,928	95	9,593
Battle Creek	3	283	10,678	56,013	177,594	153	486	5.2	12,179	32	1,445
Bay City	2	378	12,582	81,284	142,552	223	391	6.5	8,159	14	477
Detroit-Dearborn-Livonia	18	5,120	208,904	1,198,895	2,454,949	3,284	6,724	5.7	148,013	273	16,138
Flint	4	1,184	47,728	287,482	509,800	787	1,397	6	32,116	89	4,145
Grand Rapids-Wyoming-Kentwood	13	2,557	98,356	565,418	1,416,613	1,549	3,880	5.7	112,645	176	13,654
Jackson	1	383	15,428	75,092	176,997	206	485	4.9	25,587	19	1,216
Kalamazoo-Portage	2	801	36,071	188,743	433,591	517	1,188	5.2	37,197	93	4,354
Lansing-East Lansing	6	940	40,510	238,018	571,352	653	1,566	5.9	29,189	42	4,272
Midland	1	274	12,668	53,186	138,593	146	380	4.2	12,324	23	1,269
Monroe	1	238	5,815	25,841	79,176	71	217	4.4	4,124	7	584
Muskegon-Norton Shores	1	345	17,220	89,567	214,283	245	587	5.2	15,001	26	993
Niles	2	451	12,006	97,959	307,779	269	843	8.2	9,941	36	1,362
Saginaw	3	751	31,662	195,823	439,720	536	1,205	6.2	21,778	27	2,796
South Bend-Mishawaka	1	25	488	2,306	11,490	6	31	4.7	132	0	0
Traverse City	3	597	19,815	158,472	637,817	434	1,747	8	15,749	12	1,881
Warren-Troy-Farmington Hills	23	5,777	270,242	1,424,708	2,938,500	3,906	8,051	5.3	207,936	398	23,868

Note: The 2021 performance data do not reflect the full impact of the COVID-19 pandemic. Please refer to the discussion in the Introduction for more information.

TABLE 8

U.S. CENSUS DIVISION 4, EAST NORTH CENTRAL

U.S. Community Hospitals
(Nonfederal, short-term general and other special hospitals)

2022 Utilization and Personnel

OUTPATIENT VISITS		FULL-TIME EQUIVALENT PERSONNEL					FULL-TIME EQUIV. TRAINEES		
Emergency	Total	Physicians and Dentists	Registered Nurses	Licensed Practical Nurses	Other Salaried Personnel	Total Personnel	Medical and Dental Residents	Other Trainees	Total Trainees
136,969,033	799,667,133	156,181	1,595,765	81,078	3,559,675	5,392,699	127,277	15,852	143,129
21,104,862	138,249,897	18,747	154,066	20,198	443,074	636,085	3,269	858	4,127
115,864,171	661,417,236	137,434	1,441,699	60,880	3,116,601	4,756,614	124,008	14,994	139,002
21,369,744	167,508,009	28,358	244,826	10,006	571,344	854,534	22,343	3,222	25,565
4,283,719	30,337,579	3,380	27,654	2,723	79,832	113,589	409	192	601
17,086,025	137,170,430	24,978	217,172	7,283	491,512	740,945	21,934	3,030	24,964
4,969,025	39,706,797	8,799	63,686	1,822	142,397	216,704	6,936	545	7,481
852,111	5,925,937	608	6,363	698	17,804	25,473	102	19	121
4,116,914	33,780,860	8,191	57,323	1,124	124,593	191,231	6,834	526	7,360
53,950	381,851	2	651	4	1,260	1,917	12	7	19
121,418	2,243,548	36	1,992	73	3,417	5,518	119	8	127
2,596,661	21,981,636	7,053	40,588	628	88,116	136,385	5,927	323	6,250
97,246	912,904	54	732	30	1,797	2,613	0	0	0
66,988	364,517	51	396	60	1,502	2,009	15	0	15
163,523	1,468,992	274	2,161	36	4,029	6,500	7	8	15
52,866	733,552	88	463	34	1,959	2,544	34	0	34
210,210	1,323,059	308	2,366	47	4,469	7,190	16	29	45
6,656	34,998	4	41	16	156	217	0	0	0
156,062	1,331,130	135	2,317	49	5,361	7,862	329	38	367
141,943	637,845	91	1,576	26	3,375	5,068	13	24	37
113,689	727,787	0	1,554	25	3,562	5,141	335	0	335
335,702	1,639,041	95	2,486	96	5,590	8,267	27	89	116
3,547,567	21,586,248	2,176	33,033	1,610	80,988	117,807	1,539	381	1,920
760,985	5,505,497	626	4,362	492	13,182	18,662	52	35	87
2,786,582	16,080,751	1,550	28,671	1,118	67,806	99,145	1,487	346	1,833
63,103	377,158	3	679	31	1,231	1,944	0	1	1
21,086	120,964	0	152	8	277	437	0	0	0
45,265	280,079	7	331	13	1,190	1,541	0	0	0
73,914	287,904	36	807	26	1,972	2,841	11	2	13
156,256	1,109,077	157	2,474	60	4,892	7,583	70	78	148
454,041	1,633,551	44	3,271	125	5,844	9,284	42	8	50
1,002,612	6,940,883	550	11,083	385	30,303	42,321	981	203	1,184
55,896	356,498	13	281	2	631	927	0	2	2
131,683	652,406	228	1,059	59	2,538	3,884	29	3	32
364,354	2,371,532	340	4,380	190	9,217	14,127	203	36	239
99,182	553,714	58	877	86	2,192	3,213	8	4	12
69,125	285,479	26	462	33	1,099	1,620	8	2	10
56,037	230,403	1	623	16	1,367	2,007	62	5	67
99,098	344,614	42	1,296	46	2,919	4,303	47	2	49
94,930	536,489	45	896	38	2,134	3,113	26	0	26
4,493,966	37,790,055	5,110	49,904	1,449	108,801	165,264	5,053	401	5,454
732,335	5,658,123	621	4,210	354	12,485	17,670	38	21	59
3,761,631	32,131,932	4,489	45,694	1,095	96,316	147,594	5,015	380	5,395
216,156	4,844,207	32	7,386	120	14,070	21,608	121	0	121
64,622	589,581	75	489	22	1,607	2,193	0	0	0
39,354	257,966	46	656	21	2,251	2,974	22	0	22
975,250	6,875,761	1,771	9,704	244	17,735	29,454	1,644	92	1,736
176,866	866,573	23	2,234	22	3,214	5,493	406	10	416
526,753	4,625,783	532	5,602	251	15,445	21,830	588	2	590
69,961	1,027,627	130	862	46	2,143	3,181	115	23	138
126,498	1,729,655	276	1,494	32	3,300	5,102	0	2	2
227,404	1,933,242	269	1,871	31	5,131	7,302	240	43	283
37,572	341,543	9	692	20	1,459	2,180	33	0	33
36,571	203,498	0	211	27	588	826	51	0	51
81,836	1,540,644	135	848	7	2,310	3,300	77	0	77
71,104	510,310	33	625	13	1,548	2,219	66	0	66
119,744	954,111	181	1,245	28	3,773	5,227	0	2	2
7,958	37,701	0	13	0	48	61	0	0	0
71,285	758,191	84	942	30	2,717	3,773	6	35	41
912,697	5,035,539	893	10,820	181	18,977	30,871	1,646	171	1,817

Table continues

Note: The 2021 performance data do not reflect the full impact of the COVID-19 pandemic. Please refer to the discussion in the Introduction for more information.

TABLE 8 U.S. CENSUS DIVISION 4, EAST NORTH CENTRAL CONTINUED

U.S. Community Hospitals
(Nonfederal, short-term general and other special hospitals)

2022 Utilization and Personnel

CLASSIFICATION	Hospitals	Beds	Admissions	Inpatient Days	Adjusted Inpatient Days	Average Daily Census	Adjusted Average Daily Census	Average Stay (days)	Surgical Operations	NEWBORNS Bassinets	Births
Ohio	187	31,519	1,290,499	6,988,804	16,718,428	19,146	45,807	5.4	1,283,208	2,385	115,910
Nonmetropolitan	54	3,978	136,800	632,912	2,154,059	1,737	5,903	4.6	203,631	487	16,508
Metropolitan	133	27,541	1,153,699	6,355,892	14,564,369	17,409	39,904	5.5	1,079,577	1,898	99,402
Akron	7	1,910	82,257	455,834	1,011,170	1,248	2,771	5.5	76,279	188	7,063
Canton-Massillon	5	1,133	36,080	210,011	600,222	574	1,644	5.8	29,930	99	3,222
Cincinnati	18	4,501	191,661	1,051,155	2,210,111	2,880	6,055	5.5	174,390	356	20,361
Cleveland	32	7,238	310,370	1,710,696	4,310,135	4,687	11,808	5.5	346,042	314	22,534
Columbus	24	5,610	219,891	1,316,159	2,682,210	3,606	7,350	6	196,433	386	19,358
Dayton-Kettering-Beavercreek	13	2,376	112,010	586,741	1,325,277	1,607	3,632	5.2	98,825	102	10,534
Huntington-Ashland	1	8	185	499	2,841	1	8	2.7	960	0	0
Lima	5	489	24,052	108,121	246,157	295	673	4.5	13,618	64	1,819
Mansfield	3	310	12,511	63,114	158,641	173	435	5	9,681	42	1,368
Sandusky	2	280	8,349	42,423	97,731	116	268	5.1	13,709	17	1,229
Springfield	2	283	13,794	67,269	153,020	184	420	4.9	7,535	25	1,248
Toledo	10	1,831	76,198	411,793	1,026,271	1,129	2,811	5.4	72,161	153	7,193
Weirton-Steubenville	2	373	6,547	44,612	158,763	122	435	6.8	6,647	15	308
Wheeling	1	10	446	1,479	19,772	4	54	3.3	368	0	0
Youngstown-Warren	8	1,189	59,348	285,986	562,048	783	1,540	4.8	32,999	137	3,165
Wisconsin	133	11,490	464,786	2,688,800	9,224,087	7,365	25,279	5.8	624,353	994	57,220
Nonmetropolitan	59	2,280	69,220	439,737	2,524,822	1,203	6,920	6.4	130,145	247	8,478
Metropolitan	74	9,210	395,566	2,249,063	6,699,265	6,162	18,359	5.7	494,208	747	48,742
Appleton	3	332	15,211	67,540	233,524	185	640	4.4	37,657	45	1,992
Duluth	1	25	415	3,764	76,738	10	210	9.1	2,491	0	0
Eau Claire	7	488	21,268	113,402	382,564	310	1,049	5.3	37,307	48	2,240
Fond du Lac	2	145	6,471	29,994	112,788	82	309	4.6	8,730	15	716
Green Bay	6	680	28,903	156,967	682,255	431	1,870	5.4	58,374	97	4,352
Janesville-Beloit	4	303	12,952	63,676	232,910	175	639	4.9	15,430	30	1,468
Kenosha	2	366	12,382	62,286	210,003	170	575	5	13,348	36	1,760
La Crosse-Onalaska	3	415	18,349	93,473	516,903	256	1,417	5.1	26,125	20	2,262
Madison	9	1,586	69,228	423,506	1,108,221	1,161	3,035	6.1	77,179	89	7,389
Milwaukee-Waukesha	23	3,749	154,708	957,373	2,250,610	2,623	6,167	6.2	142,013	253	19,140
Minneapolis-St. Paul-Bloomington	4	76	3,608	13,106	95,326	36	262	3.6	6,674	14	906
Oshkosh-Neenah	4	370	14,912	69,950	219,019	191	601	4.7	26,723	48	2,578
Racine-Mount Pleasant	2	191	11,769	64,171	189,178	176	518	5.5	9,711	10	1,312
Sheboygan	2	165	6,775	31,438	123,822	86	339	4.6	9,718	21	1,107
Wausau	2	319	18,615	98,417	265,404	270	728	5.3	22,728	21	1,520

Note: The 2021 performance data do not reflect the full impact of the COVID-19 pandemic. Please refer to the discussion in the Introduction for more information.

TABLE 8

U.S. CENSUS DIVISION 4, EAST NORTH CENTRAL CONTINUED

U.S. Community Hospitals
(Nonfederal, short-term general and other special hospitals)

2022 Utilization and Personnel

OUTPATIENT VISITS		FULL-TIME EQUIVALENT PERSONNEL					FULL-TIME EQUIV. TRAINEES		
Emergency	Total	Physicians and Dentists	Registered Nurses	Licensed Practical Nurses	Other Salaried Personnel	Total Personnel	Medical and Dental Residents	Other Trainees	Total Trainees
6,034,098	47,317,280	11,300	70,492	4,221	170,166	256,179	7,812	1,349	9,161
1,348,559	8,302,182	919	7,948	948	22,524	32,339	104	59	163
4,685,539	39,015,098	10,381	62,544	3,273	147,642	223,840	7,708	1,290	8,998
390,367	2,734,567	1,019	4,794	348	12,548	18,709	589	28	617
127,316	1,369,698	206	2,032	290	5,737	8,265	109	8	117
784,532	6,298,883	953	9,987	281	26,306	37,527	1,700	250	1,950
1,194,281	13,494,001	3,805	18,969	1,239	45,337	69,350	3,039	757	3,796
669,127	7,090,777	3,797	12,934	394	27,947	45,072	1,505	186	1,691
671,285	2,877,418	197	5,724	183	11,801	17,905	471	31	502
1,425	5,069	0	28	2	53	83	0	0	0
87,095	715,405	42	845	154	2,106	3,147	24	7	31
75,013	404,457	44	479	26	1,140	1,689	12	4	16
73,619	404,067	50	566	27	1,308	1,951	15	6	21
78,046	390,033	35	499	23	1,093	1,650	14	3	17
252,731	1,703,522	62	3,362	127	7,256	10,807	99	2	101
32,125	418,490	68	258	44	895	1,265	69	0	69
7,033	150,321	5	33	3	122	163	0	0	0
241,544	958,390	98	2,034	132	3,993	6,257	62	8	70
2,325,088	21,107,629	973	27,711	904	68,992	98,580	1,003	546	1,549
589,729	4,945,840	606	4,771	231	13,837	19,445	113	58	171
1,735,359	16,161,789	367	22,940	673	55,155	79,135	890	488	1,378
68,047	582,450	0	744	28	1,194	1,966	0	0	0
14,152	64,536	0	61	42	223	326	0	0	0
75,879	851,032	91	1,338	40	3,939	5,408	0	10	10
40,127	258,076	0	334	9	805	1,148	0	0	0
120,861	2,149,876	159	2,016	230	4,416	6,821	0	25	25
73,097	1,390,692	0	759	17	1,872	2,648	0	0	0
90,442	720,685	0	921	10	2,367	3,298	0	16	16
93,205	1,193,550	0	1,295	64	3,472	4,831	0	0	0
234,118	2,288,326	40	3,918	35	10,545	14,538	709	65	774
674,030	4,824,470	0	8,964	108	20,449	29,521	174	345	519
31,085	271,598	15	251	10	720	996	0	0	0
64,720	463,771	0	848	51	1,810	2,709	0	8	8
67,575	546,220	0	452	16	1,083	1,551	0	1	1
37,687	183,412	1	357	8	745	1,111	0	11	11
50,334	373,095	61	682	5	1,515	2,263	7	7	14

Note: The 2021 performance data do not reflect the full impact of the COVID-19 pandemic. Please refer to the discussion in the Introduction for more information.

AHA Hospital Statistics © 2024 Health Forum LLC, an affiliate of the American Hospital Association

TABLE 8   U.S. CENSUS DIVISION 5, EAST SOUTH CENTRAL

U.S. Community Hospitals
(Nonfederal, short-term general and other special hospitals)

2022 Utilization and Personnel

CLASSIFICATION	Hospitals	Beds	Admissions	Inpatient Days	Adjusted Inpatient Days	Average Daily Census	Adjusted Average Daily Census	Average Stay (days)	Surgical Operations	NEWBORNS Bassinets	Births
UNITED STATES	5,129	784,112	31,555,807	188,912,326	427,815,753	517,547	1,172,213	6	27,415,410	52,767	3,510,787
Nonmetropolitan	1,810	101,773	2,674,924	18,315,169	70,605,601	50,170	193,475	6.8	3,612,917	8,171	329,480
Metropolitan	3,319	682,339	28,880,883	170,597,157	357,210,152	467,377	978,738	5.9	23,802,493	44,596	3,181,307
CENSUS DIVISION 5, EAST SOUTH CENTRAL	417	59,997	2,168,039	13,876,228	32,000,230	38,014	87,670	6.4	2,028,500	3,663	210,306
Nonmetropolitan	206	16,421	397,586	2,898,962	9,195,590	7,940	25,196	7.3	465,200	1,105	45,275
Metropolitan	211	43,576	1,770,453	10,977,266	22,804,640	30,074	62,474	6.2	1,563,300	2,558	165,031
Alabama	102	15,554	602,107	3,842,006	8,281,405	10,532	22,684	6.4	690,553	977	59,789
Nonmetropolitan	39	2,487	65,384	388,752	1,260,299	1,069	3,453	5.9	130,235	193	6,552
Metropolitan	63	13,067	536,723	3,453,254	7,021,106	9,463	19,231	6.4	560,318	784	53,237
Anniston-Oxford	3	429	13,626	77,686	162,956	213	446	5.7	10,535	20	1,862
Auburn-Opelika	1	544	17,956	170,304	350,068	467	959	9.5	13,526	31	2,728
Birmingham	19	4,862	198,865	1,344,680	2,595,089	3,685	7,111	6.8	206,444	249	17,907
Columbus	2	90	4,148	26,615	36,642	73	100	6.4	5,880	0	0
Daphne-Fairhope-Foley	3	352	20,746	89,712	251,351	246	688	4.3	27,988	47	2,204
Decatur	2	153	6,063	31,964	92,054	88	252	5.3	8,860	20	552
Dothan	5	826	34,196	223,902	500,595	612	1,371	6.5	31,863	57	3,371
Florence-Muscle Shoals	3	523	19,958	114,374	283,125	313	775	5.7	21,329	52	2,087
Gadsden	3	510	18,684	118,431	199,207	324	545	6.3	18,299	10	781
Huntsville	4	1,286	63,235	338,581	706,743	928	1,936	5.4	75,854	103	7,525
Mobile	6	1,569	69,076	437,332	781,385	1,199	2,140	6.3	55,513	85	5,683
Montgomery	8	1,207	46,408	306,599	605,929	841	1,659	6.6	60,340	68	5,432
Tuscaloosa	4	716	23,762	173,074	455,962	474	1,249	7.3	23,887	42	3,105
Kentucky	104	13,992	499,303	3,040,113	7,203,118	8,325	19,736	6.1	485,242	835	50,917
Nonmetropolitan	62	4,863	138,119	802,677	2,308,348	2,195	6,324	5.8	153,954	368	15,166
Metropolitan	42	9,129	361,184	2,237,436	4,894,770	6,130	13,412	6.2	331,288	467	35,751
Bowling Green	4	680	24,158	163,837	333,907	448	914	6.8	12,594	19	1,496
Cincinnati	7	970	45,846	237,479	524,711	650	1,438	5.2	37,879	38	4,180
Clarksville	2	157	5,877	34,672	99,298	95	272	5.9	4,237	18	617
Elizabethtown	2	308	15,923	70,316	276,279	193	757	4.4	21,560	26	1,237
Huntington-Ashland	2	538	18,004	147,974	290,475	405	796	8.2	10,344	18	1,989
Lexington-Fayette	10	2,300	87,629	584,370	1,218,314	1,601	3,338	6.7	74,367	124	8,521
Louisville-Jefferson County	10	3,296	127,832	809,069	1,644,912	2,218	4,507	6.3	124,347	143	13,467
Owensboro	1	362	15,392	81,794	237,467	224	651	5.3	20,446	32	2,036
Paducah	4	518	20,523	107,925	269,407	296	739	5.3	25,514	49	2,208
Mississippi	99	11,544	301,048	2,343,142	6,590,289	6,416	18,059	7.8	241,388	642	35,087
Nonmetropolitan	66	6,483	123,288	1,199,135	4,155,303	3,285	11,388	9.7	106,517	343	16,671
Metropolitan	33	5,061	177,760	1,144,007	2,434,986	3,131	6,671	6.4	134,871	299	18,416
Gulfport-Biloxi	8	1,037	36,466	203,025	460,077	556	1,259	5.6	29,871	74	4,848
Hattiesburg	3	780	31,912	171,912	305,907	471	838	5.4	16,795	29	3,624
Jackson	18	2,793	89,650	665,459	1,437,907	1,821	3,940	7.4	82,397	154	7,898
Memphis	4	451	19,732	103,611	231,095	283	634	5.3	5,808	42	2,046
Tennessee	112	18,907	765,581	4,650,967	9,925,418	12,741	27,191	6.1	611,317	1,209	64,513
Nonmetropolitan	39	2,588	70,795	508,398	1,471,640	1,391	4,031	7.2	74,494	201	6,886
Metropolitan	73	16,319	694,786	4,142,569	8,453,778	11,350	23,160	6	536,823	1,008	57,627
Chattanooga	5	1,747	74,432	460,269	884,076	1,260	2,422	6.2	87,134	113	5,694
Clarksville	1	172	9,840	41,825	86,546	115	237	4.3	6,671	30	282
Cleveland	1	182	8,810	44,574	91,148	122	250	5.1	5,409	19	892
Jackson	3	653	28,929	185,726	401,918	509	1,101	6.4	22,099	67	3,442
Johnson City	5	848	35,672	203,770	400,162	558	1,096	5.7	16,463	43	1,462
Kingsport-Bristol	6	848	39,528	194,554	418,771	532	1,147	4.9	22,639	74	860
Knoxville	11	2,527	109,132	635,811	1,474,721	1,742	4,040	5.8	91,277	126	10,874
Memphis	13	3,450	127,921	850,137	1,579,646	2,329	4,328	6.6	71,965	178	11,312
Morristown	2	179	9,508	42,515	107,264	116	294	4.5	11,184	12	793
Nashville-Davidson-Murfreesboro-Franklin	26	5,713	251,014	1,483,388	3,009,526	4,067	8,245	5.9	201,982	346	22,016

Note: The 2021 performance data do not reflect the full impact of the COVID-19 pandemic. Please refer to the discussion in the Introduction for more information.

TABLE 8

U.S. CENSUS DIVISION 5, EAST SOUTH CENTRAL

U.S. Community Hospitals
(Nonfederal, short-term general and other special hospitals)

2022 Utilization and Personnel

OUTPATIENT VISITS		FULL-TIME EQUIVALENT PERSONNEL					FULL-TIME EQUIV. TRAINEES		
Emergency	Total	Physicians and Dentists	Registered Nurses	Licensed Practical Nurses	Other Salaried Personnel	Total Personnel	Medical and Dental Residents	Other Trainees	Total Trainees
136,969,033	799,667,133	156,181	1,595,765	81,078	3,559,675	5,392,699	127,277	15,852	143,129
21,104,862	138,249,897	18,747	154,066	20,198	443,074	636,085	3,269	858	4,127
115,864,171	661,417,236	137,434	1,441,699	60,880	3,116,601	4,756,614	124,008	14,994	139,002
9,051,859	45,753,658	8,757	105,156	6,618	222,017	342,548	6,369	939	7,308
2,667,647	12,274,714	1,739	20,943	2,385	53,290	78,357	575	108	683
6,384,212	33,478,944	7,018	84,213	4,233	168,727	264,191	5,794	831	6,625
2,064,969	8,752,070	2,244	29,525	1,653	55,821	89,243	1,915	642	2,557
357,220	1,488,452	243	3,257	356	8,537	12,393	44	10	54
1,707,749	7,263,618	2,001	26,268	1,297	47,284	76,850	1,871	632	2,503
29,895	159,161	3	681	60	1,431	2,175	1	0	1
23,865	219,519	63	925	37	2,081	3,106	179	25	204
543,429	2,493,502	363	10,722	325	17,242	28,652	1,196	411	1,607
16,825	30,338	2	116	21	364	503	1	0	1
112,991	323,524	334	740	23	1,093	2,190	37	10	47
35,794	206,158	39	341	40	925	1,345	8	3	11
61,354	271,599	223	1,340	132	3,165	4,860	66	9	75
82,960	181,334	84	899	78	1,748	2,809	38	2	40
57,282	137,488	22	728	38	1,259	2,047	6	2	8
220,451	1,189,486	259	3,610	219	6,249	10,337	1	81	82
264,189	790,482	514	2,936	132	4,886	8,468	313	30	343
170,210	788,624	72	2,110	126	4,132	6,440	25	4	29
88,504	472,403	23	1,120	66	2,709	3,918	0	55	55
2,369,536	14,976,311	973	24,980	1,220	56,493	83,666	1,447	110	1,557
868,722	4,402,664	672	7,751	627	19,908	28,958	160	45	205
1,500,814	10,573,647	301	17,229	593	36,585	54,708	1,287	65	1,352
58,056	231,871	49	919	44	1,892	2,904	48	2	50
173,176	1,988,738	60	2,258	52	3,650	6,020	31	0	31
37,352	240,769	31	322	26	834	1,213	9	1	10
64,297	488,976	1	395	19	982	1,397	0	0	0
202,011	1,155,327	87	1,146	44	2,439	3,716	71	9	80
258,478	2,659,628	11	4,419	183	12,096	16,709	1,100	46	1,146
487,483	1,813,313	22	6,437	183	11,111	17,753	13	4	17
61,027	1,164,167	0	584	5	1,747	2,336	0	0	0
158,934	830,858	40	749	37	1,834	2,660	15	3	18
1,548,150	7,761,433	1,112	14,853	1,356	33,773	51,094	1,232	52	1,284
847,351	4,203,323	621	6,417	921	16,549	24,508	275	40	315
700,799	3,558,110	491	8,436	435	17,224	26,586	957	12	969
174,229	1,502,572	369	2,064	140	4,545	7,118	77	9	86
98,882	228,644	40	1,296	76	2,714	4,126	23	1	24
340,607	1,582,723	78	4,298	188	8,670	13,234	847	2	849
87,081	244,171	4	778	31	1,295	2,108	10	0	10
3,069,204	14,263,844	4,428	35,798	2,389	75,930	118,545	1,775	135	1,910
594,354	2,180,275	203	3,518	481	8,296	12,498	96	13	109
2,474,850	12,083,569	4,225	32,280	1,908	67,634	106,047	1,679	122	1,801
268,631	1,622,997	265	2,792	210	5,406	8,673	14	2	16
51,188	137,621	12	341	25	697	1,075	18	0	18
40,098	90,487	0	297	23	604	924	0	0	0
110,980	246,755	3	973	104	2,746	3,826	4	16	20
81,140	394,315	55	1,466	85	2,849	4,455	10	8	18
158,521	861,959	135	1,780	95	4,054	6,064	73	8	81
355,112	1,786,407	343	3,954	292	9,031	13,620	20	16	36
495,644	1,546,245	571	6,765	177	14,493	22,006	162	9	171
53,089	161,062	2	315	18	506	841	1	1	2
860,447	5,235,721	2,839	13,597	879	27,248	44,563	1,377	62	1,439

Note: The 2021 performance data do not reflect the full impact of the COVID-19 pandemic. Please refer to the discussion in the Introduction for more information.

AHA Hospital Statistics © 2024 Health Forum LLC, an affiliate of the American Hospital Association 187

TABLE 8

U.S. CENSUS DIVISION 6, WEST NORTH CENTRAL

U.S. Community Hospitals
(Nonfederal, short-term general and other special hospitals)

2022 Utilization and Personnel

CLASSIFICATION	Hospitals	Beds	Admissions	Inpatient Days	Adjusted Inpatient Days	Average Daily Census	Adjusted Average Daily Census	Average Stay (days)	Surgical Operations	NEWBORNS	
										Bassinets	Births
UNITED STATES	685	63,709	2,098,619	13,888,858	39,611,515	38,040	108,525	6.6	2,124,071	4,446	235,386
Nonmetropolitan	433	19,166	357,226	3,248,813	14,698,025	8,898	40,276	9.1	558,034	1,475	51,696
Metropolitan	252	44,543	1,741,393	10,640,045	24,913,490	29,142	68,249	6.1	1,566,037	2,971	183,690
CENSUS DIVISION 6, WEST NORTH CENTRAL	685	63,709	2,098,619	13,888,858	39,611,515	38,040	108,525	6.6	2,124,071	4,446	235,386
Nonmetropolitan	433	19,166	357,226	3,248,813	14,698,025	8,898	40,276	9.1	558,034	1,475	51,696
Metropolitan	252	44,543	1,741,393	10,640,045	24,913,490	29,142	68,249	6.1	1,566,037	2,971	183,690
Iowa	118	8,698	262,298	1,705,062	6,385,425	4,674	17,495	6.5	310,050	630	34,640
Nonmetropolitan	80	3,191	63,725	510,097	3,179,592	1,398	8,713	8	116,463	214	7,995
Metropolitan	38	5,507	198,573	1,194,965	3,205,833	3,276	8,782	6	193,587	416	26,645
Ames	3	305	9,157	64,369	224,698	177	615	7	12,694	30	1,481
Cedar Rapids	4	710	24,420	141,616	549,434	389	1,505	5.8	27,160	54	2,991
Davenport-Moline-Rock Island	3	483	20,915	95,122	225,886	261	619	4.5	13,268	37	2,913
Des Moines-West Des Moines	9	1,404	50,869	324,113	717,868	888	1,966	6.4	44,450	125	8,183
Dubuque	3	292	11,519	64,665	154,383	178	423	5.6	11,967	38	1,285
Iowa City	5	1,090	37,207	286,859	688,887	786	1,887	7.7	40,596	48	3,809
Omaha	3	291	11,116	50,964	137,502	139	377	4.6	12,362	28	1,087
Sioux City	2	375	15,380	82,308	157,661	225	432	5.4	7,292	14	2,216
Waterloo-Cedar Falls	6	557	17,990	84,949	349,514	233	958	4.7	23,798	42	2,680
Kansas	135	9,303	286,980	1,796,247	5,099,472	4,921	13,970	6.3	280,545	672	31,724
Nonmetropolitan	91	3,530	61,315	531,950	2,169,974	1,458	5,945	8.7	88,908	299	8,633
Metropolitan	44	5,773	225,665	1,264,297	2,929,498	3,463	8,025	5.6	191,637	373	23,091
Joplin	2	31	553	3,484	17,697	9	48	6.3	926	0	0
Kansas City	18	2,936	113,796	648,256	1,537,363	1,776	4,212	5.7	101,579	183	12,896
Lawrence	1	142	6,067	26,830	139,758	74	383	4.4	5,328	14	908
Manhattan	5	296	6,313	37,646	150,008	103	411	6	11,358	34	1,196
Topeka	5	667	28,362	158,447	395,194	434	1,083	5.6	23,620	31	2,445
Wichita	13	1,701	70,574	389,634	689,478	1,067	1,888	5.5	48,826	111	5,646
Minnesota	124	13,663	455,125	3,151,933	8,882,702	8,633	24,331	6.9	560,719	1,112	56,289
Nonmetropolitan	74	3,671	60,679	684,509	3,159,153	1,878	8,652	11.3	141,245	299	12,643
Metropolitan	50	9,992	394,446	2,467,424	5,723,549	6,755	15,679	6.3	419,474	813	43,646
Duluth	10	1,161	34,105	247,559	750,964	677	2,056	7.3	37,757	83	2,865
Grand Forks	2	95	990	15,206	90,299	42	247	15.4	518	10	142
Mankato	2	173	7,764	38,411	105,051	105	288	4.9	17,803	16	1,288
Minneapolis-St. Paul-Bloomington	27	6,270	273,219	1,593,147	3,284,130	4,361	8,996	5.8	217,357	590	32,623
Rochester	4	1,554	54,747	417,903	936,281	1,145	2,566	7.6	130,161	83	3,402
Sioux Falls	1	18	674	2,697	18,436	7	51	4	286	5	103
St. Cloud	4	721	22,947	152,501	538,388	418	1,475	6.6	15,592	26	3,223
Missouri	115	17,838	715,424	4,244,382	10,396,864	11,623	28,484	5.9	575,403	1,201	66,498
Nonmetropolitan	47	2,534	78,459	397,844	1,760,045	1,088	4,825	5.1	82,637	248	8,808
Metropolitan	68	15,304	636,965	3,846,538	8,636,819	10,535	23,659	6	492,766	953	57,690
Cape Girardeau	3	490	15,099	90,538	241,249	248	661	6	15,094	36	1,951
Columbia	4	977	39,392	245,147	474,173	671	1,298	6.2	35,017	59	3,824
Jefferson City	2	200	10,369	46,102	160,841	126	440	4.4	9,431	28	1,378
Joplin	5	676	30,032	156,011	404,178	427	1,107	5.2	16,493	56	3,039
Kansas City	21	3,714	151,345	884,926	1,946,628	2,424	5,334	5.8	105,235	185	13,088
Springfield	5	1,364	66,845	396,527	1,081,059	1,085	2,961	5.9	68,962	104	6,877
St. Joseph	1	352	13,832	70,377	187,742	193	514	5.1	9,463	28	1,316
St. Louis	27	7,531	310,051	1,956,910	4,140,949	5,361	11,344	6.3	233,071	457	26,217
Nebraska	93	6,695	183,713	1,301,588	3,332,312	3,562	9,132	7.1	212,166	479	22,824
Nonmetropolitan	66	2,799	51,105	428,470	1,520,863	1,171	4,169	8.4	74,272	249	7,078
Metropolitan	27	3,896	132,608	873,118	1,811,449	2,391	4,963	6.6	137,894	230	15,746
Grand Island	4	270	7,390	47,824	136,767	131	375	6.5	6,353	27	483
Lincoln	6	1,201	39,767	267,176	454,830	732	1,246	6.7	24,706	60	3,665
Omaha	17	2,425	85,451	558,118	1,219,852	1,528	3,342	6.5	106,835	143	11,598
North Dakota	43	3,322	87,274	713,461	2,284,843	1,953	6,259	8.2	88,156	167	11,127
Nonmetropolitan	33	1,210	12,612	224,362	975,908	613	2,673	17.8	15,834	44	1,674
Metropolitan	10	2,112	74,662	489,099	1,308,935	1,340	3,586	6.6	72,322	123	9,453
Bismarck	3	417	20,890	113,452	346,751	311	950	5.4	19,396	33	2,213
Fargo	4	759	36,287	216,621	631,585	594	1,730	6	35,560	42	3,978
Grand Forks	2	356	9,173	60,687	141,884	166	389	6.6	7,917	31	1,732
Minot	1	580	8,312	98,339	188,715	269	517	11.8	9,449	17	1,530

Note: The 2021 performance data do not reflect the full impact of the COVID-19 pandemic. Please refer to the discussion in the Introduction for more information.

188   AHA Hospital Statistics © 2024 Health Forum LLC, an affiliate of the American Hospital Association

TABLE 8

U.S. CENSUS DIVISION 6, WEST NORTH CENTRAL

U.S. Community Hospitals
(Nonfederal, short-term general and other special hospitals)

2022 Utilization and Personnel

OUTPATIENT VISITS		FULL-TIME EQUIVALENT PERSONNEL					FULL-TIME EQUIV. TRAINEES		
Emergency	Total	Physicians and Dentists	Registered Nurses	Licensed Practical Nurses	Other Salaried Personnel	Total Personnel	Medical and Dental Residents	Other Trainees	Total Trainees
8,929,279	76,460,955	14,473	120,638	8,955	287,999	432,065	4,598	1,135	5,733
2,681,465	27,191,672	3,586	25,731	4,264	75,277	108,858	153	106	259
6,247,814	49,269,283	10,887	94,907	4,691	212,722	323,207	4,445	1,029	5,474
8,929,279	76,460,955	14,473	120,638	8,955	287,999	432,065	4,598	1,135	5,733
2,681,465	27,191,672	3,586	25,731	4,264	75,277	108,858	153	106	259
6,247,814	49,269,283	10,887	94,907	4,691	212,722	323,207	4,445	1,029	5,474
1,255,943	14,903,246	1,686	15,460	1,136	40,796	59,078	894	178	1,072
496,451	7,593,773	749	5,470	749	15,920	22,888	51	56	107
759,492	7,309,473	937	9,990	387	24,876	36,190	843	122	965
42,752	371,276	23	480	21	1,299	1,823	0	0	0
125,896	1,416,962	60	1,069	31	3,069	4,229	0	11	11
90,403	302,698	4	687	5	1,077	1,773	0	0	0
176,403	1,162,392	486	2,573	54	5,877	8,990	232	0	232
49,223	239,477	4	564	12	1,182	1,762	0	0	0
88,944	1,830,270	123	2,696	58	7,139	10,016	597	111	708
48,795	180,113	10	366	11	743	1,130	0	0	0
56,445	273,250	84	639	47	1,661	2,431	0	0	0
80,631	1,533,035	143	916	148	2,829	4,036	14	0	14
1,255,041	9,968,331	2,093	15,770	1,458	38,625	57,946	47	127	174
405,507	3,969,836	517	4,080	725	12,832	18,154	15	6	21
849,534	5,998,495	1,576	11,690	733	25,793	39,792	32	121	153
8,503	56,468	5	47	9	149	210	0	0	0
386,482	3,935,443	1,134	6,460	193	13,341	21,128	2	117	119
38,106	184,471	84	271	5	1,273	1,633	0	0	0
39,417	329,942	31	334	35	708	1,108	0	0	0
89,473	396,762	246	1,310	291	4,928	6,775	0	0	0
287,553	1,095,409	76	3,268	200	5,394	8,938	30	4	34
1,908,898	11,906,059	3,669	29,614	1,579	66,581	101,443	1,257	299	1,556
537,011	4,558,789	783	4,986	903	14,678	21,350	10	16	26
1,371,887	7,347,270	2,886	24,628	676	51,903	80,093	1,247	283	1,530
239,089	1,811,835	480	2,032	63	4,558	7,133	17	7	24
9,203	41,667	12	111	19	317	459	0	0	0
39,488	284,455	46	520	34	1,268	1,868	12	3	15
897,359	3,762,449	1,435	14,615	266	29,908	46,224	509	125	634
109,138	854,054	892	6,053	225	13,044	20,214	685	109	794
3,951	48,141	9	28	12	98	147	0	0	0
73,659	544,669	12	1,269	57	2,710	4,048	24	39	63
2,770,889	26,669,337	3,196	35,220	2,573	84,556	125,545	2,151	341	2,492
576,763	5,806,297	643	4,063	940	12,493	18,139	43	1	44
2,194,126	20,863,040	2,553	31,157	1,633	72,063	107,406	2,108	340	2,448
65,938	1,360,520	224	944	173	3,391	4,732	0	0	0
113,237	1,690,648	4	1,708	239	5,091	7,042	434	15	449
62,277	703,600	92	471	84	1,142	1,789	10	0	10
147,857	1,129,152	203	1,287	78	3,104	4,672	38	0	38
649,055	4,098,048	607	7,221	356	18,225	26,409	273	193	466
164,755	3,224,568	925	4,038	365	13,778	19,106	30	0	30
48,659	1,051,096	174	688	164	2,355	3,381	0	0	0
942,348	7,605,408	324	14,800	174	24,977	40,275	1,323	132	1,455
947,142	6,790,502	1,393	11,831	901	28,040	42,165	81	70	151
400,765	3,041,327	455	3,869	585	10,867	15,776	25	10	35
546,377	3,749,175	938	7,962	316	17,173	26,389	56	60	116
41,570	190,648	19	365	29	884	1,297	1	1	2
115,187	517,560	42	1,585	81	3,867	5,575	16	6	22
389,620	3,040,967	877	6,012	206	12,422	19,517	39	53	92
457,849	2,776,264	1,205	6,040	549	13,044	20,838	142	24	166
100,836	607,738	132	1,226	115	3,297	4,770	7	6	13
357,013	2,168,526	1,073	4,814	434	9,747	16,068	135	18	153
64,225	388,104	263	1,353	108	2,835	4,559	11	2	13
96,107	566,352	656	2,173	282	4,072	7,183	6	0	6
112,269	581,662	47	573	24	1,296	1,940	17	4	21
84,412	632,408	107	715	20	1,544	2,386	101	12	113

Table continues

Note: The 2021 performance data do not reflect the full impact of the COVID-19 pandemic. Please refer to the discussion in the Introduction for more information.

TABLE 8

U.S. CENSUS DIVISION 6, WEST NORTH CENTRAL CONTINUED

U.S. Community Hospitals
(Nonfederal, short-term general and other special hospitals)

2022 Utilization and Personnel

CLASSIFICATION	Hospitals	Beds	Admissions	Inpatient Days	Adjusted Inpatient Days	Average Daily Census	Adjusted Average Daily Census	Average Stay (days)	Surgical Operations	NEWBORNS	
										Bassinets	Births
South Dakota	57	4,190	107,805	976,185	3,229,897	2,674	8,854	9.1	97,032	185	12,284
Nonmetropolitan	42	2,231	29,331	471,581	1,932,490	1,292	5,299	16.1	38,675	122	4,865
Metropolitan	15	1,959	78,474	504,604	1,297,407	1,382	3,555	6.4	58,357	63	7,419
Rapid City	5	586	22,485	146,791	346,287	402	948	6.5	10,691	24	1,943
Sioux City	1	40	1,160	5,657	15,503	15	42	4.9	923	0	0
Sioux Falls	9	1,333	54,829	352,156	935,617	965	2,565	6.4	46,743	39	5,476

Note: The 2021 performance data do not reflect the full impact of the COVID-19 pandemic. Please refer to the discussion in the Introduction for more information.

TABLE 8

U.S. CENSUS DIVISION 6, WEST NORTH CENTRAL CONTINUED

U.S. Community Hospitals
(Nonfederal, short-term general and other special hospitals)

2022 Utilization and Personnel

OUTPATIENT VISITS		FULL-TIME EQUIVALENT PERSONNEL					FULL-TIME EQUIV. TRAINEES		
Emergency	Total	Physicians and Dentists	Registered Nurses	Licensed Practical Nurses	Other Salaried Personnel	Total Personnel	Medical and Dental Residents	Other Trainees	Total Trainees
333,517	3,447,216	1,231	6,703	759	16,357	25,050	26	96	122
164,132	1,613,912	307	2,037	247	5,190	7,781	2	11	13
169,385	1,833,304	924	4,666	512	11,167	17,269	24	85	109
66,783	671,394	168	824	103	3,217	4,312	24	0	24
7,165	23,077	1	51	7	132	191	0	0	0
95,437	1,138,833	755	3,791	402	7,818	12,766	0	85	85

Note: The 2021 performance data do not reflect the full impact of the COVID-19 pandemic. Please refer to the discussion in the Introduction for more information.

TABLE 8 — U.S. CENSUS DIVISION 7, WEST SOUTH CENTRAL

U.S. Community Hospitals
(Nonfederal, short-term general and other special hospitals)

2022 Utilization and Personnel

CLASSIFICATION	Hospitals	Beds	Admissions	Inpatient Days	Adjusted Inpatient Days	Average Daily Census	Adjusted Average Daily Census	Average Stay (days)	Surgical Operations	NEWBORNS Bassinets	NEWBORNS Births
UNITED STATES	5,129	784,112	31,555,807	188,912,326	427,815,753	517,547	1,172,213	6	27,415,410	52,767	3,510,787
Nonmetropolitan	1,810	101,773	2,674,924	18,315,169	70,605,601	50,170	193,475	6.8	3,612,917	8,171	329,480
Metropolitan	3,319	682,339	28,880,883	170,597,157	357,210,152	467,377	978,738	5.9	23,802,493	44,596	3,181,307
CENSUS DIVISION 7, WEST SOUTH CENTRAL	886	101,418	4,022,285	22,552,597	47,507,026	61,789	130,150	5.6	3,395,780	7,143	525,555
Nonmetropolitan	281	12,140	327,898	1,695,686	6,098,085	4,647	16,707	5.2	325,147	1,030	42,886
Metropolitan	605	89,278	3,694,387	20,856,911	41,408,941	57,142	113,443	5.6	3,070,633	6,113	482,669
Arkansas	93	9,546	351,584	1,933,644	4,453,594	5,302	12,196	5.5	304,786	694	33,726
Nonmetropolitan	50	2,999	84,496	458,290	1,519,822	1,257	4,163	5.4	70,996	245	8,007
Metropolitan	43	6,547	267,088	1,475,354	2,933,772	4,045	8,033	5.5	233,790	449	25,719
Fayetteville-Springdale-Rogers	10	1,240	52,289	238,810	513,772	655	1,405	4.6	52,713	85	7,730
Fort Smith	7	899	32,447	179,600	380,288	494	1,042	5.5	35,442	50	3,325
Hot Springs	5	495	20,487	111,195	200,933	305	550	5.4	16,803	27	1,335
Jonesboro	4	751	33,159	190,404	440,019	522	1,205	5.7	17,108	46	2,722
Little Rock-North Little Rock-Conway	15	3,126	128,225	753,848	1,378,309	2,065	3,775	5.9	111,665	241	10,607
Memphis	1	11	379	1,242	17,943	3	49	3.3	59	0	0
Texarkana	1	25	102	255	2,508	1	7	2.5	0	0	0
Louisiana	159	14,643	512,575	2,965,012	7,370,394	8,124	20,195	5.8	475,852	897	62,123
Nonmetropolitan	41	1,870	46,370	264,807	935,961	728	2,568	5.7	51,429	110	4,988
Metropolitan	118	12,773	466,205	2,700,205	6,434,433	7,396	17,627	5.8	424,423	787	57,135
Alexandria	6	792	27,533	166,181	330,154	455	905	6	13,803	52	4,004
Baton Rouge	21	2,252	79,367	452,896	1,149,718	1,241	3,149	5.7	75,416	155	10,735
Hammond	8	428	13,433	85,624	198,773	235	545	6.4	16,384	14	972
Houma-Bayou Cane-Thibodaux	7	467	16,752	87,845	337,816	239	926	5.2	22,011	43	2,845
Lafayette	13	1,211	45,834	275,269	625,986	753	1,714	6	37,451	89	6,109
Lake Charles	10	818	25,038	146,921	403,863	404	1,107	5.9	24,950	66	4,853
Monroe	13	989	31,351	180,706	388,671	494	1,064	5.8	19,740	64	5,363
New Orleans-Metairie	20	3,598	122,388	778,333	1,796,574	2,133	4,923	6.4	123,357	176	12,994
Shreveport-Bossier City	11	1,602	77,343	384,890	828,070	1,055	2,266	5	58,852	95	5,904
Slidell-Mandeville-Covington	9	616	27,166	141,540	374,808	387	1,028	5.2	32,459	33	3,426
Oklahoma	125	11,155	392,881	2,291,171	5,348,703	6,278	14,655	5.8	415,576	708	45,588
Nonmetropolitan	62	2,675	75,637	405,776	1,294,422	1,112	3,546	5.4	83,894	217	10,896
Metropolitan	63	8,480	317,244	1,885,395	4,054,281	5,166	11,109	5.9	331,682	491	34,692
Enid	2	279	6,731	39,323	106,214	108	291	5.8	6,846	16	1,207
Fort Smith	1	41	533	1,931	9,319	5	26	3.6	706	0	0
Lawton	2	515	13,904	102,994	274,386	283	752	7.4	11,304	28	1,993
Oklahoma City	33	4,604	162,876	1,000,758	2,131,314	2,740	5,838	6.1	197,912	288	18,940
Tulsa	25	3,041	133,200	740,389	1,533,048	2,030	4,202	5.6	114,914	159	12,552
Texas	509	66,074	2,765,245	15,362,770	30,334,335	42,085	83,104	5.6	2,199,566	4,844	384,118
Nonmetropolitan	128	4,596	121,395	566,813	2,347,880	1,550	6,430	4.7	118,828	458	18,995
Metropolitan	381	61,478	2,643,850	14,795,957	27,986,455	40,535	76,674	5.6	2,080,738	4,386	365,123
Abilene	4	696	23,237	129,882	247,557	356	679	5.6	16,690	11	2,678
Amarillo	5	931	38,205	204,896	356,911	562	979	5.4	25,952	54	4,389
Austin-Round Rock-San Marcos	35	3,874	182,142	1,019,527	1,801,124	2,791	4,935	5.6	139,495	357	30,294
Beaumont-Port Arthur	10	1,084	35,698	204,310	448,344	561	1,229	5.7	32,423	77	4,973
Brownsville-Harlingen	6	1,069	46,394	249,701	388,427	685	1,066	5.4	26,885	88	6,647
College Station-Bryan	7	539	27,580	131,495	302,994	360	828	4.8	22,145	62	3,866
Corpus Christi	7	1,222	51,678	321,373	550,987	880	1,510	6.2	44,586	73	6,230
Dallas-Plano-Irving	78	10,899	460,755	2,680,155	4,925,971	7,340	13,494	5.8	360,049	807	67,187
Eagle Pass	1	60	4,161	15,374	33,842	42	93	3.7	3,255	14	967
El Paso	11	2,074	87,558	480,680	848,315	1,317	2,323	5.5	57,367	195	13,857
Fort Worth-Arlington-Grapevine	37	5,638	267,086	1,413,797	2,437,491	3,872	6,678	5.3	194,386	410	34,954
Houston-Pasadena-The Woodlands	79	16,249	697,838	4,012,651	8,106,536	10,992	22,208	5.8	539,115	1,110	95,928
Killeen-Temple	7	1,010	43,728	245,150	629,992	672	1,724	5.6	42,235	66	5,155
Laredo	4	570	21,577	119,990	237,221	329	650	5.6	21,734	66	4,990
Longview	5	697	31,206	149,516	323,523	410	886	4.8	27,977	77	4,597
Lubbock	12	1,403	55,009	302,253	579,199	830	1,587	5.5	39,180	85	6,001
McAllen-Edinburg-Mission	8	2,182	87,725	454,784	834,972	1,244	2,287	5.2	103,907	186	15,579
Midland	3	396	13,883	81,910	156,171	225	428	5.9	9,787	30	2,514
Odessa	3	599	17,532	102,731	184,578	282	506	5.9	12,542	56	4,025
San Angelo	1	368	16,621	85,367	230,173	234	631	5.1	17,185	35	1,914
San Antonio-New Braunfels	25	5,769	268,920	1,483,883	2,489,650	4,067	6,822	5.5	206,555	340	32,552
Sherman-Denison	5	592	25,954	152,189	242,069	417	664	5.9	26,500	30	1,232
Texarkana	5	657	21,259	116,744	249,040	319	682	5.5	10,719	33	2,406
Tyler	8	1,259	54,824	307,174	690,458	843	1,893	5.6	52,613	28	4,180
Victoria	5	591	15,885	98,773	202,282	270	554	6.2	12,723	30	1,961
Waco	4	602	30,391	137,504	310,462	377	851	4.5	19,908	46	4,169
Wichita Falls	6	448	17,004	94,148	178,166	258	487	5.5	14,825	20	1,878

Note: The 2021 performance data do not reflect the full impact of the COVID-19 pandemic. Please refer to the discussion in the Introduction for more information.

192 AHA Hospital Statistics © 2024 Health Forum LLC, an affiliate of the American Hospital Association

TABLE 8

U.S. CENSUS DIVISION 7, WEST SOUTH CENTRAL

U.S. Community Hospitals
(Nonfederal, short-term general and other special hospitals)

2022 Utilization and Personnel

OUTPATIENT VISITS		FULL-TIME EQUIVALENT PERSONNEL					FULL-TIME EQUIV. TRAINEES		
Emergency	Total	Physicians and Dentists	Registered Nurses	Licensed Practical Nurses	Other Salaried Personnel	Total Personnel	Medical and Dental Residents	Other Trainees	Total Trainees
136,969,033	799,667,133	156,181	1,595,765	81,078	3,559,675	5,392,699	127,277	15,852	143,129
21,104,862	138,249,897	18,747	154,066	20,198	443,074	636,085	3,269	858	4,127
115,864,171	661,417,236	137,434	1,441,699	60,880	3,116,601	4,756,614	124,008	14,994	139,002
18,366,124	74,959,893	9,670	185,210	15,133	366,932	576,945	6,312	1,740	8,052
2,679,468	12,129,760	1,107	15,919	4,021	44,601	65,648	228	29	257
15,686,656	62,830,133	8,563	169,291	11,112	322,331	511,297	6,084	1,711	7,795
1,446,356	6,207,820	1,531	15,068	1,787	30,760	49,146	367	42	409
540,643	2,219,582	332	3,566	960	10,072	14,930	132	3	135
905,713	3,988,238	1,199	11,502	827	20,688	34,216	235	39	274
233,121	778,486	168	2,250	182	4,218	6,818	8	2	10
128,192	497,039	66	993	158	1,973	3,190	31	0	31
63,206	249,065	107	593	57	1,086	1,843	11	0	11
94,911	540,975	51	1,201	59	2,196	3,507	63	34	97
364,611	1,882,894	806	6,398	363	11,067	18,634	122	3	125
17,908	27,336	0	42	0	65	107	0	0	0
3,764	12,443	1	25	8	83	117	0	0	0
2,635,771	11,863,651	2,501	24,951	3,217	58,350	89,019	657	85	742
350,447	1,440,297	213	2,574	528	7,021	10,336	30	5	35
2,285,324	10,423,354	2,288	22,377	2,689	51,329	78,683	627	80	707
134,256	488,951	14	1,094	104	1,936	3,148	10	3	13
397,358	1,318,086	504	4,145	408	9,554	14,611	104	3	107
83,605	522,340	123	672	93	2,254	3,142	0	1	1
134,616	865,220	114	847	122	2,485	3,568	24	1	25
239,529	737,399	131	2,029	324	4,280	6,764	1	2	3
122,502	646,193	94	1,570	116	3,171	4,951	48	5	53
139,225	583,672	95	1,295	221	2,881	4,492	8	8	16
660,352	2,688,285	738	6,448	718	14,588	22,492	411	35	446
243,485	1,754,856	329	2,950	416	7,216	10,911	21	21	42
130,396	818,352	146	1,327	167	2,964	4,604	0	1	1
1,906,646	7,867,172	1,212	17,803	1,826	38,948	59,789	243	125	368
561,363	2,447,293	272	3,375	755	9,758	14,160	58	4	62
1,345,283	5,419,879	940	14,428	1,071	29,190	45,629	185	121	306
35,047	151,647	0	275	34	552	861	0	0	0
1,503	11,519	4	30	7	96	137	0	0	0
69,132	270,091	108	373	141	1,321	1,943	28	0	28
807,137	3,365,264	775	8,994	587	17,464	27,820	149	121	270
432,464	1,621,358	53	4,756	302	9,757	14,868	8	0	8
12,377,351	49,021,250	4,426	127,388	8,303	238,874	378,991	5,045	1,488	6,533
1,227,015	6,022,588	290	6,404	1,778	17,750	26,222	8	17	25
11,150,336	42,998,662	4,136	120,984	6,525	221,124	352,769	5,037	1,471	6,508
99,814	410,300	1	1,380	116	2,535	4,032	0	256	256
133,423	364,818	0	1,423	89	2,264	3,776	0	3	3
794,026	2,307,356	3	6,981	277	9,398	16,659	32	26	58
192,589	689,285	4	1,693	206	2,473	4,376	34	0	34
194,294	350,596	0	1,055	166	2,151	3,372	0	0	0
120,478	931,700	0	1,012	74	1,946	3,032	0	1	1
228,734	683,553	100	2,171	117	5,099	7,487	51	5	56
2,011,089	6,158,654	223	24,363	732	40,186	65,504	1,732	96	1,828
22,446	49,776	0	79	2	223	304	0	0	0
394,409	1,576,323	64	3,621	147	6,048	9,880	0	11	11
1,275,529	3,359,374	3	12,504	539	19,295	32,341	369	114	483
2,706,044	12,649,970	2,375	37,180	1,313	76,865	117,733	1,240	840	2,080
216,592	2,424,031	581	2,069	287	4,543	7,480	476	20	496
112,015	297,221	0	599	43	1,205	1,847	0	2	2
165,610	522,172	9	1,196	32	1,388	2,625	0	0	0
158,340	1,009,372	11	3,230	211	4,840	8,292	0	0	0
369,641	1,060,095	152	2,777	338	6,759	10,026	0	0	0
70,684	177,804	5	437	57	1,583	2,082	0	80	80
80,145	380,895	0	647	90	1,566	2,303	0	0	0
60,707	288,803	0	474	45	1,479	1,998	0	0	0
1,081,951	3,928,826	165	9,268	837	17,115	27,385	946	13	959
97,559	189,954	71	913	89	1,663	2,736	24	0	24
93,638	359,983	0	800	73	1,297	2,170	0	1	1
189,806	1,798,895	312	2,743	363	4,481	7,899	109	2	111
71,317	248,808	45	670	159	1,513	2,387	24	0	24
129,077	556,941	11	952	53	1,469	2,485	0	1	1
80,379	223,157	1	747	70	1,740	2,558	0	0	0

Note: The 2021 performance data do not reflect the full impact of the COVID-19 pandemic. Please refer to the discussion in the Introduction for more information.

TABLE 8 — U.S. CENSUS DIVISION 8, MOUNTAIN

U.S. Community Hospitals
(Nonfederal, short-term general and other special hospitals)

2022 Utilization and Personnel

CLASSIFICATION	Hospitals	Beds	Admissions	Inpatient Days	Adjusted Inpatient Days	Average Daily Census	Adjusted Average Daily Census	Average Stay (days)	Surgical Operations	NEWBORNS Bassinets	NEWBORNS Births
UNITED STATES	5,129	784,112	31,555,807	188,912,326	427,815,753	517,547	1,172,213	6	27,415,410	52,767	3,510,787
Nonmetropolitan	1,810	101,773	2,674,924	18,315,169	70,605,601	50,170	193,475	6.8	3,612,917	8,171	329,480
Metropolitan	3,319	682,339	28,880,883	170,597,157	357,210,152	467,377	978,738	5.9	23,802,493	44,596	3,181,307
CENSUS DIVISION 8, MOUNTAIN	456	50,822	1,998,233	11,337,363	25,756,803	31,062	70,580	5.7	1,708,744	4,203	248,784
Nonmetropolitan	196	7,647	164,115	1,198,588	4,869,974	3,278	13,348	7.3	289,512	799	29,823
Metropolitan	260	43,175	1,834,118	10,138,775	20,886,829	27,784	57,232	5.5	1,419,232	3,404	218,961
Arizona	87	14,673	639,833	3,424,355	6,507,224	9,385	17,830	5.4	478,192	879	74,855
Nonmetropolitan	8	282	13,450	46,277	162,983	127	447	3.4	19,322	48	1,473
Metropolitan	79	14,391	626,383	3,378,078	6,344,241	9,258	17,383	5.4	458,870	831	73,382
Flagstaff	4	382	14,535	79,245	160,468	217	440	5.5	15,480	32	1,401
Lake Havasu City-Kingman	4	512	21,024	105,098	242,113	289	663	5	19,972	27	3,048
Phoenix-Mesa-Chandler	50	9,932	444,638	2,434,607	4,460,736	6,672	12,221	5.5	314,975	539	52,335
Prescott Valley-Prescott	3	321	17,201	75,688	165,368	208	454	4.4	11,031	68	1,958
Sierra Vista-Douglas	4	160	5,559	21,985	93,956	60	258	4	7,106	10	548
Tucson	12	2,641	106,062	583,555	1,022,308	1,599	2,801	5.5	79,494	121	11,159
Yuma	2	443	17,364	77,900	199,292	213	546	4.5	10,812	34	2,933
Colorado	92	11,192	434,715	2,468,885	5,730,317	6,761	15,703	5.7	378,638	979	59,069
Nonmetropolitan	40	1,465	30,363	216,135	922,172	592	2,528	7.1	63,121	141	6,562
Metropolitan	52	9,727	404,352	2,252,750	4,808,145	6,169	13,175	5.6	315,517	838	52,507
Boulder	5	654	29,581	127,049	306,811	348	841	4.3	24,021	131	5,739
Colorado Springs	5	1,125	52,935	280,291	593,784	767	1,627	5.3	42,695	94	7,967
Denver-Aurora-Centennial	28	6,020	253,850	1,461,365	2,891,912	4,002	7,926	5.8	188,625	436	29,113
Fort Collins-Loveland	5	695	26,716	152,364	435,062	418	1,191	5.7	21,403	74	4,191
Grand Junction	3	403	13,138	73,855	195,943	202	537	5.6	11,493	46	1,723
Greeley	4	496	12,545	72,128	170,121	198	466	5.7	9,617	32	1,987
Pueblo	2	334	15,587	85,698	214,512	234	587	5.5	17,663	25	1,787
Idaho	47	3,588	127,568	650,271	1,813,299	1,780	4,967	5.1	131,693	336	18,946
Nonmetropolitan	25	727	14,919	93,119	481,834	254	1,320	6.2	36,172	91	3,629
Metropolitan	22	2,861	112,649	557,152	1,331,465	1,526	3,647	4.9	95,521	245	15,317
Boise City	10	1,456	57,759	295,295	713,560	809	1,955	5.1	52,796	125	8,988
Coeur d'Alene	4	467	20,415	101,633	240,039	278	658	5	17,838	27	2,116
Idaho Falls	3	345	11,374	62,707	130,778	172	358	5.5	5,936	35	855
Lewiston	1	123	5,164	18,218	43,582	50	119	3.5	2,237	22	371
Logan	1	43	543	1,900	11,417	5	31	3.5	951	5	89
Pocatello	1	178	8,341	39,437	94,282	108	258	4.7	6,220	15	1,049
Twin Falls	2	249	9,053	37,962	97,807	104	268	4.2	9,543	16	1,849
Montana	59	3,598	93,985	746,527	2,463,383	2,044	6,753	7.9	109,627	242	11,009
Nonmetropolitan	44	1,771	27,705	309,459	1,271,825	846	3,487	11.2	40,602	106	3,679
Metropolitan	15	1,827	66,280	437,068	1,191,558	1,198	3,266	6.6	69,025	136	7,330
Billings	6	676	27,875	156,051	341,172	428	935	5.6	26,875	57	2,695
Bozeman	2	132	6,250	24,542	91,724	67	252	3.9	6,947	21	1,053
Great Falls	2	500	12,048	139,401	388,479	382	1,064	11.6	17,448	15	1,292
Helena	2	148	6,153	35,218	122,906	97	337	5.7	4,703	12	667
Missoula	3	371	13,954	81,856	247,277	224	678	5.9	13,052	31	1,623
Nevada	46	6,476	256,447	1,616,921	3,041,774	4,433	8,333	6.3	145,616	314	22,272
Nonmetropolitan	10	323	8,176	47,704	198,674	131	544	5.8	9,693	34	1,050
Metropolitan	36	6,153	248,271	1,569,217	2,843,100	4,302	7,789	6.3	135,923	280	21,222
Carson City	1	211	10,754	53,535	135,370	147	371	5	8,285	12	1,058
Las Vegas-Henderson-North Las Vegas	27	4,820	187,597	1,224,323	2,139,116	3,357	5,859	6.5	91,220	193	15,042
Reno	8	1,122	49,920	291,359	568,614	798	1,559	5.8	36,418	75	5,122
New Mexico	43	3,669	172,571	885,056	2,121,145	2,424	5,814	5.1	153,075	572	15,420
Nonmetropolitan	25	1,003	34,664	141,725	494,859	387	1,356	4.1	56,936	143	5,102
Metropolitan	18	2,666	137,907	743,331	1,626,286	2,037	4,458	5.4	96,139	429	10,318
Albuquerque	10	1,905	99,702	561,508	1,194,160	1,539	3,272	5.6	58,828	357	7,583
Farmington	1	130	8,048	40,041	98,087	110	269	5	5,448	22	846
Las Cruces	5	420	19,315	87,633	200,293	240	550	4.5	25,046	36	1,023
Santa Fe	2	211	10,842	54,149	133,746	148	367	5	6,817	14	866

Note: The 2021 performance data do not reflect the full impact of the COVID-19 pandemic. Please refer to the discussion in the Introduction for more information.

TABLE 8 — U.S. CENSUS DIVISION 8, MOUNTAIN

U.S. Community Hospitals
(Nonfederal, short-term general and other special hospitals)

2022 Utilization and Personnel

OUTPATIENT VISITS		FULL-TIME EQUIVALENT PERSONNEL					FULL-TIME EQUIV. TRAINEES		
Emergency	Total	Physicians and Dentists	Registered Nurses	Licensed Practical Nurses	Other Salaried Personnel	Total Personnel	Medical and Dental Residents	Other Trainees	Total Trainees
136,969,033	799,667,133	156,181	1,595,765	81,078	3,559,675	5,392,699	127,277	15,852	143,129
21,104,862	138,249,897	18,747	154,066	20,198	443,074	636,085	3,269	858	4,127
115,864,171	661,417,236	137,434	1,441,699	60,880	3,116,601	4,756,614	124,008	14,994	139,002
8,789,979	47,797,284	8,895	100,290	4,080	214,700	327,965	4,135	636	4,771
1,510,823	9,722,781	1,982	11,707	1,157	36,515	51,361	82	39	121
7,279,156	38,074,503	6,913	88,583	2,923	178,185	276,604	4,053	597	4,650
2,156,190	6,627,349	3,408	28,105	883	52,290	84,686	1,683	227	1,910
66,923	313,831	64	640	61	1,679	2,444	9	5	14
2,089,267	6,313,518	3,344	27,465	822	50,611	82,242	1,674	222	1,896
63,743	155,393	94	730	19	1,929	2,772	2	1	3
97,123	393,803	67	1,009	88	2,369	3,533	40	2	42
1,428,480	4,076,338	1,143	19,710	481	33,338	54,672	773	186	959
50,085	148,262	79	555	17	1,402	2,053	14	2	16
67,007	314,025	29	308	30	906	1,273	10	0	10
316,055	731,033	1,818	4,503	179	8,842	15,342	810	25	835
66,774	494,664	114	650	8	1,825	2,597	25	6	31
2,358,403	11,883,661	1,734	23,829	684	50,936	77,183	575	65	640
340,754	2,275,356	651	2,618	294	8,855	12,418	8	3	11
2,017,649	9,608,305	1,083	21,211	390	42,081	64,765	567	62	629
139,091	700,340	112	1,381	8	2,961	4,462	2	0	2
291,961	1,172,907	1	2,463	6	4,053	6,523	0	0	0
1,143,927	5,385,800	783	13,688	289	27,216	41,976	445	59	504
175,290	1,158,893	18	1,490	27	3,116	4,651	22	0	22
67,894	377,639	38	828	23	1,711	2,600	28	3	31
95,399	519,887	23	634	30	1,287	1,974	40	0	40
104,087	292,839	108	727	7	1,737	2,579	30	0	30
943,798	6,785,715	1,122	8,306	636	20,586	30,650	145	110	255
181,996	1,337,101	201	1,328	177	4,258	5,964	5	5	10
761,802	5,448,614	921	6,978	459	16,328	24,686	140	105	245
416,688	3,371,045	593	4,121	189	9,166	14,069	82	44	126
60,828	684,496	215	952	75	3,162	4,404	21	54	75
94,378	246,545	21	682	51	1,211	1,965	11	2	13
29,492	157,496	21	222	12	545	800	7	1	8
3,960	4,843	7	30	7	87	131	0	0	0
110,570	297,273	13	357	26	732	1,128	19	1	20
45,886	686,916	51	614	99	1,425	2,189	0	3	3
441,258	5,285,004	1,242	6,191	410	17,016	24,859	36	19	55
182,484	2,026,511	529	2,109	161	7,432	10,231	1	10	11
258,774	3,258,493	713	4,082	249	9,584	14,628	35	9	44
92,716	1,242,233	337	1,627	114	3,774	5,852	30	5	35
42,650	575,533	95	456	7	1,116	1,674	0	3	3
43,484	738,634	177	748	66	2,295	3,286	0	0	0
26,094	276,239	75	437	43	1,185	1,740	5	0	5
53,830	425,854	29	814	19	1,214	2,076	0	1	1
798,210	2,945,061	299	9,334	479	18,225	28,337	445	22	467
80,073	440,833	21	442	57	1,451	1,971	5	1	6
718,137	2,504,228	278	8,892	422	16,774	26,366	440	21	461
39,193	323,747	1	337	2	885	1,225	0	0	0
483,074	1,366,348	257	6,528	374	12,131	19,290	424	19	443
195,870	814,133	20	2,027	46	3,758	5,851	16	2	18
945,647	4,029,913	538	8,517	398	19,237	28,690	108	104	212
372,613	1,359,809	225	1,811	169	5,183	7,388	24	7	31
573,034	2,670,104	313	6,706	229	14,054	21,302	84	97	181
290,017	1,316,074	115	4,909	124	9,850	14,998	14	92	106
163,783	874,653	34	360	21	877	1,292	11	1	12
70,269	235,091	89	834	54	1,719	2,696	43	1	44
48,965	244,286	75	603	30	1,608	2,316	16	3	19

Table continues

Note: The 2021 performance data do not reflect the full impact of the COVID-19 pandemic. Please refer to the discussion in the Introduction for more information.

TABLE 8   U.S. CENSUS DIVISION 8, MOUNTAIN CONTINUED

U.S. Community Hospitals
(Nonfederal, short-term general and other special hospitals)

2022 Utilization and Personnel

CLASSIFICATION	Hospitals	Beds	Admissions	Inpatient Days	Adjusted Inpatient Days	Average Daily Census	Adjusted Average Daily Census	Average Stay (days)	Surgical Operations	NEWBORNS Bassinets	Births
Utah	54	5,734	235,181	1,200,362	2,983,897	3,292	8,177	5.1	272,871	714	42,053
Nonmetropolitan	20	688	14,607	88,886	428,203	244	1,174	6.1	34,403	110	4,959
Metropolitan	34	5,046	220,574	1,111,476	2,555,694	3,048	7,003	5	238,468	604	37,094
Logan	2	161	6,855	20,704	81,866	57	225	3	10,279	36	2,277
Ogden	7	1,011	38,504	204,787	435,018	561	1,192	5.3	34,083	119	6,530
Provo-Orem-Lehi	8	793	36,931	160,418	354,349	439	971	4.3	43,913	145	9,271
Salt Lake City-Murray	16	2,787	119,540	653,838	1,501,488	1,794	4,114	5.5	133,833	274	16,301
St. George	1	294	18,744	71,729	182,973	197	501	3.8	16,360	30	2,715
Wyoming	28	1,892	37,933	344,986	1,095,764	943	3,003	9.1	39,032	167	5,160
Nonmetropolitan	24	1,388	20,231	255,283	909,424	697	2,492	12.6	29,263	126	3,369
Metropolitan	4	504	17,702	89,703	186,340	246	511	5.1	9,769	41	1,791
Casper	3	306	8,953	47,384	92,569	130	254	5.3	5,426	25	800
Cheyenne	1	198	8,749	42,319	93,771	116	257	4.8	4,343	16	991

Note: The 2021 performance data do not reflect the full impact of the COVID-19 pandemic. Please refer to the discussion in the Introduction for more information.

TABLE 8

U.S. CENSUS DIVISION 8, MOUNTAIN CONTINUED

U.S. Community Hospitals
(Nonfederal, short-term general and other special hospitals)

2022 Utilization and Personnel

OUTPATIENT VISITS		FULL-TIME EQUIVALENT PERSONNEL					FULL-TIME EQUIV. TRAINEES		
Emergency	Total	Physicians and Dentists	Registered Nurses	Licensed Practical Nurses	Other Salaried Personnel	Total Personnel	Medical and Dental Residents	Other Trainees	Total Trainees
945,016	8,963,953	297	13,560	412	29,639	43,908	1,116	87	1,203
153,363	963,781	67	1,091	81	2,829	4,068	3	6	9
791,653	8,000,172	230	12,469	331	26,810	39,840	1,113	81	1,194
42,425	441,715	2	332	10	655	999	0	3	3
154,046	928,887	63	1,603	106	3,574	5,346	57	6	63
158,707	1,143,935	30	1,792	47	3,148	5,017	44	12	56
371,648	4,657,608	135	8,020	151	17,907	26,213	1,012	49	1,061
64,827	828,027	0	722	17	1,526	2,265	0	11	11
201,457	1,276,628	255	2,448	178	6,771	9,652	27	2	29
132,617	1,005,559	224	1,668	157	4,828	6,877	27	2	29
68,840	271,069	31	780	21	1,943	2,775	0	0	0
31,287	112,707	3	375	12	678	1,068	0	0	0
37,553	158,362	28	405	9	1,265	1,707	0	0	0

CBSAs

Note: The 2021 performance data do not reflect the full impact of the COVID-19 pandemic. Please refer to the discussion in the Introduction for more information.

TABLE 8 — U.S. CENSUS DIVISION 9, PACIFIC

U.S. Community Hospitals
(Nonfederal, short-term general and other special hospitals)

2022 Utilization and Personnel

CLASSIFICATION	Hospitals	Beds	Admissions	Inpatient Days	Adjusted Inpatient Days	Average Daily Census	Adjusted Average Daily Census	Average Stay (days)	Surgical Operations	NEWBORNS Bassinets	Births
UNITED STATES	5,129	784,112	31,555,807	188,912,326	427,815,753	517,547	1,172,213	6	27,415,410	52,767	3,510,787
Nonmetropolitan	1,810	101,773	2,674,924	18,315,169	70,605,601	50,170	193,475	6.8	3,612,917	8,171	329,480
Metropolitan	3,319	682,339	28,880,883	170,597,157	357,210,152	467,377	978,738	5.9	23,802,493	44,596	3,181,307
CENSUS DIVISION 9, PACIFIC	551	97,923	4,170,341	24,500,694	48,655,221	67,122	133,285	5.9	3,223,176	6,669	562,902
Nonmetropolitan	108	4,551	144,036	881,907	3,338,607	2,416	9,147	6.1	210,851	396	21,827
Metropolitan	443	93,372	4,026,305	23,618,787	45,316,614	64,706	124,138	5.9	3,012,325	6,273	541,075
Alaska	20	1,639	51,306	418,838	1,146,973	1,149	3,141	8.2	55,477	170	7,522
Nonmetropolitan	14	535	10,661	122,348	526,470	336	1,442	11.5	21,886	40	1,744
Metropolitan	6	1,104	40,645	296,490	620,503	813	1,699	7.3	33,591	130	5,778
Anchorage	5	887	36,081	251,909	510,115	691	1,397	7	29,775	114	4,718
Fairbanks-College	1	217	4,564	44,581	110,388	122	302	9.8	3,816	16	1,060
California	355	73,877	3,169,185	18,351,352	34,183,760	50,271	93,644	5.8	2,196,265	4,709	423,912
Nonmetropolitan	30	1,411	45,859	279,439	892,789	764	2,445	6.1	55,678	89	6,126
Metropolitan	325	72,466	3,123,326	18,071,913	33,290,971	49,507	91,199	5.8	2,140,587	4,620	417,786
Anaheim-Santa Ana-Irvine	27	6,119	265,763	1,352,317	2,579,109	3,704	7,066	5.1	184,717	347	38,154
Bakersfield-Delano	11	1,659	65,623	359,841	773,348	986	2,119	5.5	37,295	106	10,897
Chico	3	569	30,996	140,104	298,295	384	816	4.5	19,335	28	3,002
El Centro	2	268	9,503	48,117	132,996	132	364	5.1	8,472	24	2,587
Fresno	10	2,010	100,999	591,816	1,169,398	1,622	3,202	5.9	56,055	147	12,558
Hanford-Corcoran	1	173	7,902	36,932	90,471	101	248	4.7	6,625	20	2,260
Los Angeles-Long Beach-Glendale	85	20,672	887,281	5,047,686	8,880,323	13,824	24,327	5.7	547,294	1,183	105,922
Merced	2	224	12,506	54,039	104,452	148	286	4.3	7,080	39	2,958
Modesto	6	1,312	52,096	374,386	684,770	1,026	1,876	7.2	37,839	87	6,458
Napa	2	218	9,493	42,824	98,180	117	269	4.5	11,206	12	690
Oakland-Fremont-Berkeley	19	4,565	184,756	1,142,946	2,114,698	3,131	5,793	6.2	134,548	337	27,889
Oxnard-Thousand Oaks-Ventura	6	1,222	62,232	331,435	607,226	909	1,663	5.3	33,031	111	7,990
Redding	5	563	22,380	147,184	303,739	403	832	6.6	16,169	31	1,698
Riverside-San Bernardino-Ontario	40	8,071	366,640	1,961,356	3,518,541	5,370	9,640	5.3	221,881	575	48,042
Sacramento-Roseville-Folsom	17	4,103	188,788	1,102,903	1,998,554	3,021	5,474	5.8	172,754	314	26,822
Salinas	4	719	34,608	175,063	332,262	480	912	5.1	17,781	71	4,986
San Diego-Chula Vista-Carlsbad	20	5,978	284,780	1,628,390	2,795,697	4,461	7,660	5.7	192,062	342	37,945
San Francisco-San Mateo-Redwood City	16	4,565	130,054	1,161,154	2,062,822	3,182	5,651	8.9	124,869	186	14,691
San Jose-Sunnyvale-Santa Clara	11	3,507	162,397	1,008,676	1,914,777	2,766	5,245	6.2	128,382	235	23,251
San Luis Obispo-Paso Robles	3	309	14,185	63,465	161,559	173	443	4.5	9,879	30	2,559
San Rafael	3	352	14,254	72,237	159,802	198	438	5.1	15,114	8	1,511
Santa Cruz-Watsonville	3	325	14,513	71,771	183,922	197	503	4.9	13,585	41	2,743
Santa Maria-Santa Barbara	5	980	38,024	235,929	447,678	646	1,227	6.2	20,945	35	5,921
Santa Rosa-Petaluma	8	885	34,281	205,043	451,746	562	1,237	6	30,060	52	4,452
Stockton-Lodi	7	1,137	57,393	253,641	497,512	696	1,363	4.4	43,627	107	10,530
Vallejo	4	676	27,477	147,410	307,235	404	842	5.4	27,267	73	4,554
Visalia	3	905	32,327	208,498	438,918	571	1,202	6.4	16,429	67	4,899
Yuba City	2	380	12,075	106,790	182,941	293	501	8.8	6,286	12	1,817
Hawaii	23	2,946	105,662	726,778	1,542,768	1,990	4,226	6.9	110,654	200	13,176
Nonmetropolitan	8	558	19,823	132,041	410,038	362	1,124	6.7	17,699	45	2,499
Metropolitan	15	2,388	85,839	594,737	1,132,730	1,628	3,102	6.9	92,955	155	10,677
Kahului-Wailuku	4	490	9,553	88,191	175,153	241	479	9.2	6,163	20	1,320
Urban Honolulu	11	1,898	76,286	506,546	957,577	1,387	2,623	6.6	86,792	135	9,357
Oregon	61	7,027	319,666	1,753,762	4,201,884	4,807	11,511	5.5	323,607	650	38,760
Nonmetropolitan	24	875	35,731	153,639	671,338	421	1,840	4.3	46,858	117	4,980
Metropolitan	37	6,152	283,935	1,600,123	3,530,546	4,386	9,671	5.6	276,749	533	33,780
Albany	2	95	3,862	18,460	79,716	51	218	4.8	6,795	18	670
Bend	4	407	20,428	96,988	210,843	266	578	4.7	26,798	33	2,268
Corvallis	1	185	7,924	43,961	95,335	120	261	5.5	9,904	20	950
Eugene-Springfield	5	631	33,260	165,971	347,894	455	952	5	23,870	56	3,282
Grants Pass	1	123	7,171	26,694	70,092	73	192	3.7	5,759	14	685
Medford	3	526	21,437	140,953	286,677	386	785	6.6	20,733	29	2,225
Portland-Vancouver-Hillsboro	17	3,598	157,779	954,832	2,102,328	2,618	5,760	6.1	164,779	304	19,143
Salem	4	587	32,074	152,264	337,661	417	925	4.7	18,111	59	4,557

Note: The 2021 performance data do not reflect the full impact of the COVID-19 pandemic. Please refer to the discussion in the Introduction for more information.

198   AHA Hospital Statistics © 2024 Health Forum LLC, an affiliate of the American Hospital Association

TABLE 8

U.S. CENSUS DIVISION 9, PACIFIC

U.S. Community Hospitals
(Nonfederal, short-term general and other special hospitals)

2022 Utilization and Personnel

OUTPATIENT VISITS		FULL-TIME EQUIVALENT PERSONNEL					FULL-TIME EQUIV. TRAINEES		
Emergency	Total	Physicians and Dentists	Registered Nurses	Licensed Practical Nurses	Other Salaried Personnel	Total Personnel	Medical and Dental Residents	Other Trainees	Total Trainees
136,969,033	799,667,133	156,181	1,595,765	81,078	3,559,675	5,392,699	127,277	15,852	143,129
21,104,862	138,249,897	18,747	154,066	20,198	443,074	636,085	3,269	858	4,127
115,864,171	661,417,236	137,434	1,441,699	60,880	3,116,601	4,756,614	124,008	14,994	139,002
18,332,720	90,056,566	17,731	225,263	9,781	465,494	718,269	18,549	1,347	19,896
1,203,293	9,462,979	1,129	9,373	765	29,317	40,584	86	39	125
17,129,427	80,593,587	16,602	215,890	9,016	436,177	677,685	18,463	1,308	19,771
237,702	1,278,759	306	3,272	170	8,331	12,079	92	15	107
55,238	488,954	111	894	82	3,079	4,166	4	6	10
182,464	789,805	195	2,378	88	5,252	7,913	88	9	97
150,369	638,703	132	1,974	79	4,097	6,282	88	9	97
32,095	151,102	63	404	9	1,155	1,631	0	0	0
13,103,190	55,960,281	11,986	170,064	7,898	340,499	530,447	14,019	1,000	15,019
440,030	2,806,712	213	3,123	271	7,824	11,431	56	9	65
12,663,160	53,153,569	11,773	166,941	7,627	332,675	519,016	13,963	991	14,954
935,827	5,251,582	1,096	14,237	623	28,422	44,378	1,029	57	1,086
276,146	859,968	150	3,022	241	7,212	10,625	43	11	54
203,820	1,082,960	55	1,563	73	3,706	5,397	18	6	24
86,785	401,407	54	473	47	1,251	1,825	13	2	15
320,384	1,331,756	309	4,216	182	9,886	14,593	411	64	475
46,474	248,189	15	159	10	386	570	5	0	5
3,071,885	12,015,980	3,850	47,945	2,494	94,374	148,663	3,647	580	4,227
94,096	206,124	0	571	33	940	1,544	32	0	32
203,282	549,658	72	2,552	97	4,267	6,988	34	7	41
36,660	252,770	13	479	12	894	1,398	1	1	2
993,496	3,416,106	417	9,382	442	19,504	29,745	526	19	545
215,226	957,585	70	2,734	99	5,033	7,936	179	13	192
61,090	257,906	23	1,259	78	1,986	3,346	45	1	46
1,394,538	5,003,373	358	17,063	1,146	32,135	50,702	1,034	59	1,093
1,009,344	3,210,383	1,002	12,168	289	22,643	36,102	1,027	25	1,052
181,184	723,874	51	1,623	31	3,620	5,325	33	0	33
1,022,016	4,111,294	173	15,677	554	26,952	43,356	927	43	970
567,001	4,470,865	3,110	9,208	340	21,080	33,738	1,881	11	1,892
594,452	3,760,554	612	10,784	404	24,614	36,414	2,403	28	2,431
51,202	205,679	30	693	58	1,564	2,345	23	1	24
84,722	189,350	0	697	2	1,744	2,443	0	0	0
55,316	313,297	42	568	25	1,273	1,908	11	4	15
140,182	545,934	77	1,679	54	3,802	5,612	118	2	120
180,150	726,687	13	1,833	51	2,949	4,846	56	0	56
393,649	930,152	40	2,694	105	4,713	7,552	149	25	174
220,029	740,363	0	1,386	37	2,984	4,407	27	0	27
162,811	1,273,898	101	1,596	78	3,876	5,651	291	32	323
61,393	115,875	40	680	22	865	1,607	0	0	0
460,850	3,073,014	478	5,490	428	11,093	17,489	32	29	61
89,204	450,046	67	818	62	2,028	2,975	8	8	16
371,646	2,622,968	411	4,672	366	9,065	14,514	24	21	45
57,631	99,487	7	579	6	1,100	1,692	0	0	0
314,015	2,523,481	404	4,093	360	7,965	12,822	24	21	45
1,548,211	12,086,420	1,986	17,463	211	37,035	56,695	1,424	104	1,528
302,012	2,782,199	396	2,287	68	8,163	10,914	10	11	21
1,246,199	9,304,221	1,590	15,176	143	28,872	45,781	1,414	93	1,507
44,836	542,321	89	398	15	1,111	1,613	0	21	21
94,629	333,140	143	1,082	8	1,337	2,570	0	15	15
31,871	418,123	119	435	5	1,089	1,648	106	16	122
163,321	525,199	48	1,711	19	2,779	4,557	2	0	2
45,321	298,351	24	178	12	571	785	0	1	1
87,879	854,480	47	984	22	2,173	3,226	0	7	7
615,217	5,518,014	897	8,986	49	16,167	26,099	1,305	33	1,338
163,125	814,593	223	1,402	13	3,645	5,283	1	0	1

Table continues

Note: The 2021 performance data do not reflect the full impact of the COVID-19 pandemic. Please refer to the discussion in the Introduction for more information.

TABLE 8 U.S. CENSUS DIVISION 9, PACIFIC CONTINUED

U.S. Community Hospitals
(Nonfederal, short-term general and other special hospitals)

2022 Utilization and Personnel

CLASSIFICATION	Hospitals	Beds	Admissions	Inpatient Days	Adjusted Inpatient Days	Average Daily Census	Adjusted Average Daily Census	Average Stay (days)	Surgical Operations	NEWBORNS	
										Bassinets	Births
Washington	92	12,434	524,522	3,249,964	7,579,836	8,905	20,763	6.2	537,173	940	79,532
Nonmetropolitan	32	1,172	31,962	194,440	837,972	533	2,296	6.1	68,730	105	6,478
Metropolitan	60	11,262	492,560	3,055,524	6,741,864	8,372	18,467	6.2	468,443	835	73,054
Bellingham	1	274	13,588	72,602	142,421	199	390	5.3	7,334	13	1,881
Bremerton-Silverdale-Port Orchard	1	248	13,026	75,926	171,043	208	469	5.8	11,293	10	2,065
Everett	4	884	37,185	247,485	441,285	677	1,209	6.7	31,358	53	5,914
Kennewick-Richland	4	492	23,733	115,387	287,983	316	789	4.9	21,107	43	3,087
Lewiston	1	25	1,228	4,661	25,139	13	69	3.8	2,646	0	0
Longview-Kelso	1	180	6,280	33,644	83,025	92	227	5.4	4,603	14	780
Mount Vernon-Anacortes	3	205	10,699	53,069	167,889	145	460	5	10,573	27	1,467
Olympia-Lacey-Tumwater	2	423	20,787	133,465	236,391	366	648	6.4	31,309	43	2,054
Portland-Vancouver-Hillsboro	2	607	29,502	167,135	342,550	457	938	5.7	19,194	64	5,365
Seattle-Bellevue-Kent	18	4,269	175,486	1,169,990	2,570,386	3,208	7,041	6.7	158,738	269	28,103
Spokane-Spokane Valley	8	1,440	50,106	338,090	666,077	926	1,824	6.7	75,009	111	6,910
Tacoma-Lakewood	7	1,545	80,632	494,088	1,052,731	1,354	2,885	6.1	54,464	103	9,648
Walla Walla	1	129	4,940	23,549	71,256	65	195	4.8	4,804	15	848
Wenatchee-East Wenatchee	4	230	11,215	58,754	254,858	161	697	5.2	16,962	23	1,666
Yakima	3	311	14,153	67,679	228,830	185	626	4.8	19,049	47	3,266

Note: The 2021 performance data do not reflect the full impact of the COVID-19 pandemic. Please refer to the discussion in the Introduction for more information.

TABLE 8

U.S. CENSUS DIVISION 9, PACIFIC CONTINUED

U.S. Community Hospitals
(Nonfederal, short-term general and other special hospitals)

2022 Utilization and Personnel

OUTPATIENT VISITS		FULL-TIME EQUIVALENT PERSONNEL					FULL-TIME EQUIV. TRAINEES		
Emergency	Total	Physicians and Dentists	Registered Nurses	Licensed Practical Nurses	Other Salaried Personnel	Total Personnel	Medical and Dental Residents	Other Trainees	Total Trainees
2,982,767	17,658,092	2,975	28,974	1,074	68,536	101,559	2,982	199	3,181
316,809	2,935,068	342	2,251	282	8,223	11,098	8	5	13
2,665,958	14,723,024	2,633	26,723	792	60,313	90,461	2,974	194	3,168
61,345	166,077	6	780	4	1,144	1,934	1	0	1
65,204	403,374	46	534	22	1,263	1,865	22	2	24
139,671	865,323	10	1,451	19	3,120	4,600	0	32	32
205,507	929,602	111	1,441	95	3,300	4,947	67	4	71
18,962	119,482	14	99	10	301	424	1	3	4
50,381	154,098	4	387	3	730	1,124	2	7	9
163,366	960,281	86	807	86	2,133	3,112	14	5	19
88,383	624,307	59	968	26	1,699	2,752	18	0	18
142,885	408,731	66	1,698	10	2,881	4,655	17	0	17
775,883	5,812,243	1,324	11,018	218	27,212	39,772	2,262	120	2,382
254,745	1,289,276	174	2,637	20	4,733	7,564	284	8	292
444,392	1,167,345	521	2,976	176	6,074	9,747	251	4	255
30,465	199,240	31	351	20	856	1,258	10	1	11
92,169	1,072,662	17	720	52	2,335	3,124	0	0	0
132,600	550,983	164	856	31	2,532	3,583	25	8	33

Note: The 2021 performance data do not reflect the full impact of the COVID-19 pandemic. Please refer to the discussion in the Introduction for more information.

AHA Hospital Statistics © 2024 Health Forum LLC, an affiliate of the American Hospital Association

Statistics for Health Care Systems and their Hospitals

The following tables describing health care systems refers to information in section B of the 2024 *AHA Guide*. Table 1 shows the number of health care systems by type of control. Table 2 provides a breakdown of the number of systems that own, lease, sponsor or contract manage hospitals within each control category. Table 3 gives the number of hospitals and beds in each control category as well as total hospitals and beds. Finally, Table 4 shows the percentage of hospitals and beds in each control category.

For more information on health care systems, please write to the American Hospital Association at support@aha.org.

Table 1. Multihospital Health Care Systems, by Type of Organizaton Control

Type of Control	Code	Number of Systems
Catholic (Roman) church–related	CC	26
Other church–related	CO	7
Subtotal, church–related		33
Other not–for–profit	NP	310
Subtotal, not–for–profit		343
Investor Owned	IO	80
Federal Government	FG	5
Total		428

Table 2. Multihospital Health Care Systems, by Type of Ownership and Control

Type of Ownership	Catholic Church–Related (CC)	Other Church–Related (CO)	Total Church–Related (CC + CO)	Other Not–for–Profit (NP)	Total Not–for–Profit (CC, CO, + NP)	Investor–Owned (IO)	Federal Govern–ment (FG)	All Systems
Systems that only own, lease or sponsor	18	6	24	185	209	17	4	230
Systems that only contract–manage	0	0	0	13	13	5	0	18
Systems that manage, own, lease, or sponsor	8	1	9	112	121	58	1	180
Total	26	7	33	310	343	80	5	428

Table 3. Hospitals and Beds in Multihospital Health Care Systems, by Type of Ownership and Control

Type of Ownership	Catholic Church–Related (CC) H	B	Other Church–Related (CO) H	B	Total Church–Related (CC + CO) H	B	Other Not–for–Profit (NP) H	B	Total Not–for–Profit (CC, CO, + NP) H	B	Investor–Owned (IO) H	B	Federal Govern–ment (FG) H	B	All Systems H	B
Owned, leased or sponsored	572	102,790	79	18,194	651	120,984	1,661	354,862	2,312	475,846	1,365	164,493	203	38,668	3,880	679,007
Contract–managed	43	2,442	3	485	46	2,927	128	9,283	174	12,210	104	5,712	0	0	278	17,922
Total	615	105,232	82	18,679	697	123,911	1,789	364,145	2,486	488,056	1,469	170,205	203	38,668	4,158	696,929

H = hospitals; **B** = beds.

Table 4. Hospitals and Beds in Multihospital Health Care Systems, by Type of Ownership and Control as a Percentage of All Systems

Type of Ownership	Catholic Church–Related (CC) H	B	Other Church–Related (CO) H	B	Total Church–Related (CC + CO) H	B	Other Not–for–Profit (NP) H	B	Total Not–for–Profit (CC, CO, + NP) H	B	Investor–Owned (IO) H	B	Federal Govern–ment (FG) H	B	All Systems H	B
Owned, leased or sponsored	14.7	15.1	2.0	2.7	16.8	17.8	42.8	52.3	59.6	70.1	35.2	24.2	5.2	5.7	99.9	100
Contract managed	15.5	13.6	1.1	2.7	16.6	16.3	46.0	52.3	62.6	68.1	37.4	24.2	0	5.7	100	98.5
Total	10.8	15.1	1.4	2.7	12.3	17.8	58.4	52.3	70.6	70.0	25.8	24.2	3.6	5.7	100	100

H = hospitals; **B** = beds.

*Please note that figures may not always equal the provided subtotal or total percentages due to rounding.

Note: The 2021 performance data do not reflect the full impact of the COVID-19 pandemic. Please refer to the discussion in the Introduction for more information.

Glossary

This glossary explains specific terms as they are used in the tables and text of AHA Hospital Statistics.

Ablation of Barrett's esophagus: A premalignant condition that can lead to adenocarcinoma of the esophagus. The nonsurgical ablation of the premalignant tissue in Barrett's esophagus by the application of thermal energy or light through an endoscope passed from the mouth into the esophagus.

Acute long-term care: Provider-specialized acute hospital care to medically complex patients who are critically ill, have multisystem complications and/or failure, and require hospitalization averaging 25 days, in a facility offering specialized treatment programs and therapeutic intervention on a 24 hour/7day-a-week basis.

Adjusted admission: An aggregate measure of workload reflecting the sum of admissions and equivalent admissions attributed to outpatient services. The number of equivalent admissions attributed to outpatient services is derived by multiplying admissions by the ratio of outpatient revenue to inpatient revenue.

$$\frac{\text{Adjusted}}{\text{admissions}} = \text{admissions} + [\text{admissions} * \left(\frac{\text{outpatient revenue}}{\text{inpatient revenue}}\right)]$$

Adjusted average daily census: An estimate of the average number of patients (both inpatients and outpatients) receiving care each day during the reporting period, which is usually 12 months. The figure is derived by dividing the number of inpatient day equivalents (also called ***adjusted inpatient days***) by the number of days in the reporting period.

Adjusted inpatient days: An aggregate measure of workload reflecting the sum of inpatient days and equivalent patient days attributed to outpatient services. The number of equivalent patient days attributed to outpatient services is derived by multiplying inpatient days by the ratio of outpatient revenue to inpatient revenue.

$$\frac{\text{Adjusted}}{\text{inpatient days}} = \text{inpatient days} + [\text{inpatient days} * \left(\frac{\text{outpatient revenue}}{\text{inpatient revenue}}\right)]$$

Admissions: The number of patients, excluding newborns, accepted for inpatient service during the reporting period; the number includes patients who visit the emergency room and are later admitted for inpatient service.

Adult cardiac surgery: Includes minimally invasive procedures that include surgery done with only a small incision or no incision at all, such as through a laparoscope or an endoscope, and more invasive major surgical procedures that include open chest and open heart surgery.

Adult cardiology services: An organized clinical service offering diagnostic and interventional procedures to manage the full range of adult heart conditions.

Adult day care program: A program providing supervision, medical and psychological care, and social activities for older adults who live at home or in another family setting but cannot be alone or prefer to be with others during the day. May include intake assessment, health monitoring, occupational therapy, personal care, noon meal, and transportation services.

Adult diagnostic/invasive catheterization: Also called *coronary angiography* or *coronary arteriography*, used to assist in diagnosing complex heart conditions. Coronary angiography involves the insertion of a tiny catheter into the artery in the groin, then carefully threading the catheter up into the aorta where the coronary arteries originate. Once the catheter is in place, a dye is injected to allow the cardiologist to see the size, shape, and distribution of the coronary arteries. These images are used to diagnose heart disease and to determine, among other things, whether or not surgery is indicated.

Adult Interventional cardiac catheterization: A nonsurgical procedure that utilizes the same basic principles as diagnostic catheterization and then uses advanced techniques to improve the heart's function. It can be a less-invasive alternative to heart surgery.

Air ambulance services: Aircraft and especially a helicopter equipped for transporting the injured or sick. Most air ambulances carry critically ill or injured patients, whose condition could rapidly change for the worse.

Airborne infection isolation room: A single-occupancy room for patient care where environmental factors are controlled in an effort to minimize the transmission of those infectious agents usually spread person to person by droplet nuclei associated with coughing and inhalation. Such rooms typically have specific ventilation requirements for controlled ventilation, air pressure, and filtration.

Alcoholism-chemical dependency partial hospitalization services: Organized hospital services providing intensive day/evening outpatient services of three or more hours' duration, distinguished from other outpatient visits of 1 hour.

Alcoholism-chemical dependency pediatric services: Provides diagnosis and therapeutic services to pediatric patients with alcoholism or other drug dependencies. Includes care for inpatient/residential treatment for patients whose course of treatment involves more intensive care than provided in an outpatient setting or where patient requires supervised withdrawal.

Alcoholism/drug abuse or dependency inpatient care: Provides diagnosis and therapeutic services to patients with alcoholism or other drug dependencies. Includes care for inpatient/residential treatment for patients whose course of treatment involves more intensive care than provided in an outpatient setting or where patient requires supervised withdrawal.

Alcoholism/drug abuse or dependency outpatient services: Organized hospital services that provide medical care and/or rehabilitative treatment services to outpatients for whom the primary diagnosis is alcoholism or other chemical dependency.

Alzheimer center: A facility that offers care to persons with Alzheimer's disease and their families through an integrated program of clinical services, research, and education.

Ambulance services: The provision of ambulance services to the ill and injured who require medical attention on a scheduled or unscheduled basis.

Ambulatory surgery center: A facility that provides care to patients requiring surgery who are admitted and discharged on the same day. Ambulatory surgery centers are distinct from same day surgical units within the hospital outpatient departments for purposes of Medicare payments.

Arthritis treatment center: Specifically equipped and staffed center for the diagnosis and treatment of arthritis and other joint disorders.

Assisted living: A special combination of housing, supportive services, personalized assistance, and health care designed to respond to the individual needs of those who need help in activities of daily living and instrumental activities of daily living. Supportive services are available, 24 hours a day, to meet scheduled and unscheduled needs in a way that promotes maximum independence and dignity for each resident and encourages the involvement of a resident's family, neighbor, and friends.

Assistive technology center: A program providing access to specialized hardware and software with adaptations allowing individuals greater independence with mobility, dexterity, or increased communication options.

Auxiliary: A volunteer community organization formed to assist the hospital in carrying out its purpose and to serve as a link between the institution and the community.

Average daily census: The average number of people served on an inpatient basis on a single day during the reporting period; the figure is calculated by dividing the number of inpatient days by the number of days in the reporting period.

Bariatric/weight control services: Referred to as Bariatrics, the medical practice of weight reduction.

Beds: The number of beds regularly maintained (set up and staffed for use) for inpatients as of the close of the reporting period. Excludes newborn bassinets.

Bed-size category: Relates to the number of beds a hospital has set up and staffed for use at the end of the reporting period. The 8 categories in *AHA Hospital Statistics* are 6 to 24 beds; 25 to 49; 50 to 99; 100 to 199; 200 to 299; 300 to 399; 400 to 499; and 500 or more.

Biocontainment patient care unit: A permanent unit that provides the first line of treatment for people affected by bioterrorism or highly hazardous communicable diseases. The unit is equipped to safely care for anyone exposed to a highly contagious and dangerous disease.

Birthing room, LDR room, and LDRP room: A single-room type of maternity care with a more homelike setting for families than the traditional 3-room unit (labor/ delivery/recovery) with a separate postpartum area. A *birthing room* combines labor and delivery in one room. An *LDR room* accommodates 3 stages in the birthing process: labor, delivery, and recovery. An *LDRP room* accommodates all 4 stages of the birthing process: labor, delivery, recovery, and postpartum.

Births: The total number of infants born in the hospital during the reporting period. Births do not include infants transferred from other institutions and exclude them from admission and discharge figures.

Blood donor center: A facility that engages in or is responsible for the collection, processing, testing, or distribution of blood and components.

Bone marrow transplant: See *transplant services*.

Breast cancer screening/mammograms: Mammography screening—the use of breast x-ray to detect unsuspected breast cancer in asymptomatic. women. Diagnostic mammography is the x-ray imaging of breast tissue in symptomatic women who are considered to have a substantial likelihood of having breast cancer already.

Burn care: Provides care to severely burned patients. Severely burned patients are those with any of the following: (1) second-degree burns of more than 25% total body surface area for adults or 20% total body surface area for children; (2) third-degree burns of more than 10% total body surface area; (3) any severe burns of the hands, face, eyes, ears, or feet; and (4) all inhalation injuries, electrical burns, complicated burn injuries involving fractures and other major traumas, and all other poor-risk factors.

Cardiac electrophysiology: The evaluation and management of patients with complex rhythm or conduction abnormalities including diagnostic testing, treatment of arrhythmias by catheter ablation or drug therapy, and pacemaker/defibrillator implantation and follow-up.

Cardiac intensive care: Provides patient care of a more specialized nature than the usual medical and surgical care, on the basis of physicians' orders and approved nursing care plans. The unit is staffed with specially trained nursing personnel and contains monitoring and specialized support or treatment equipment for patients who, because of heart seizure, open-heart surgery, or other life-threatening conditions, require intensified, comprehensive observation and care. May include myocardial infarction, pulmonary care, and heart transplant units.

Cardiac rehabilitation: A medically supervised program to help heart patients recover quickly and improve their overall physical and mental functioning.

The goal is to reduce risk of another cardiac event or to keep an already present heart condition from getting worse. Cardiac rehabilitation programs include counseling to patients, establishing an exercise program, helping patients modify risk factors such as smoking and high blood pressure, providing vocational guidance to enable the patient to return to work, supplying information on physical limitations, and lending emotional support.

Case management: A system of assessment, treatment planning, referral, and follow-up that ensures the provision of comprehensive and continuous services and the coordination of payment and reimbursement for care.

Chaplaincy/pastoral care services: A service ministering religious activities and providing pastoral counseling to patients, their families, and the staff of a health care organization.

Chemotherapy: An organized program for the treatment of cancer by the use of drugs or chemicals.

Children's wellness program: A program that encourages improved health status and a healthful lifestyle of children through health education, exercise, and nutrition and health promotion.

Chiropractic services: An organized clinical service including spinal manipulation or adjustment and related diagnostic and therapeutic services.

Community health education: Education that provides health information to individuals and populations, as well as support for personal, family and community health decisions with the objective of improving health status.

Community hospitals: All nonfederal, short-term general and special hospitals whose facilities and services are available to the public. Special hospitals include obstetrics and gynecology; eye, ear, nose, and throat; rehabilitation; orthopedic; and other individually described specialty services. Short-term general and special children's hospitals are also considered to be community hospitals.

A hospital may include a nursing-home-type unit and still be classified as short-term, provided that the majority of its patients are admitted to units where the average length of stay is less than 30 days. Therefore, statistics for community hospitals often include some data about such nursing-home-type units. An example is furnished by Montana, where in 1995 63.6 percent of all hospitals classified as community hospitals include nursing-home type units.

Note that before 1972, hospital units of institutions such as prison and college infirmaries were included in the category of community hospitals. Including these units made this category equivalent to the short-term general and other special hospitals category. Although these hospital units are few in number and small in size, this change in definition should be taken into consideration when comparing data.

Community outreach: A program that systematically interacts with the community to identify those in need of services, alerting persons and their families to the availability of services, locating needed services, and enabling persons to enter the service delivery system.

Complementary and alternative medicine services: Organized hospital services or formal arrangements to providers that provide care or treatment not based solely on traditional Western allopathic medical teachings as instructed in most US medical schools. Services include any of the following: acupuncture, chiropractic, homeopathy, osteopathy, diet and lifestyle changes, herbal medicine, and message therapy, among others.

Computer-assisted orthopedic surgery (CAOS): Orthopedic surgery using computer technology, enabling three-dimensional graphic models to visualize a patient's anatomy.

Control: The type of organization responsible for establishing policy concerning the overall operation of hospitals. The 3 major categories are government (including federal, state, and local); nongovernment (nonprofit); and investor-owned (for-profit).

Crisis prevention: Services provided to promote physical and mental well-being and the early identification of disease and ill health prior to the onset and recognition of symptoms so as to permit early treatment.

CT scanner: Computed tomographic scanner for head or whole body scans.

Dental services: An organized dental service or dentists on staff, not necessarily involving special facilities, providing dental or oral services to inpatients or outpatients.

Diabetes prevention program: A program to prevent or delay the onset of type 2 diabetes by offering evidence based lifestyle changes based on research studies, which showed that modest behavior changes helped individuals with prediabetes reduce their risk of developing type 2 diabetes.

Diagnostic radioisotope facility: The use of radioactive isotopes (radiopharmaceuticals) as tracers or indicators to detect an abnormal condition or disease.

Electrodiagnostic services: Diagnostic testing services for nerve and muscle function, including services such as nerve conduction studies and needle electromyography.

Electron beam computed tomography (EBCT): A high-tech computed tomography scan used to detect coronary artery disease by measuring coronary calcifications. This imaging procedure uses electron beams that are magnetically steered to produce a visual of the coronary artery, and the images are produced faster than with conventional CT scans.

Emergency department: Hospital facilities for the provision of unscheduled outpatient services to patients whose conditions require immediate care.

Emergency room visits: The number of visits to the emergency unit. When emergency outpatients are admitted to the inpatient areas of the hospital, they are counted as emergency room visits and subsequently as inpatient admissions.

Emergency services: Health services that are provided after the onset of a medical condition that manifests itself by symptoms of sufficient severity, including severe pain, that the absence of immediate medical attention could reasonably be expected by a prudent layperson, who possesses an average knowledge of health and medicine, to result in placing the patient's health in serious jeopardy.

Employment support services: Services designed to support individuals with significant disabilities to seek and maintain employment.

Enabling services: A program that is designed to help the patient access health care services by offering transportation services and/or referrals to local social services agencies.

Endoscopic retrograde cholangiopancreatography (ERCP): A procedure in which a catheter is introduced through an endoscope into the bile ducts and pancreatic ducts. Injection of contrast materials permits detailed x-ray of these structures. The procedure is used diagnostically as well as therapeutically to relieve obstruction or remove stones.

Endoscopic ultrasound: A specially designed endoscope that incorporates an ultrasound transductor used to obtain detailed images of organs in the chest and abdomen. The endoscope can be passed through the mouth or the anus. When combined with needle biopsy, the procedure can assist in diagnosis and staging of cancer.

Enrollment (insurance) assistance services: A program that provides enrollment assistance for patients who are potentially eligible for public health insurance programs such as Medicaid, State Children's Health Insurance, or local/state indigent care programs. The specific services offered could include explaining benefits, assisting applicants in completing the application and locating all relevant documents, conducting eligibility interviews, and/or forwarding applications and documentation to state/local social service or health agency.

Esophageal impedance study: A test in which a catheter is placed through the nose into the esophagus to measure whether gas or liquids are passing from the stomach into the esophagus and causing symptoms.

Extracorporeal shock wave lithotripter (ESWL): A medical device used for treating stones in the kidney or urethra. The device disintegrates kidney stones noninvasively through the transmission of acoustic shock waves directed at the stones.

Fertility clinic: A specialized program set in an infertility center that provides counseling and education as well as advanced reproductive techniques such as injectable therapy, reproductive surgeries, treatment for endometriosis, male factor infertility, tubal reversals, in vitro fertilization (IVF), and donor eggs to help patients achieve successful pregnancies.

Fitness center: Provides exercise, testing, or evaluation programs and fitness activities to the community and hospital employees.

Freestanding outpatient care center: A facility owned and operated by the hospital but is physically separate from the hospital and provides various medical treatments and diagnostic services on an outpatient basis only. Laboratory and radiology services are usually available.

Full-field digital mammography (FFDM): Combines the x-ray generators and tubes used in analog screen-film mammography (SFM) with a detector plate that converts the x-rays into a digital signal.

Full-time equivalent employees (FTE): Full-time personnel on payroll plus one-half of the part-time personnel on payroll. For purposes of *AHA Hospital*

---

208   AHA Hospital Statistics © 2024 Health Forum LLC, an affiliate of the American Hospital Association

Statistics, full-time and part-time medical and dental residents/interns and other trainees are excluded from the calculation.

General medical-surgical care: Provides acute care to patients in medical and surgical units on the basis of physicians' orders and approved nursing care plans.

Genetic testing/counseling: A service equipped with adequate laboratory facilities and directed by a qualified physician to advise parents and prospective parents on potential problems in cases of genetic defects.

A genetic test is the analysis of human DNA, RNA, chromosomes, proteins, and certain metabolites in order to detect heritable disease-related genotypes, mutations, phenotypes, or karyotypes for clinical purposes. Genetic tests can have diverse purposes, including the diagnosis of genetic diseases in newborns, children, and adults; the identification of future health risks; the prediction of drug responses; and the assessment of risks to future children.

Geriatric services: The branch of medicine dealing with the physiology of aging and the diagnosis and treatment of disease affecting the aged. Services could include adult day care, Alzheimer's diagnostic-assessment services, comprehensive geriatric assessment, emergency response system, geriatric acute care unit, and/or geriatric clinics.

Government, nonfederal, state, local: Control by an agency of state, county, or city government.

Group purchasing organization: An organization whose primary function is to negotiate contracts for the purpose of purchasing for members of the group or has a central supply site for its members.

Health fair: Community health education events that focus on the prevention of disease and promotion of health through such activities as audiovisual exhibits and free diagnostic services.

Health research: An organized hospital research program in any of the following areas: basic research, clinical research, community health research, and/or research on innovative health care delivery.

Health screening: A preliminary procedure such as a test or examination to detect the most characteristic sign or signs of a disorder that may require further investigation.

Heart transplant: See *transplant services.*

Hemodialysis: Provision of equipment and personnel for the treatment of renal insufficiency on an inpatient or outpatient basis.

HIV-AIDS services: Could include an *HIV-AIDS unit* is a special unit or team designated and equipped specifically for diagnosis, treatment, continuing care planning, and counseling services for HIV-AIDS patients

and their families. *General inpatient care for HIV-AIDS* provides inpatient diagnosis and treatment for human immunodeficiency virus and acquired immunodeficiency syndrome patients, but dedicated unit is not available. *Specialized outpatient program for HIV-AIDS* is a special outpatient program providing diagnostic, treatment, continuing care planning, and counseling for HIV-AIDS patients and their families.

Home health services: Service providing nursing, therapy, and health-related homemaker or social services in the patient's home.

Hospice: A program providing palliative care, chiefly medical relief of pain and supportive services, addressing the emotional, social, financial, and legal needs of terminally ill patients and their families. Care can be provided in a variety of settings, both inpatient and at home.

Hospital unit: The hospital operation, excluding activity pertaining to nursing-home-type unit (as described below), for the following items: admissions, beds, FTEs (full-time, part-time, and total), inpatient days, length of stay.

Hospital unit of institutions: A hospital unit that is not open to the public and is contained within a nonhospital unit. An example is an infirmary that is contained within a college.

Hospitals in a network: Hospitals participating in a group that may include other hospitals, physicians, other providers, insurers, and/or community agencies that work together to coordinate and deliver a broad spectrum of services to the community.

Hospitals in a system: Hospitals belonging to a corporate body that owns and/or manages health provider facilities or health-related subsidiaries; the system may also own non-health-related facilities.

Image-guided radiation therapy (IGRT): An automated system for IGRT that enables clinicians to obtain high-resolution x-ray images to pinpoint tumor sites, adjust patient positioning when necessary, and complete a treatment, all within the standard treatment time slot, allowing for more effective cancer treatments.

Immunization program: Plans, coordinates, and conducts immunization services in the community.

Indigent care clinic: Health care services for uninsured and underinsured persons where care is free of charge or charged on a sliding scale. This includes "free clinics" staffed by volunteer practitioners, but free clinics could also be staffed by employees with sponsoring health care organizations subsidizing the cost of service.

Inpatient days: The number of adult and pediatric days of care, excluding newborn days of care, rendered during the entire reporting period.

AHA Hospital Statistics © 2024 Health Forum LLC, an affiliate of the American Hospital Association **209**

Inpatient palliative care unit: A physically discreet, inpatient nursing unit where the focus is palliative care. The patient care focus is on symptom relief for complex patients who may be continuing to undergo primary treatment. Care is delivered by palliative medicine specialists.

Inpatient surgeries: Surgical services provided to patients who remain in the hospital overnight.

Intensity-modulated radiation therapy (IMRT): A type of three-dimensional radiation therapy, which improves the targeting of treatment delivery in a way that is likely to decrease damage to normal tissues and allows varying intensities.

Intermediate nursing care: Provides health-related services (skilled nursing care and social services) to residents with a variety of physical conditions or functional disabilities. These residents do not require the care provided by a hospital or skilled nursing facility, but they do need supervision and support services.

Intraoperative magnetic resonance imaging: An integrated surgery system which provides a magnetic resonance imaging (MRI) system in an operating room. The interoperative MRI system allows for immediate evaluation of the degree to tumor resection while the patient is undergoing a surgical resection.

Intraoperative MRI exists when an MRI (low-field or high-field) is placed in the operating theater and is used during surgical resection without moving the patient from the operating room to the diagnostic imaging suite.

Investor-owned, for-profit: Hospitals controlled on a for-profit basis by an individual, partnership, or profit-making corporation.

Kidney transplant: See *transplant services*.

Length of stay (LOS): The average number of days a patient stays at the facility. Short-term hospitals are those where the average LOS is less than 30 days. Long-term hospitals are those where the average LOS is 30 days or more. The figure is derived by dividing the number of inpatient days by the number of admissions.

Note that this publication carries two LOS variables: *total facility length of stay* and *hospital unit length of stay*. *Total facility* includes admissions and inpatient days from nursing-home-type units under control of the hospital. In *hospital unit length of stay*, nursing home use is subtracted.

Licensed practical nurse (LPN): A nurse who has graduated from an approved school of practical (vocational) nursing and works under the supervision of registered nurses and/or physicians.

Linguistic/translation services: Services provided by the hospital designed to make health care more accessible to non-English-speaking patients and their physicians.

Liver transplant: See *transplant services*.

Long-term: A hospital classification measure. Hospitals are classified either short-term or long-term according to the average length of stay (LOS). A long-term hospital is one in which the average LOS is 30 days or more.

Lung transplant: See *transplant services*.

Magnetic resonance imaging (MRI): The use of a uniform magnetic field and radio frequencies to study tissue and structure of the body. This procedure enables the visualization of biochemical activity of the cell in vivo without the use of ionizing radiation, radio-isotopic substances, or high-frequency sound.

Magnetoencephalography (MEG): A noninvasive neurophysiological measurement tool used to study magnetic fields generated by neuronal activity of the brain. The primary uses of MEG include assisting surgeons in localizing the source of epilepsy, sensory mapping, and the study of brain function. When MEG is combined with structural imaging, it is known as *magnetic source imaging (MSI)*.

Meals on wheels: A hospital-sponsored program that delivers meals to people, usually the elderly, who are unable to prepare their own meals. Low-cost, nutritional meals are delivered to individuals' homes on a regular basis.

Medical surgical intensive care: Provides patient care of a more intensive nature than the usual medical and surgical care, on the basis of physicians' orders and approved nursing care plans. These units are staffed with specially trained nursing personnel and contain monitoring and specialized support equipment for patients who, because of shock, trauma, or other life-threatening conditions, require intensified, comprehensive observation and care. Includes mixed intensive care units.

Mobile health services: Services using vans and other vehicles to deliver primary care services.

Multislice spiral computed tomography (<64 slice CT): A specialized computed tomography procedure that provides three-dimensional processing and allows narrower and multiple slices with increased spatial resolution and faster scanning times as compared with a regular computed tomography scan.

Multislice spiral computed tomography (64+ slice CT): Involves the acquisition of volumetric tomographic x-ray absorption data expressed in Hounsfield units using multiple rows of detectors. 64+ systems reconstruct the equivalent of 64 or greater slices to cover the imaged volume.

Neonatal intensive care (NICU): A unit that must be separate from the newborn nursery providing intensive care to all sick infants, including those with the very lowest birth weights (less than 1500 grams). NICU has potential for providing mechanical ventilation, neonatal surgery, and special care for the sickest infants born in the hospital or transferred from another institution. A full-time neonatologist serves as director of the NICU.

Neonatal intermediate care: A unit that must be separate from the normal newborn nursery and that provides intermediate and/or recovery care and some specialized services, including immediate resuscitation, intravenous therapy, and capacity for prolonged oxygen therapy and monitoring.

Neurological services: Services provided by the hospital dealing with the operative and nonoperative management of disorders of the central, peripheral, and autonomic nervous system.

Nongovernment, nonprofit: Hospitals that are nongovernment, nonprofit are controlled by not-for-profit organizations, including religious organizations (Catholic hospitals, for example), fraternal societies, and others.

Nursing-home-type unit/facility: A unit or facility that primarily offers the following type of services to a majority of all admissions:

- *Skilled nursing:* the provision of medical and nursing care services, health-related services, and social services under the supervision of a registered nurse on a 24-hour basis.

- *Intermediate care:* the provision, on a regular basis, of health-related care and services to individuals who do not require the degree of care or treatment that a skilled nursing unit is designed to provide.

- *Personal care:* the provision of general supervision and direct personal care services for residents who require assistance in activities of daily living but who do not need nursing services or inpatient care. Medical and nursing services are available as needed.

- *Sheltered/residential care:* the provision of general supervision and protective services for residents who do not need nursing services or continuous personal care services in the conduct of daily life. Medical and nursing services are available as needed.

Nutrition programs: Those services within a health care facility that are designed to provide inexpensive, nutritionally sound meals to patients.

Obstetrics: Organizes levels of care as follows: (1) unit provides services for uncomplicated maternity and newborn cases; (2) unit provides services for uncomplicated cases, the majority of complicated problems, and special neonatal services; and (3) unit provides services for all serious illnesses and abnormalities and is supervised by a full time maternal/fetal specialist.

Occupational health services: Includes services designed to protect the safety of employees from hazards in the work environment.

Off-campus emergency department: A facility owned and operated by the hospital but physically separate from the hospital for the provision of unscheduled outpatient services to patients whose conditions require immediate care. A freestanding emergency department is not physically connected to a hospital but has all the necessary emergency staffing and equipment on site.

Oncology services: Inpatient and outpatient services for patients with cancer, including comprehensive care, support, and guidance in addition to patient education and prevention, chemotherapy, counseling, and other treatment methods.

Optical colonoscopy: An examination of the interior of the colon using a long, flexible, lighted tube with a small built-in camera.

Orthopedic services: Services provided for the prevention or correction of injuries or disorders of the skeletal system and associated muscles, joints, and ligaments.

Osteopathic hospitals: Practice osteopathic medicine, a medical practice based on a theory that diseases are caused chiefly by a loss of structural integrity, which can be restored by manipulation of the neuromuscular and skeletal systems, supplemented by therapeutic measures such as medicine or surgery.

Other intensive care: A specially staffed, specialty equipped separate section of a hospital dedicated to the observation, care, and treatment of patients with life-threatening illnesses, injuries, or complications from which recovery is possible. It provides special expertise and facilities for the support of vital function and utilizes the skill of medical nursing and other staff experienced in the management of these problems.

Other long-term care: The provision of long-term care other than skilled nursing care or intermediate care for those who do not require daily medical or nursing services but may require some assistance in the activities of daily living. This can include residential care, elderly care, or sheltered-care facilities for developmentally disabled.

Other special care: Provides care to patients requiring care more intensive than that provided in the acute area, yet not sufficiently intensive to require admission to an intensive care unit. Patients admitted to this area are usually transferred here from an intensive care unit once their condition has improved. These units are sometimes referred to as definitive observation, step-down, or progressive care units.

Other transplant: See *transplant services.*

AHA Hospital Statistics © 2024 Health Forum LLC, an affiliate of the American Hospital Association **211**

Outpatient care: Treatment provided to patients who do not remain in the hospital for overnight care. Hospitals may deliver outpatient care on site or through a facility owned and operated by the hospital but physically separate from the hospital. In addition to treating minor illnesses or injuries, a freestanding center will stabilize seriously ill or injured patients before transporting them to a hospital. Laboratory and radiology services are usually available.

Outpatient care center (freestanding): A facility owned and operated by the hospital, but physically separate from the hospital, that provides various medical treatments on an outpatient basis only. In addition to treating minor illnesses or injuries, the center will stabilize seriously ill or injured patients before transporting them to a hospital. Laboratory and radiology services are usually available.

Outpatient care center services (hospital-based): Organized hospital health care services offered by appointment on an ambulatory basis. Services may include outpatient surgery, examination, diagnosis, and treatment of a variety of medical conditions on a nonemergency basis, and laboratory and other diagnostic testing as ordered by staff or outside physician referral.

Outpatient surgery: Scheduled surgical services provided to patients who do not remain in the hospital overnight. The surgery may be performed in operating suites also used for inpatient surgery, specially designated surgical suites for outpatient surgery, or procedure rooms within an outpatient care facility.

Outpatient visit: A visit by a patient who is not lodged in the hospital while receiving medical, dental, or other services. Each visit an outpatient makes to a discrete unit constitutes one visit regardless of the number of diagnostic and/or therapeutic treatments the patient receives. Total outpatient visits should include all clinic visits, referred visits, observation services, outpatient surgeries, and emergency room visits.

Pain management program: A recognized clinical service or program providing specialized medical care, drugs, or therapies for the management of acute or chronic pain or other distressing symptom, administered by specially trained physicians and other clinicians, to patients suffering from acute illness of diverse causes.

Palliative care inpatient unit: A physically discreet, inpatient nursing unit where the focus is palliative care. The patient care focus is on symptom relief for complex patients who may be continuing to undergo primary treatment. Care is delivered by palliative medicine specialists.

Palliative care program: An organized program providing specialized medical care and drugs or therapies for the management of acute or chronic pain and/or the control of symptoms administered by specially trained physicians and other clinicians. Also, supportive care services such as counseling on advanced directives, spiritual care, and social services are provided to patients with advanced disease and their families.

Patient-controlled analgesia (PCA): Intravenously administered pain medicine under the patient's control. The PCA patient has a button on the end of a cord that can be pushed at will whenever more pain medicine is desired. This button will deliver more pain medicine only at predetermined intervals, as programmed by the doctor's order.

Patient education center: Provides written goals and objectives for the patient and/or family related to therapeutic regimens, medical procedures, and self-care.

Patient representative services: Organized hospital services providing personnel through whom patients and staff can seek solutions to institutional problems affecting the delivery of high-quality care and services.

Pediatric cardiac surgery: Includes minimally invasive procedures that include surgery done with only a small incision or no incision at all, such as through a laparoscope or an endoscope, and more invasive major surgical procedures that include open chest and open heart surgery.

Pediatric cardiology services: An organized clinical service offering diagnostic and interventional procedures to manage the full range of pediatric heart conditions.

Pediatric diagnostic/invasive catheterization: Also called *cardiac angiography* or *coronary arteriography*, used to assist in diagnosing complex heart conditions. Cardiac angiography involves the insertion of a tiny catheter into the artery in the groin, then carefully threading the catheter up into the aorta where the coronary arteries originate. Once the catheter is in place, a dye is injected to allow the cardiologist to see the size, shape, and distribution of the coronary arteries. These images are used to diagnose heart disease and to determine, among other things, whether or not surgery is indicated.

Pediatric intensive care: Provides care to pediatric patients that is of a more intensive nature than that usually provided to pediatric patients. The unit is staffed with specially trained personnel and contains monitoring and specialized support equipment for treatment of patients who, because of shock, trauma, or other life-threatening conditions, require intensified, comprehensive observation and care.

Pediatric interventional cardiac catheterization: Nonsurgical procedure that utilizes the same basic principles as diagnostic catheterization and then uses advanced techniques to improve the heart's function. It can be a less-invasive alternative to heart surgery.

Pediatric medical-surgical care: Provides acute care to pediatric patients on the basis of physicians' orders and approved nursing care plans.

Personnel: Number of persons on the hospital payroll at the end of the reporting period. Personnel are recorded in *AHA Hospital Statistics* as full-time equivalents (FTEs), which are calculated by adding the number of full-time personnel to one-half the number of part-time personnel, excluding medical and dental residents, interns, and other trainees. *Per-100 adjusted census* indicates the ratio of personnel to adjusted average daily census, calculated on a per-100 basis.

Physical rehabilitation inpatient care: Provides care encompassing a comprehensive array of restoration services for the disabled and all support services necessary to help patients attain their maximum functional capacity.

Physical rehabilitation outpatient services: An outpatient program providing medical, health-related therapy and social and/or vocational services to help disabled persons attain or retain their maximum functional capacity.

Population: Refers to the residential population of the United States. This includes both civilian and military personnel. Note that this population is being used to calculate the values *for community health indicators per 1000 population.*

Positron emission tomography/CT (PET/CT): Provides metabolic functional information for the monitoring of chemotherapy, radiotherapy, and surgical planning.

Positron emission tomography scanner (PET): A nuclear medicine imaging technology that uses radioactive (positron-emitting) isotopes, created in a cyclotron or generator, and computers to produce composite pictures of the brain and heart at work. PET scanning produces sectional images depicting metabolic activity or blood flow rather than anatomy.

Primary care department: A unit or clinic within the hospital that provides primary care services (eg, general pediatric care, general internal medicine, family practice, gynecology) through hospital-salaried medical and/or nursing staff, focusing on evaluating and diagnosing medical problems and providing medical treatment on an outpatient basis.

Prosthetic and orthotic services: Services providing comprehensive prosthetic and orthotic evaluation, fitting, and training.

Proton beam therapy: A form of radiation therapy which administers proton beams. While producing the same biologic effects as x-ray beams, the energy distribution of protons differs from conventional x-ray beams in that they can be more precisely focused in tissue volumes in a three-dimensional pattern resulting in less surrounding tissue damage than through conventional radiation therapy and permitting administration of higher doses.

Psychiatric pediatric care: The branch of medicine focused on the diagnosis, treatment, and prevention of mental, emotional, and behavioral disorders in pediatric patients.

Psychiatric consultation-liaison services: Provides organized psychiatric consultation/liaison services to nonpsychiatric hospital staff and/or departments on psychological aspects of medical care that may be generic or specific to individual patients.

Psychiatric education services: Provides psychiatric educational services to community agencies and workers such as schools, police, courts, public health nurses, welfare agencies, and clergy. The purpose is to expand the mental health knowledge and competence of personnel not working in the mental health field and to promote good mental health through improved understanding, attitudes, and behavioral patterns.

Psychiatric emergency services: Services of facilities available on a 24-hour basis to provide immediate, unscheduled outpatient care, diagnosis, evaluation, crisis intervention, and assistance to persons suffering acute emotional or mental distress.

Psychiatric geriatric services: Provides care to emotionally disturbed elderly patients, including those admitted for diagnosis and those admitted for treatment.

Psychiatric inpatient care: Provides acute or long-term care to emotionally disturbed patients, including patients admitted for diagnosis and those admitted for treatment of psychiatric problems, on the basis of physicians' orders and approved nursing care plans. Long-term care may include intensive supervision to the chronically mentally ill, mentally disordered, or other mentally incompetent persons.

Psychiatric intensive outpatient services: A prescribed course of treatment in which the patient receives outpatient care no less than 3 times a week, which may include more than 1 service per day.

Psychiatric outpatient services: Provides medical care, including diagnosis and treatment, of psychiatric outpatients.

Psychiatric partial hospitalization program: Organized hospital services of intensive day/evening outpatient services of 3 or more hours' duration, distinguished from other outpatient visits of 1 hour.

Psychiatric residential treatment: Overnight psychiatric care in conjunction with an intensive treatment program in a setting other than a hospital.

Radiology, diagnostic: The branch of radiology that deals with the utilization of all modalities of radiant energy in medical diagnoses and therapeutic procedures using radiologic guidance. This includes, but is not restricted to, imaging techniques and methodologies utilizing radiation emitted by x-ray tubes, radionuclides,

---

AHA Hospital Statistics © 2024 Health Forum LLC, an affiliate of the American Hospital Association **213**

and ultrasonographic devices and the radiofrequency electromagnetic radiation emitted by atoms.

Radiology, therapeutic: The branch of medicine concerned with radioactive substances and using various techniques of visualization, with the diagnosis and treatment of disease using any of the various sources of radiant energy. Services could include megavoltage radiation therapy, radioactive implants, stereotactic radiosurgery, therapeutic radioisotop facility, and/or x-ray radiation therapy.

Registered nurse (RN): A nurse who has graduated from an approved school of nursing and who is currently registered by the state. RNs are responsible for the nature and quality of all nursing care that patients receive. In Tables 1 and 2, the number of RNs does not include those registered nurses more appropriately reported in other occupational categories, such as facility administrators, which are listed under *all other personnel.*

Rehabilitation services: A wide array of restoration services for disabled and recuperating patients, including all support services necessary to help them attain their maximum functional capacity.

Retirement housing: A facility that provides social activities to senior citizens, usually retired persons, who do not require health care but may be provided with some short-term skilled nursing care. A retirement center may furnish housing and may also have acute hospital and long-term care facilities, or it may arrange for acute and long-term care through affiliated institutions.

Robot-assisted walking therapy: A form of physical therapy that uses a robotic device to assist patients who are relearning how to walk.

Robotic surgery: The use of mechanical guidance devices to remotely manipulate surgical instrumentation.

Rural: Describes a hospital located outside a metropolitan statistical area (MSA), as designated by the US Office of Management and Budget (0MB) effective June 6, 2003. An urban area is a geographically defined, integrated social and economic unit with a large population nucleus. Micropolitan areas, which were new to the 0MB June 6, 2003, definitions, continue to be classified as rural for purposes of this publication.

Rural health clinic: A clinic located in a rural, medically underserved area in the United States that has a separate reimbursement structure from that of the standard medical office under the Medicare and Medicaid programs.

Shaped-beam radiation system: A precise, noninvasive treatment that involves targeting beams of radiation that mirror the exact size and shape of a tumor at a specific area of a tumor to shrink or destroy cancerous cells. This procedure delivers a therapeutic dose of radiation

that conforms precisely to the shape of the tumor, thus minimizing the risk to nearby tissues.

Simulated rehabilitation environment: Rehabilitation focused on retraining functional skills in a contextually appropriate environment such as simulated home and community settings or in a traditional setting, such as a gymnasium, using motor learning principles.

Single-photon emission computerized tomography (SPECT): A nuclear medicine imaging technology that combines existing technology of gamma camera imaging with computed tomographic imaging technology to provide a more precise and clear image.

Skilled nursing care: Provides nonacute medical and skilled nursing care services, therapy, and social services under the supervision of a licensed registered nurse on a 24-hour basis.

Sleep center: Specially equipped and staffed center for the diagnosis and treatment of sleep disorders.

Social work services: Organized services that are properly directed and sufficiently staffed by qualified individuals who provide assistance and counseling to patients and their families in dealing with social, emotional, and environmental problems associated with illness or disability, often in the context of financial or discharge planning coordination.

Sports medicine: The provision of diagnostic screening and assessment and clinical and rehabilitation services for the prevention and treatment of sports-related injuries.

Stereotactic radiosurgery (SRS): A radiotherapy modality that delivers a high dosage of radiation to a discrete treatment area in as few as one treatment session. SRS may include gamma knife, cyberknife, and so on.

Support groups: Hospital-sponsored programs that allow groups of individuals with the same or similar problems to meet periodically to share experiences, problems, and solutions in order to support each other.

Supportive housing services: A hospital program that provides decent, safe, affordable, community-based housing with flexible support services designed to help the individual or family stay housed and live a more productive life in the community.

Surgical operations: Those surgical operations, whether major or minor, performed in the operating room(s). A surgical operation involving more than one surgical procedure is still considered only one surgical operation.

Swing bed services: Provides hospital beds that can be used to provide either acute care or long-term care depending on community or patient needs. To be eligible a hospital must have a Medicare provider agreement in place, have fewer than 100 beds, and be located in a rural area. It must not have a 24-hour nursing service

214   AHA Hospital Statistics © 2024 Health Forum LLC, an affiliate of the American Hospital Association

waiver in effect nor have not been terminated from the program in the prior 2 years. It must, in addition, meet various service conditions.

Teen outreach services: A program focusing on the teenager that encourages an improved health status and a healthful lifestyle that includes physical, emotional, mental, social, spiritual, and economic health through education, exercise, and nutrition and health promotion.

Telehealth: A broad variety of technologies and tactics to deliver virtual medical, public health, and health education delivery and support services using telecommunications technologies. Telehealth is used more commonly to describe the wide range of diagnosis and management, education, and other related fields of health care. These include but are not limited to dentistry, counseling, physical and occupational therapy, home health, chronic disease monitoring and management, disaster management and consumer and professional education, and remote patient monitoring.

Tissue transplant: See *transplant services*.

Tobacco treatment/cessation program: Organized hospital services with the purpose of ending tobacco use habits of patients addicted to tobacco/nicotine.

Transplant services: The branch of medicine that transfers an organ or tissue from one person to another or from one body part to another to replace a diseased structure or to restore function or to change appearance. Services could include a bone marrow transplant program or heart, lung, kidney, intestine, or tissue transplant. Services other than bone marrow, heart, kidney, liver, lung, and tissue transplants may involve heart/lung or other multitransplant surgeries.

Transportation to health facilities: A long-term care support service designed to assist the mobility of the elderly. Some programs offer improved financial access by offering reduced rates and barrier-free buses or vans with ramps and lifts to assist the elderly or handicapped; others offer subsidies for public transport systems or operate minibus services for use exclusively by senior citizens.

Trauma center (certified): A facility to provide emergency and specialized intensive care to critically ill and injured patients. **Level 1:** a regional resource trauma center, which is capable of providing total care for every aspect of injury and plays a leadership role in trauma research and education. **Level 2:** a community trauma center, which is capable of providing trauma care to all but the most severely injured patients who require highly specialized care. **Level 3:** a rural trauma hospital, which is capable of providing care to a large number of injury victims and can resuscitate and stabilize more severely injured patients so that they can be transported to level 1 or 2 facilities.

Ultrasound: The use of acoustic waves above the range of 20,000 cycles per second to visualize internal body structures.

Urban: Describes a hospital located inside a metropolitan statistical area (MSA), designated by the US Office of Management and Budget (OMB) effective June 6, 2003. An urban areas is a geographically defined, integrated social and economic unit with a large population base. Micropolitan areas, which were new to the 0MB June 6, 2003, definitions, are not considered to be urban for purposes of this publication.

Urgent care center: A facility that provides care and treatment for problems that are not life-threatening but require attention over the short-term.

Violence prevention program for the workplace: A violence prevention program with goals and objectives for preventing workplace violence against staff and patients.

Violence prevention program for the community: An organized program that attempts to make a positive impact on the type(s) of violence a community is experiencing. For example, it can assist victims of violent crimes (eg, rape) or incidents (eg, bullying) to hospital or to community services to prevent further victimization or retaliation. A program that targets the underlying circumstances that contribute to violence (eg, poor housing, insufficient job training, and/or substance abuse) through means such as direct involvement and support, education, mentoring, anger management, crisis intervention, and training programs would also qualify.

Virtual colonoscopy: Noninvasive screening procedure used to visualize, analyze, and detect cancerous or potentially cancerous polyps in the colon.

Volunteer services department: An organized hospital department responsible for coordinating the services of volunteers working within the institution.

Women's health center/services: An area set aside for coordinated education and treatment services specifically for and promoted to women as provided by this special unit. Services may or may not include obstetrics but do include a range of other services.

Wound management services: Services for patients with chronic wounds and nonhealing wounds often resulting from diabetes, poor circulation, improper seating, and immunocompromising conditions. The goals are to progress chronic wounds through stages of healing, reduce and eliminate infections, and increase physical function to minimize complications from current wounds and to prevent future chronic wounds. Wound management services are provided on an inpatient or outpatient basis, depending on the intensity of service needed.

AHA Hospital Statistics © 2024 Health Forum LLC, an affiliate of the American Hospital Association **215**

2022 AHA Annual Survey
American Hospital Association

HOSPITAL NAME: _____

CITY & STATE: _____

> **Please return to:**
> **AHA Annual Survey**
> **155 N Wacker Drive**
> **Suite 400**
> **Chicago IL 60606**

A. REPORTING PERIOD (please refer to the instructions and definitions at the end of this questionnaire)

Report data for a full 12-month period, preferably your last completed fiscal year (365 days). Be consistent in using the same reporting period for responses throughout various sections of this survey.

1. Reporting Period used (beginning and ending date) ...... __ __ / __ __ / __ __ __ __ to __ __ / __ __ / __ __ __ __

                                                                Month Day   Year   Month Day   Year

2. a. Were you in operation 12 full months at the end of your reporting period? .... YES ☐ NO ☐

   b. Number of days open during reporting period .... _____

3. Indicate the beginning of your current fiscal year .... __ __ / __ __ / __ __ __ __

                                                         Month Day   Year

B. ORGANIZATIONAL STRUCTURE

1. CONTROL

Indicate the type of organization that is responsible for establishing policy for overall operation of your hospital. CHECK ONLY ONE:

Government, nonfederal
- ☐ 12 State
- ☐ 13 County
- ☐ 14 City
- ☐ 15 City-County
- ☐ 16 Hospital district or authority

Nongovernment, not-for-profit (NFP)
- ☐ 21 Church-operated
- ☐ 23 Other not-for-profit (including NFP Corporation)

Investor-owned, for-profit
- ☐ 31 Individual
- ☐ 32 Partnership
- ☐ 33 Corporation

Government, federal
- ☐ 40 Department of Defense
- ☐ 44 Public Health Service
- ☐ 45 Veterans' Affairs
- ☐ 46 Federal other than 40-45 or 47-48
- ☐ 47 PHS Indian Service
- ☐ 48 Department of Justice

2. SERVICE

Indicate the ONE category that BEST describes your hospital or the type of service it provides to the MAJORITY of patients:

- ☐ 10 General medical and surgical
- ☐ 11 Hospital unit of an institution (prison hospital, college infirmary)
- ☐ 12 Hospital unit within a facility for persons with intellectual disabilities
- ☐ 13 Surgical
- ☐ 22 Psychiatric
- ☐ 33 Tuberculosis and other respiratory diseases
- ☐ 41 Cancer
- ☐ 42 Heart
- ☐ 44 Obstetrics and gynecology
- ☐ 45 Eye, ear, nose, and throat

- ☐ 46 Rehabilitation
- ☐ 47 Orthopedic
- ☐ 48 Chronic disease
- ☐ 62 Intellectual disabilities
- ☐ 80 Acute long-term care hospital
- ☐ 82 Substance use disorder
- ☐ 49 Other - specify treatment area: _____

AHA Hospital Statistics © 2024 Health Forum LLC, an affiliate of the American Hospital Association **217**

B. ORGANIZATIONAL STRUCTURE (continued)

3. OTHER

    a. Does your hospital restrict admissions primarily to children? .... YES ☐   NO ☐

    b. Does the hospital itself operate subsidiary corporations? .... YES ☐   NO ☐

    c. Is the hospital contract managed? If yes, please provide the name, city, and state of the organization.... YES ☐   NO ☐

        Name: _____   City: _____   State: _____

    d. Is your hospital owned in whole or in part by physicians or a physician group?... YES ☐   NO ☐

    e. If you checked 80 Acute long-term care hospital (LTCH) in Section B2 (Service), please indicate if you are a freestanding LTCH or a LTCH arranged within a general acute care hospital.

        ☐ Free standing LTCH   ☐ LTCH arranged in a general acute care hospital

        If you are arranged in a general acute care hospital, what is your host hospital's name?

        Name_____ City_____ State_____

    f. Are any other types of hospitals co-located in your hospital?   YES ☐   NO ☐

    g. If you checked yes for 3f, what type of hospital is co-located? (Check all that apply)

        1. ☐ Cancer

        2. ☐ Cardiac

        3. ☐ Orthopedic

        4. ☐ Pediatric

        5. ☐ Psychiatric

        6. ☐ Surgical

        7. ☐ Other _____

    h. Is your hospital designated as a state, jurisdiction, or federal Ebola or other Special Pathogens facility? (Check all that apply)

        1. ☐ Federal designation: Regional Emerging Special Pathogen Treatment Center

        2. ☐ State/Jurisdiction designation: Special Pathogen Treatment Center

        3. ☐ State/Jurisdiction designation: Special Pathogen Assessment Hospital

        4. ☐ Frontline facility

        5. ☐ None of the above

C. FACILITIES AND SERVICES

For each service or facility listed below, please check all the categories that describe how each item is provided **as of the last day of the reporting period**. Check all categories that apply for an item. If you check column (1) C1-20, please include the number of **staffed beds**.
The sum of the beds reported in 1-20 should equal Section E (1b), beds set up and staffed on page 14.

	(1) Owned or provided by my hospital or its subsidiary	(2) Provided by my Health System (in my local community)	(3) Provided through a formal contractual arrangement or joint venture with another provider that is not in my system (in my local community)	(4) Do Not Provide
1. General medical-surgical care ....(#Beds_____)	☐	☐	☐	☐
2. Pediatric medical-surgical care ....(#Beds_____)	☐	☐	☐	☐
3. Obstetrics..............[Hospital level of unit (1-3):(____)] (#Beds_____)	☐	☐	☐	☐
4. Medical-surgical intensive care....................(#Beds_____)	☐	☐	☐	☐
5. Cardiac intensive care ....(#Beds_____)	☐	☐	☐	☐
6. Neonatal intensive care ....(#Beds_____)	☐	☐	☐	☐
7. Neonatal intermediate care..........................(#Beds_____)	☐	☐	☐	☐
8. Pediatric intensive care...............................(#Beds_____)	☐	☐	☐	☐
9. Burn care..(#Beds_____)	☐	☐	☐	☐
10. Other special care _____ ....(#Beds_____)	☐	☐	☐	☐
11. Other intensive care_____ ....(#Beds_____)	☐	☐	☐	☐
12. Physical rehabilitation ....(#Beds_____)	☐	☐	☐	☐
13. Substance use disorder care ....(#Beds_____)	☐	☐	☐	☐
14. Psychiatric care ....(#Beds_____)	☐	☐	☐	☐
15. Skilled nursing care ....(#Beds_____)	☐	☐	☐	☐
16. Intermediate nursing care..........................(#Beds_____)	☐	☐	☐	☐
17. Acute long-term care ....(#Beds_____)	☐	☐	☐	☐
18. Other long-term care ....(#Beds_____)	☐	☐	☐	☐
19. Biocontainment patient care unit ....(#Beds_____)	☐	☐	☐	☐
20. Other care _____ ....(#Beds_____)	☐	☐	☐	☐
21. Adult day care program	☐	☐	☐	☐
22. Airborne infection isolation room............................(#rooms_____)	☐	☐	☐	☐
23. Alzheimer center..	☐	☐	☐	☐
24. Ambulance services	☐	☐	☐	☐
25. Air Ambulance services	☐	☐	☐	☐
26. Ambulatory surgery center................................	☐	☐	☐	☐
27. Arthritis treatment center..................................	☐	☐	☐	☐
28. Auxiliary...	☐	☐	☐	☐
29. Bariatric/weight control services........................	☐	☐	☐	☐
30. Birthing room/LDR room/LDRP room...................	☐	☐	☐	☐
31. Blood donor center	☐	☐	☐	☐
32. Breast cancer screening/mammograms...............	☐	☐	☐	☐
33. Cardiology and cardiac surgery services				
a. Adult cardiology services	☐	☐	☐	☐
b. Pediatric cardiology services................................	☐	☐	☐	☐
c. Adult diagnostic catheterization............................	☐	☐	☐	☐
d. Pediatric diagnostic catheterization......................	☐	☐	☐	☐
e. Adult interventional cardiac catheterization	☐	☐	☐	☐
f. Pediatric interventional cardiac catheterization	☐	☐	☐	☐
g. Adult cardiac surgery	☐	☐	☐	☐
h. Pediatric cardiac surgery.....................................	☐	☐	☐	☐
i. Adult cardiac electrophysiology	☐	☐	☐	☐
j. Pediatric cardiac electrophysiology	☐	☐	☐	☐
k. Cardiac rehabilitation	☐	☐	☐	☐

AHA Hospital Statistics © 2024 Health Forum LLC, an affiliate of the American Hospital Association **219**

C. FACILITIES AND SERVICES (continued)

	(1) Owned or provided by my hospital or its subsidiary	(2) Provided by my Health System (in my local community)	(3) Provided through a formal contractual arrangement or joint venture with another provider that is not in my system (in my local community)	(4) Do Not Provide
34. Case management	☐	☐	☐	☐
35. Chaplaincy/pastoral care services	☐	☐	☐	☐
36. Chemotherapy	☐	☐	☐	☐
37. Children's wellness program	☐	☐	☐	☐
38. Chiropractic services	☐	☐	☐	☐
39. Community outreach	☐	☐	☐	☐
40. Complementary and alternative medicine services	☐	☐	☐	☐
41. Computer assisted orthopedic surgery (CAOS)	☐	☐	☐	☐
42. Crisis prevention	☐	☐	☐	☐
43. Dental services	☐	☐	☐	☐
44. Diabetes prevention program	☐	☐	☐	☐
45. Emergency services				
a. On-campus emergency department	☐	☐	☐	☐
b. Off-campus emergency department	☐	☐	☐	☐
c. Pediatric emergency department	☐	☐	☐	☐
d. Trauma center (certified) [Hospital level of unit (1-3) _____]	☐	☐	☐	☐
e. If column(1) is checked for 45d (Trauma center), does your hospital own the trauma certification?	Yes ☐	No ☐		
46. Enabling services	☐	☐	☐	☐
47. Endoscopic services				
a. Optical colonoscopy	☐	☐	☐	☐
b. Endoscopic ultrasound	☐	☐	☐	☐
c. Ablation of Barrett's esophagus	☐	☐	☐	☐
d. Esophageal impedance study	☐	☐	☐	☐
e. Endoscopic retrograde cholangiopancreatography (ERCP)	☐	☐	☐	☐
48. Enrollment (insurance) assistance services	☐	☐	☐	☐
49. Employment support services	☐	☐	☐	☐
50. Extracorporeal shock wave lithotripter (ESWL)	☐	☐	☐	☐
51. Fertility clinic	☐	☐	☐	☐
52. Fitness center	☐	☐	☐	☐
53. Freestanding outpatient care center	☐	☐	☐	☐
54. Geriatric services	☐	☐	☐	☐
55. Health fair	☐	☐	☐	☐
56. Community health education	☐	☐	☐	☐
57. Genetic testing/counseling	☐	☐	☐	☐
58. Health screenings	☐	☐	☐	☐
59. Health research	☐	☐	☐	☐
60. Hemodialysis	☐	☐	☐	☐
61. HIV/AIDS services	☐	☐	☐	☐
62. Home health services	☐	☐	☐	☐
63. Hospice program	☐	☐	☐	☐
64. Hospital-based outpatient care center services	☐	☐	☐	☐

C. FACILITIES AND SERVICES (continued)

	(1) Owned or provided by my hospital or its subsidiary	(2) Provided by my Health System (in my local community)	(3) Provided through a formal contractual arrangement or joint venture with another provider that is not in my system (in my local community)	(4) Do Not Provide
65. Housing services				
a. Assisted living	☐	☐	☐	☐
b. Retirement housing	☐	☐	☐	☐
c. Supportive housing services	☐	☐	☐	☐
66. Immunization program	☐	☐	☐	☐
67. Indigent care clinic	☐	☐	☐	☐
68. Linguistic/translation services	☐	☐	☐	☐
69. Meal delivery services	☐	☐	☐	☐
70. Mobile health services	☐	☐	☐	☐
71. Neurological services	☐	☐	☐	☐
72. Nutrition program	☐	☐	☐	☐
73. Occupational health services	☐	☐	☐	☐
74. Oncology services	☐	☐	☐	☐
75. Orthopedic services	☐	☐	☐	☐
76. Outpatient surgery	☐	☐	☐	☐
77. Pain management program	☐	☐	☐	☐
78. Palliative care program	☐	☐	☐	☐
79. Palliative care inpatient unit	☐	☐	☐	☐
80. Patient controlled analgesia (PCA)	☐	☐	☐	☐
81. Patient education center	☐	☐	☐	☐
82. Patient representative services	☐	☐	☐	☐
83. Physical rehabilitation services				
a. Assistive technology center	☐	☐	☐	☐
b. Electrodiagnostic services	☐	☐	☐	☐
c. Physical rehabilitation outpatient services	☐	☐	☐	☐
d. Prosthetic and orthotic services	☐	☐	☐	☐
e. Robot-assisted walking therapy	☐	☐	☐	☐
f. Simulated rehabilitation environment	☐	☐	☐	☐
84. Primary care department	☐	☐	☐	☐
85. Psychiatric services				
a. Psychiatric consultation-liaison services	☐	☐	☐	☐
b. Psychiatric pediatric care .... (#Beds_____)	☐	☐	☐	☐
c. Psychiatric geriatric care .... (#Beds_____)	☐	☐	☐	☐
d. Psychiatric education services	☐	☐	☐	☐
e. Psychiatric emergency services	☐	☐	☐	☐
f. Psychiatric outpatient services	☐	☐	☐	☐
g. Psychiatric intensive outpatient services	☐	☐	☐	☐
h. Social and community psychiatric services	☐	☐	☐	☐
i. Forensic psychiatric services	☐	☐	☐	☐
j. Prenatal and postpartum psychiatric services	☐	☐	☐	☐
k. Psychiatric partial hospitalization services – adult	☐	☐	☐	☐
l. Psychiatric partial hospitalization services – pediatric	☐	☐	☐	☐
m. Psychiatric residential treatment – adult	☐	☐	☐	☐
n. Psychiatric residential treatment – pediatric	☐	☐	☐	☐
o. Suicide prevention services	☐	☐	☐	☐

AHA Hospital Statistics © 2024 Health Forum LLC, an affiliate of the American Hospital Association

C. FACILITIES AND SERVICES (continued)

	(1) Owned or provided by my hospital or its subsidiary	(2) Provided by my Health System (in my local community)	(3) Provided through a formal contractual arrangement or joint venture with another provider that is not in my system (in my local community)	(4) Do Not Provide
86. Radiology, diagnostic				
a. CT Scanner	☐	☐	☐	☐
b. Diagnostic radioisotope facility	☐	☐	☐	☐
c. Electron beam computed tomography (EBCT)	☐	☐	☐	☐
d. Full-field digital mammography (FFDM)	☐	☐	☐	☐
e. Magnetic resonance imaging (MRI)	☐	☐	☐	☐
f. Intraoperative magnetic resonance imaging	☐	☐	☐	☐
g. Magnetoencephalography (MEG)	☐	☐	☐	☐
h. Multi-slice spiral computed tomography (<64+ slice CT)	☐	☐	☐	☐
i. Multi-slice spiral computed tomography (64+ slice CT)	☐	☐	☐	☐
j. Positron emission tomography (PET)	☐	☐	☐	☐
k. Positron emission tomography/CT (PET/CT)	☐	☐	☐	☐
l. Single photon emission computerized tomography (SPECT)	☐	☐	☐	☐
m. Ultrasound	☐	☐	☐	☐
87. Radiology, therapeutic				
a. Image-guided radiation therapy (IGRT)	☐	☐	☐	☐
b. Intensity-modulated radiation therapy (IMRT)	☐	☐	☐	☐
c. Proton beam therapy	☐	☐	☐	☐
d. Shaped beam radiation system	☐	☐	☐	☐
e. Stereotactic radiosurgery	☐	☐	☐	☐
f. Basic interventional radiology	☐	☐	☐	☐
88. Robotic surgery	☐	☐	☐	☐
89. Rural health clinic	☐	☐	☐	☐
90. Sleep center	☐	☐	☐	☐
91. Social work services	☐	☐	☐	☐
92. Sports medicine	☐	☐	☐	☐
93. Substance use disorder services				
a. Substance use disorder pediatric services .... (#Beds_____)	☐	☐	☐	☐
b. Substance use disorder outpatient services	☐	☐	☐	☐
c. Substance use disorder partial hospitalization services	☐	☐	☐	☐
d. Medication assisted treatment for Opioid Use Disorder	☐	☐	☐	☐
e. Medication assisted treatment for other substance use disorders	☐	☐	☐	☐
94. Support groups	☐	☐	☐	☐
95. Swing bed services	☐	☐	☐	☐
96. Teen outreach services	☐	☐	☐	☐
97. Tobacco treatment/cessation program	☐	☐	☐	☐
98. Telehealth				
a. Consultation and office visits	☐	☐	☐	☐
b. eICU	☐	☐	☐	☐
c. Stroke care	☐	☐	☐	☐
d. Psychiatric and addiction treatment	☐	☐	☐	☐

C. FACILITIES AND SERVICES (continued)

	(1) Owned or provided by my hospital or its subsidiary	(2) Provided by my Health System (in my local community)	(3) Provided through a formal contractual arrangement or joint venture with another provider that is not in my system (in my local community)	(4) Do Not Provide
98. Telehealth services (continued)				
e. Remote patient monitoring				
1. Post-discharge	☐	☐	☐	☐
2. Ongoing chronic care management	☐	☐	☐	☐
3. Other remote patient monitoring	☐	☐	☐	☐
f. Other telehealth	☐	☐	☐	☐
99. Transplant services				
a. Bone marrow	☐	☐	☐	☐
b. Heart	☐	☐	☐	☐
c. Kidney	☐	☐	☐	☐
d. Liver	☐	☐	☐	☐
e. Lung	☐	☐	☐	☐
f. Tissue	☐	☐	☐	☐
g. Other	☐	☐	☐	☐
100. Transportation to health services (non-emergency)	☐	☐	☐	☐
101. Urgent care center	☐	☐	☐	☐
102. Violence prevention programs				
a. For the workplace	☐	☐	☐	☐
b. For the community	☐	☐	☐	☐
103. Virtual colonoscopy	☐	☐	☐	☐
104. Volunteer services department	☐	☐	☐	☐
105. Women's health center/services	☐	☐	☐	☐
106. Wound management services	☐	☐	☐	☐

107a. Does your organization routinely offer **psychiatric consultation & liaison services** in the following care areas?
Consultation-liaison psychiatrists, medical physicians, or advanced practice providers (APPs) work to help people suffering from a combination of mental and physical illness by consulting with them and liaising with other members of their care team.

	Yes	No
1. Emergency services	☐	☐
2. Primary care services	☐	☐
3. Acute inpatient care	☐	☐
4. Extended care	☐	☐

107b. Does your organization routinely offer **addiction/substance use disorder consultation & liaison services** in the following care areas?

	Yes	No
1. Emergency services	☐	☐
2. Primary care services	☐	☐
3. Acute inpatient care	☐	☐
4. Extended care	☐	☐

C. FACILITIES AND SERVICES (continued)

107c. Does your organization routinely screen for **psychiatric disorders** in the following care areas?
Screens can include but are not limited to the PHQ-2 and PHQ9 depression screen, the Columbia DISC Depression Scale, and/or the GAD-2 and GAD-7 for anxiety disorders.

	Yes	No
1. Emergency services	☐	☐
2. Primary care services	☐	☐
3. Acute inpatient care	☐	☐
4. Extended care	☐	☐

107d. Does your organization routinely screen for **substance use disorders** in the following care areas?
Screens can include but are not limited to the CAGE Substance Abuse Screening Tool; NIDA's drug screening tool; and/or TAPS: Tobacco, Alcohol, Prescription medication, and other Substance use Tool

	Yes	No
1. Emergency services	☐	☐
2. Primary care services	☐	☐
3. Acute inpatient care	☐	☐
4. Extended care	☐	☐

108a. For each of the physician-organization arrangements, please report the number of physicians involved in these arrangements.

	Number of Involved Physicians	(1) My Hospital	(2) My Health System	(3) Do Not Provide
1. Independent Practice Association (IPA)	_____	☐	☐	☐
2. Group practice without walls	_____	☐	☐	☐
3. Open Physician-Hospital Organization (PHO)	_____	☐	☐	☐
4. Closed Physician-Hospital Organization (PHO)	_____	☐	☐	☐
5. Management Service Organization (MSO)	_____	☐	☐	☐
6. Integrated Salary Model	_____	☐	☐	☐
7. Equity Model	_____	☐	☐	☐
8. Foundation	_____	☐	☐	☐
9. Other, please specify _____	_____	☐	☐	☐

108b. For those arrangements reported in 108a, please report the approximate ownership share.

	Hospital ownership share	Physician ownership share	Parent corporation ownership share	Insurance ownership share
1. Independent Practice Association (IPA)	_____ %	_____ %	_____ %	_____ %
2. Group practice without walls	_____ %	_____ %	_____ %	_____ %
3. Open Physician-Hospital Organization (PHO)	_____ %	_____ %	_____ %	_____ %
4. Closed Physician-Hospital Organization (PHO)	_____ %	_____ %	_____ %	_____ %
5. Management Service Organization (MSO)	_____ %	_____ %	_____ %	_____ %
6. Integrated Salary Model	_____ %	_____ %	_____ %	_____ %
7. Equity Model	_____ %	_____ %	_____ %	_____ %
8. Foundation	_____ %	_____ %	_____ %	_____ %
9. Other, specified above	_____ %	_____ %	_____ %	_____ %

108c. If the hospital owns physician practices, how are they organized?

	Percent	Number of physicians
1. Solo practice	_____ %	_____
2. Single specialty group	_____ %	_____
3. Multi-specialty group	_____ %	_____

224 AHA Hospital Statistics © 2024 Health Forum LLC, an affiliate of the American Hospital Association

C. FACILITIES AND SERVICES (continued)

108d. Of the physician practices owned by the hospital, what percentage are primary care? _____%

108e. Of the physician practices owned by the hospital, what percentage are specialty care? _____%

109. Looking across all the relationships identified in question 108a, what is the total number of physicians (count each physician only once) that are engaged in an arrangement with your hospital that allows for joint contracting with payers or shared responsibility for financial risk or clinical performance between the hospital and physician? (Arrangement may be any type of ownership.)

_____ Number of physicians

110a. Does your hospital participate in any joint venture arrangements with physicians or physician groups? Yes ☐ No ☐

110b. If your hospital participates in any joint ventures with physicians or physician groups, please indicate which types of services are involved in those joint ventures. (Check all that apply)

    1. ☐ Limited service hospital

    2. ☐ Ambulatory surgical centers

    3. ☐ Imaging centers

    4. ☐ Other _____

110c. If you selected '1. Limited service hospital' above, please tell us what type(s) of services are provided. (Check all that apply)

    1. ☐ Cardiac

    2. ☐ Orthopedic

    3. ☐ Surgical

    4. ☐ Other _____

110d. Does your hospital participate in joint venture arrangements with organizations other than physician groups? Yes ☐ No ☐

111. Bed Changes

    a. Was there a temporary **increase** in the total number of **beds set up and staffed** for use during the reporting period? Yes ☐ No ☐

    b. Was there a temporary **increase** in the total number of **ICU beds set up and staffed** for use during the reporting period? Yes ☐ No ☐

112. Airborne infection isolation rooms

    a. Please indicate the total number of airborne infection isolation rooms set up and staffed at the start of the reporting period. _____

    b. Please indicate the total number of airborne infection isolation rooms set up and staffed at the end of the reporting period. _____

    c. Please indicate how many rooms not set up and staffed as airborne infection isolation rooms at the end of the reporting period can be converted to airborne infection isolation rooms. _____

113. Temporary spaces

    Please indicate if any temporary spaces such as tents or other spaces not typically used for clinical purposes were set up for using in triage, testing or treatment during the reporting period. Yes ☐ No ☐

AHA Hospital Statistics © 2024 Health Forum LLC, an affiliate of the American Hospital Association **225**

C. FACILITIES AND SERVICES (continued)

114. Ventilators

    a. How many **adult** (in use and not in use) mechanical ventilators were there in your facility at the start of the reporting period? _____

    b. How many **adult** (in use and not in use) mechanical ventilators were there in your facility at the end of the reporting period? _____

    c. How many **pediatric/NICU** (in use and not in use) mechanical ventilators were there in your facility at the start of the reporting period? _____

    d. How many **pediatric/NICU** (in use and not in use) mechanical ventilators were there in your facility at the end of the reporting period? _____

115. Emergency Departments

    Was there a temporary **increase** in the total number of **emergency department beds set up and staffed** for use during the reporting period?   Yes ☐   No ☐

D. INSURANCE AND ALTERNATIVE PAYMENT MODELS

INSURANCE

1. Does your hospital own or jointly own a health plan? Yes ☐ No ☐

    a. If yes, in what states? States: _____

2. Does your system own or jointly own a health plan? Yes ☐ No ☐

    a. If yes, in what states? States: _____

3. Does your hospital/system have a significant partnership with an insurer or an insurance company/health plan? Yes ☐ No ☐

    a. If yes, in what states? States: _____

4. If yes to 1, 2 and/or 3 above, please indicate the insurance product(s). (Check all that apply)

Insurance Products	Hospital	System	JV	No	Do not know
a. Medicare Advantage	☐	☐	☐	☐	☐
b. Medicaid Managed Care	☐	☐	☐	☐	☐
c. Health Insurance Marketplace ("exchange")	☐	☐	☐	☐	☐
d. Other Individual Market	☐	☐	☐	☐	☐
e. Small Group	☐	☐	☐	☐	☐
f. Large Group	☐	☐	☐	☐	☐
g. Other _____	☐	☐	☐	☐	☐

If you have answered 'no' to all parts of questions 1, 2 and 3, please skip to question 8.

5. Does your **health plan** make capitated payments to physicians either within or outside of your network for specific groups or enrollees?

    a. Physicians within your network Yes ☐ No ☐ Do not know ☐

    b. Physicians outside your network Yes ☐ No ☐ Do not know ☐

    c. If yes, which specialties? _____

6. Does your **health plan** make bundled payments to providers in your network or to outside providers?

    a. Providers within your network Yes ☐ No ☐ Do not know ☐

    b. Providers outside your network Yes ☐ No ☐ Do not know ☐

    c. If yes, which specialties? _____

7. Does your **health plan** offer other shared risk contracts to either providers in your network or to outside providers? (i.e., other than capitation or bundled payment.)

    a. Providers within your network Yes ☐ No ☐ Do not know ☐

    b. Providers outside your network Yes ☐ No ☐ Do not know ☐

    c. If yes, which specialties? _____

8. Does your hospital or health system fund the health benefits for your employees? Yes ☐ No ☐

    a. If yes, does the hospital or health system also administer the benefits (as opposed to contracting with a third party administrator)? Yes ☐ No ☐

D. INSURANCE AND ALTERNATIVE PAYMENT MODELS (continued)

9. What percentage of your **hospital's** patient revenue is paid on a capitated basis? _____%

    a. In total, how many patients do you serve under capitated contracts? Total patients: _____

10. Does your **hospital** participate in any bundled payment arrangements? Yes ☐ No ☐ (skip to 12)

10a. If yes, for which of the following payers and medical/surgical conditions does your **hospital** have a bundled payment arrangement? (Check all that apply)

	(a) Traditional Medicare	(b) Medicare Advantage Plan	(c) Commercial Insurance Plan (including ACA participants, individual, group or employer markets)	(d) Medicaid
1. Cardiovascular	☐	☐	☐	☐
2. Orthopedic	☐	☐	☐	☐
3. Oncologic	☐	☐	☐	☐
4. Neurology	☐	☐	☐	☐
5. Hematology	☐	☐	☐	☐
6. Gastrointestinal	☐	☐	☐	☐
7. Pulmonary	☐	☐	☐	☐
8. Infectious disease	☐	☐	☐	☐
9. Hospitalist	☐	☐	☐	☐
10. Nephrology	☐	☐	☐	☐
11. Obstetrics	☐	☐	☐	☐
12. Endocrinology	☐	☐	☐	☐
13. Psychiatric disorders	☐	☐	☐	☐
14. Substance use disorders	☐	☐	☐	☐
15. Other:_____	☐	☐	☐	☐

10b. What percentage of the **hospital's** patient revenue is paid through bundled payment arrangements? _____%

11. Does your **hospital** participate in a bundled payment program involving care settings outside of the hospital (e.g., physician, outpatient, post-acute)? Yes ☐ No ☐

    a. If yes, does your **hospital** share upside or downside risk for any of those outside providers? Yes ☐ No ☐

12. What percentage of your **hospital's** patient revenue is paid on a shared risk basis (other than capitated or bundled payments)? _____%

13. Does your **hospital** contract directly with employers or a coalition of employers to provide care on a capitated, predetermined, or shared risk basis? Yes ☐ No ☐

14. Does your **hospital** have contracts with commercial payers where payment is tied to performance on quality/safety metrics? Yes ☐ No ☐

15a. Has your **hospital** or **health care system** established an accountable care organization (ACO)?
    1. ☐ My hospital/system currently leads an ACO **(Skip to 15b)**
    2. ☐ My hospital/system currently participates in an ACO (but is not its leader) **(Skip to 17)**
    3. ☐ My hospital/system previously led or participated in an ACO but is no longer doing so **(Skip to 17)**
    4. ☐ My hospital/system has never participated or led an ACO **(Skip to 16)**

15b. With which of the following types of payers does your hospital/system have an accountable care contract? (Check all that apply)
    1. ☐ Traditional Medicare (MSSP and NextGen) **(Skip to 15c)**
    2. ☐ A Medicare Advantage plan **(Skip to 15d)**
    3. ☐ A commercial insurance plan (including ACO participants, individual, group, and employer markets) **(Skip to 15d)**
    4. ☐ Medicaid **(Skip to 15d)**

---

228   AHA Hospital Statistics © 2024 Health Forum LLC, an affiliate of the American Hospital Association

D. INSURANCE AND ALTERNATIVE PAYMENT MODELS (continued)

15c. If you selected Traditional Medicare, in which of the following Medicare programs is your hospital/system participating? (Check all that apply)

1. ☐ MSSP BASIC Track, Level A

2. ☐ MSSP BASIC Track, Level B

3. ☐ MSSP BASIC Track, Level C

4. ☐ MSSP BASIC Track, Level D

5. ☐ MSSP BASIC Track, Level E

6. ☐ MSSP ENHANCED Track

7. ☐ Original MSSP program, Tracks 1, 1+, 2 or 3

8. ☐ Comprehensive ESRD Care

15d. What percentage of your hospital's/system's patients are covered by accountable care contracts? _____%

15e. What percentage of your hospital's/system's patient revenue came from ACO contracts in 2022? _____% **(Skip to 17)**

16. Has your hospital/system ever considered participating in an ACO?

a. ☐ Yes, and we are planning to join one

b. ☐ Yes, but we are not planning to join one

c. ☐ No, we have not even considered it

17. Do any hospitals and/or physician groups with your system, or the system itself, plan to participate in any of the following risk arrangements in the next three years? (Check all that apply)

a. ☐ Shared savings/losses

b. ☐ Bundled payment

c. ☐ Capitation

d. ☐ ACO (ownership)

e. ☐ ACO (joint venture)

f. ☐ Health plan (ownership)

g. ☐ Health plan (joint venture)

h. ☐ Primary care transformation, including direct contracting

i. ☐ Other, please specify: _____

j. ☐ None

18. Does your hospital/system have an established medical home program?

a. Hospital   Yes ☐   No ☐

b. System   Yes ☐   No ☐

E. TOTAL FACILITY BEDS, UTILIZATION, FINANCES, AND STAFFING

Please report beds, utilization, financial, and staffing data for the 12-month period that is consistent with the period reported on page 1. Report financial data for reporting period only. Include within your operations all activities that are wholly owned by the hospital, including subsidiary corporations regardless of where the activity is physically located. Please do not include within your operations distinct and separate divisions that may be owned by your hospital's parent corporation. If final figures are not available, please estimate. Round to the nearest dollar. Report all personnel who were on the payroll and whose payroll expenses are reported in E3f. (Please refer to specific definitions on pages 37-39.)

> **Fill out column (2) if hospital owns and operates a nursing home type unit/facility. Column (1) should be the combined total of hospital plus nursing home unit/facility.**

1. BEDS AND UTILIZATION

	(1) Total Facility	(2) Nursing Home Unit/Facility
a. Total licensed beds	_____	_____
b. Beds set up and staffed for use at the end of the reporting period	_____	_____
c. Bassinets set up and staffed for use at the end of the reporting period	_____	
d. Births (exclude fetal deaths)	_____	
e. Admissions (exclude newborns; include neonatal & swing admissions)	_____	_____
f. Inpatient days (exclude newborns; include neonatal & swing days)	_____	_____
g. Emergency department visits	_____	
h. Total outpatient visits (include emergency department visits & outpatient surgeries)	_____	
i. Inpatient surgical operations	_____	
j. Number of operating rooms	_____	
k. Outpatient surgical operations	_____	

2. UTILIZATION BY PAYER

	(1) Total Facility	(2) Nursing Home Unit/Facility
a1. Total Medicare (Title XVIII) inpatient discharges (including Medicare Managed Care)	_____	_____
a2. How many Medicare inpatient discharges were Medicare Managed Care?	_____	_____
b1. Total Medicare (Title XVIII) inpatient days (including Medicare Managed Care)	_____	_____
b2. How many Medicare inpatient days were Medicare Managed Care?	_____	_____
c1. Total Medicaid (Title XIX) inpatient discharges (including Medicaid Managed Care)	_____	_____
c2. How many Medicaid inpatient discharges were Medicaid Managed Care?	_____	_____
d1. Total Medicaid (Title XIX) inpatient days (including Medicaid Managed Care)	_____	_____
d2. How many Medicaid inpatient days were Medicaid Managed Care?	_____	_____
e1. Total self-pay inpatient discharges	_____	_____
e2. Total self-pay inpatient days	_____	_____
f1. Total third-party (non-Medicare, non-Medicaid) inpatient discharges	_____	_____
f2. Total third-party (non-Medicare, non-Medicaid) inpatient days	_____	_____
g1. Other payer (government and non-government) inpatient discharges	_____	_____
g2. Other payer (government and non-government) inpatient days	_____	_____
h. Total inpatient discharges (all payers) (add a1,c1,e1,f1,g1)	_____	_____

E. TOTAL FACILITY BEDS, UTILIZATION, FINANCES, AND STAFFING (continued)

3. FINANCIAL

	(1) Total Facility	(2) Nursing Home Unit/Facility
*a. Net patient revenue (treat bad debt as a deduction from gross revenue)...............	.00	.00
*b. Tax appropriations...	.00	
*c. Other operating revenue...	.00	
*d. Nonoperating revenue..	.00	
*e. TOTAL REVENUE (add 3a thru 3d)...	.00	.00
f. Payroll expense (only)	.00	.00
g. Employee benefits..	.00	.00
h. Depreciation expense (for reporting period only)............................	.00	
i. Interest expense..	.00	
j. Pharmacy expense...	.00	
k. Supply expense (other than pharmacy)......................................	.00	
l. All other expenses...	.00	
m. TOTAL EXPENSES (add 3f thru 3l. Exclude bad debt)......................	.00	.00

n. Do your total expenses (E3.m) reflect full allocation from your corporate office?   Yes ☐   No ☐

4. REVENUE BY TYPE

*a. Total gross inpatient revenue..	.00
*b. Total gross outpatient revenue..	.00
*c. Total gross patient revenue	.00

5. UNCOMPENSATED CARE & PROVIDER TAXES

*a. Bad debt (Revenue forgone at full established rates. Include in gross revenue.).. .00

   *1. Are you able to distinguish bad debt derived from patients with or without insurance?   Yes ☐   No ☐

   *2. If yes, how much is from patients with insurance?... .00

*b. Financial assistance (Includes charity care) (Revenue forgone at full-established rates. Include in gross revenue.).. .00

*c. Is your bad debt (5a) reported on the basis of full charges?   Yes ☐   No ☐

*d. Does your state have a provider Medicaid tax/assessment program?   Yes ☐   No ☐

*e. If yes, please report the total gross amount paid into the program. .... .00

*f. Due to differing accounting standards, please indicate whether the provider tax/assessment amount is included in:

   *1. Total expenses   Yes ☐   No ☐

   *2. Deductions from net patient revenue   Yes ☐   No ☐

E. TOTAL FACILITY BEDS, UTILIZATION, FINANCES, AND STAFFING (continued)

6. REVENUE BY PAYER (report total facility gross & net figures)

	(1) Gross	(2) Net
*a. GOVERNMENT		
(1) Medicare:		
a. Fee for service patient revenue	.00	.00
b. Managed care revenue	.00	.00
c. **Total (a + b)**	.00	.00
(2) Medicaid:		
a. Fee for service patient revenue	.00	.00
b. Managed care revenue	.00	.00
c. Medicaid Graduate Medical Education (GME) payments		.00
d. Medicaid Disproportionate Share Hospital Payments (DSH)		.00
e. Medicaid Supplemental Payments (not including Medicaid DSH Payments)		.00
f. Other Medicaid		.00
g. **Total (a thru f)**	.00	.00
(3) Other government	.00	.00
*b. NONGOVERNMENT		
(1) Self-pay	.00	.00
(2) Third-party payers:		
a. Managed care (includes HMO and PPO)	.00	.00
b. Other third-party payers	.00	.00
c. **Total third-party payers (a + b)**	.00	.00
(3) All other nongovernment	.00	.00
*c. TOTAL	.00	.00

(Total gross should equal 4c on page15. Total net should equal 3a on page 15.)

	(1) Inpatient	(2) Outpatient
*d. If you report Medicaid Supplemental Payments on line 6a (2) e, please break the payment total into inpatient and outpatient care.	.00	.00

*e. If you are a government owned facility (control codes 12-16), does your facility participate in the Medicaid intergovernmental transfer or certified public expenditures program? Yes ☐ No ☐

	(1) Gross	(2) Net
*f. If yes, please report gross and net revenue.	.00	.00

7. COVID RELIEF FUNDS

Include all funds received from federal and state governments for COVID relief, such as CARES Act Provider Relief Fund payments. Do not include any funds that constitute a loan and may be on the balance sheet as a liability.

*a. Provider/COVID Relief Funds recognized as revenue in **2022** _____.00

*b. On which survey line did you report this revenue?

    *1. Net patient revenue   Yes ☐ No ☐

    *2. Other operating revenue   Yes ☐ No ☐

    *3. Nonoperating revenue   Yes ☐ No ☐

*c. Provider/COVID Relief Funds recognized as revenue in **2021** _____.00
(please do not include these dollars in 7a)

*d. Did you include these funds as revenue on the **2021** survey?   Yes ☐ No ☐

*e. If yes, on which survey line did you report this revenue

    *1. Net patient revenue   Yes ☐ No ☐

    *2. Other operating revenue   Yes ☐ No ☐

    *3. Nonoperating revenue   Yes ☐ No ☐

E. TOTAL FACILITY BEDS, UTILIZATION, FINANCES, AND STAFFING (continued)

8. FINANCIAL PERFORMANCE – MARGIN

*a. Total Margin _____%

*b. Operating Margin _____%

*c. EBITDA Margin _____%

*d. Medicare Margin _____%

*e. Medicaid Margin _____%

9. FIXED ASSETS

a. Property, plant and equipment at <u>cost</u>.. _____.00

b. Accumulated <u>depreciation</u>.. _____.00

c. Net property, plant and equipment (a–b)... _____.00

d. Total gross square feet of your physical plant used for or in support of your healthcare activities....................... _____

10. TOTAL CAPITAL EXPENSES

Include all expenses used to acquire assets, including buildings, remodeling projects, equipment, or property .... _____.00

11. INFORMATION TECHNOLOGY AND CYBERSECURITY

If you are part of larger health system, report the overall system cyber budget and related numbers, unless each hospital in the system has their own independent cyber budget.

*a. Overall IT Budget _____.00

*b. Number of internal IT staff (in FTEs) _____

*c. What percent of your IT budget is spent on cybersecurity? _____%

*d. Number of internal staff devoted to cybersecurity (in FTEs) _____

*e. Number of outsourced staff devoted to cybersecurity (in FTEs) _____

*f. What position does your cybersecurity lead report to? _____

*g. Does your organization rank cybersecurity as an enterprise risk issue? Yes ☐ No ☐

*h. If yes, what priority number rank it as? _____

*i. How often is the board briefed on cybersecurity?

☐ Quarterly   ☐ Semi-annually   ☐ Yearly   ☐ Never   ☐ Other _____

*j. What do you view as your biggest cybersecurity threat? (Please rank the choices 1-9, with 1 being the biggest threat)

*1. Ransomware which may disrupt and delay patient care delivery _____

*2. Ransomware which may disrupt business operations _____

*3. Theft of sensitive patient data such as Protected Health Information (PHI) or Personally identifiable Information (PII) _____

*4. Theft of medical research or intellectual property _____

*5. Cyber risk exposure through business associates. Business associate as conduit for cyber attacks or theft of your data stored by third parties. _____

*6. Software and supply chain cyber risk _____

*7. Medical device cyber risk _____

*8. Phishing emails or other social engineering attacks which may result in the delivery of malware or ransomware into the organization. _____

*9. Phishing emails or other social engineering attacks which may result in the theft of funds _____

E. TOTAL FACILITY BEDS, UTILIZATION, FINANCES, AND STAFFING (continued)

INFORMATION TECHNOLOGY AND CYBERSECURITY (continued)

*k. Does your organization use any of the following cybersecurity techniques?

*1. Enterprise wide multi-factor authentication for all remote access to networks, data and applications. Yes ☐ No ☐

*2. Network segmentation Yes ☐ No ☐

*3. Off line, network segmented, redundant network and data back ups Yes ☐ No ☐

*4. Immutable backups Yes ☐ No ☐

*5. Intrusion detection systems Yes ☐ No ☐

*6. Employee cybersecurity education including phishing email simulations Yes ☐ No ☐

*7. 24/7 Security Operations Center (SOC) monitoring all cyber incidents and events Yes ☐ No ☐

*8. Highly efficient and effective patch management program Yes ☐ No ☐

*9. Forced password change every 90 days or less Yes ☐ No ☐

*10. Integration of cyber incident response plans with emergency management plans Yes ☐ No ☐

*11. Cross function cyber incident response exercise for all leaders Yes ☐ No ☐

*12. Relationship with local FBI and CISA offices Yes ☐ No ☐

*13. Third Party Risk Management Program which assesses business associate access to networks and bulk sensitive data; mission criticality and life criticality of third party Yes ☐ No ☐

*l. How confident are you in the organization's ability to sustain care delivery through manual downtime procedures for up to four weeks, without the benefit of network and internet connected technology?

☐ Confident ☐ Somewhat confident ☐ Uncertain ☐ Somewhat not confident ☐ Not confident

*m. What do you view as your biggest challenges in improving your organization's cybersecurity posture? (Please rank the choices 1-6, with 1 being the biggest challenge)

*1. Funding _____

*2. Staffing _____

*3. Legacy insecure technology _____

*4. Leadership support _____

*5. Organizational culture _____

*6. Non-compliant third parties/business associates _____

Are the financial data on pages 15-17 from your audited financial statement? Yes ☐ No ☐

---

* These data will be treated as confidential and not released without written permission. AHA will however, share these data with your respective state hospital association and, if requested, with your appropriate metropolitan/regional association.

For members of the Catholic Health Association of the United States (CHA), AHA will also share these data with CHA unless there are objections expressed by checking this box ☐

The state/metropolitan/regional associations and CHA may not release these data without written permission from the hospital.

234 AHA Hospital Statistics © 2024 Health Forum LLC, an affiliate of the American Hospital Association

E. TOTAL FACILITY BEDS, UTILIZATION, FINANCES, AND STAFFING (continued)

12. STAFFING

Report full-time (35 hours or more) and part-time (less than 35 hours) personnel who were on the hospital/facility **payroll at the end of your reporting period.** Include members of religious orders for whom dollar equivalents were reported. Exclude private-duty nurses, volunteers, and all personnel whose salary is financed entirely by outside research grants. Exclude physicians and dentists who are paid on a fee basis. **FTE** is the total number of hours **worked** (excluding non-worked hours such as PTO, etc.) by all employees over the full (12 month) reporting period divided by the normal number of hours worked by a full-time employee for that same time period. For example, if your hospital considers a normal workweek for a full-time employee to be 40 hours, a total of 2,080 would be worked over a full year (52 weeks). If the total number of hours worked by all employees on the payroll is 208,000, then the number of Full-Time Equivalents (FTE) is 100 (employees). The FTE calculation for a specific occupational category such as registered nurses is exactly the same. The calculation for each occupational category should be based on the number of hours worked by staff employed in that specific category.

For each occupational category, please report the number of staff vacancies as of the last day of your reporting period. A vacancy is defined as a budgeted staff position which is unfilled as of the last day of the reporting period and for which the hospital is actively seeking either a full-time or part-time permanent replacement. Personnel who work in more than one area should be included only in the category of their primary responsibility and should be counted only once.

	(1) Full-Time (35 hr/wk or more) On Payroll (Headcount)	(2) Part-Time (Less than 35hr/wk) On Payroll (Headcount)	(3) FTE	(4) Vacancies (Headcount)
a. Physicians	_____	_____	_____	_____
b. Dentists	_____	_____	_____	_____
c. Medical residents/interns	_____	_____	_____	_____
d. Dental residents/interns	_____	_____	_____	_____
e. Other trainees	_____	_____	_____	_____
f. Registered nurses	_____	_____	_____	_____
g. Licensed practical (vocational) nurses	_____	_____	_____	_____
h. Nursing assistive personnel	_____	_____	_____	_____
i. Radiology technicians	_____	_____	_____	_____
j. Laboratory technicians	_____	_____	_____	_____
k. Pharmacists licensed	_____	_____	_____	_____
l. Pharmacy technicians	_____	_____	_____	_____
m. Respiratory therapists	_____	_____	_____	_____
n. All other personnel	_____	_____	_____	_____
o. Total facility personnel (add 12a through 12n)	_____	_____	_____	_____

(Total facility personnel (a-o) should include hospital and nursing home type unit/facility, if applicable.

Nursing home type unit/facility personnel should also be reported separately in 12p and 12q.)

p. Nursing home type unit/facility registered nurses	_____	_____	_____	_____
q. Total nursing home type unit/facility personnel	_____	_____	_____	_____

r. For your employed RN FTEs reported above (E.12f, column 3) please report the number of full-time equivalents who are involved in direct patient care.   _____ Number of direct patient care FTEs

s. For your medical residents/interns reported above (E.12c. column 1) please indicate the number of full-time on payroll by specialty.

    Full-Time (35 hr/wk or more) On Payroll (Headcount)

    1. Primary care (general practitioner, general internal medicine, family practice, general pediatrics, geriatrics)   _____

    2. Other specialties   _____

E. TOTAL FACILITY BEDS, UTILIZATION, FINANCES, AND STAFFING (continued)

13. CONTRACTED STAFF

Please report the number of contracted FTEs for each occupational category. <u>Personnel that are on the hospitals payroll and reported in E(12) should not be reported here.</u>

CONTRACTED FTEs

a. Registered nurses _____

b. Radiology technicians _____

c. Laboratory technicians _____

d. Pharmacists licensed _____

e. Pharmacy technicians _____

f. Respiratory therapists _____

g. All other contracted staff _____

14. PRIVILEGED PHYSICIANS

Report the total number of physicians with privileges at your hospital by type of relationship with the hospital. <u>The sum of the physicians reported in 14a-14g should equal the total number of privileged physicians (14h) in the hospital.</u>

	(1) Total Employed	(2) Total Individual Contract	(3) Total Group Contract	(4) Not Employed or Under Contract	(5) Total Privileged (add columns 1-4)
a. Primary care (general practitioner, general internal medicine, family practice, general pediatrics).......	_____	_____	_____	_____	_____
b. Obstetrics/gynecology	_____	_____	_____	_____	_____
c. Emergency medicine	_____	_____	_____	_____	_____
d. Hospitalist....................................	_____	_____	_____	_____	_____
e. Intensivist	_____	_____	_____	_____	_____
f. Radiologist/pathologist/anesthesiologist	_____	_____	_____	_____	_____
g. Other specialist................................	_____	_____	_____	_____	_____
h. Total (add 14a-14g).........................	_____	_____	_____	_____	_____

15. HOSPITALISTS

a. Do hospitalists provide care for patients in your hospital? (if no, please skip to 16)................. Yes ☐ No ☐ (If yes, please report in E.14d)

b. If yes, please report the total number of full-time equivalent (FTE) hospitalists .... _____FTE

16. INTENSIVISTS

a. Do intensivists provide care for patients in your hospital? (if no, please skip to17)................. Yes ☐ No ☐ (If yes, please report in E.14e)

b. If yes, please report the total number of FTE intensivists and assign them to the following areas. Please indicate whether the intensive care area is closed to intensivists. (Meaning that only intensivists are authorized to care for ICU patients.)

		FTE	Closed to Intensivists
1.	Medical-surgical intensive care	_____	☐
2.	Cardiac intensive care	_____	☐
3.	Neonatal intensive care	_____	☐
4.	Pediatric intensive care	_____	☐
5.	Other intensive care	_____	☐
6.	**Total**	_____	

236 AHA Hospital Statistics © 2024 Health Forum LLC, an affiliate of the American Hospital Association

E. TOTAL FACILITY BEDS, UTILIZATION, FINANCES, AND STAFFING (continued)

17. ADVANCED PRACTICE REGISTERED NURSES/PHYSICIAN ASSISTANTS

a. Do advanced practice nurses/physician assistants provide care for patients in your hospital? (If no, please skip to 18)   YES ☐   NO ☐

b. If yes, please report the number of full time, part time and FTE advanced practice nurses and physician assistants who provide care for patients in your hospital.

Advanced Practice Registered Nurses   _____ Full-time   _____ Part-time   _____ FTE

Physician Assistants   _____ Full-time   _____ Part-time   _____ FTE

c. If yes, please indicate the type of service(s) provided. (check all that apply)

1. ☐ Primary care   **2.** ☐ Anesthesia services (Certified registered nurse anesthetist)   **3.** ☐ Emergency department care

4. ☐ Other specialty care   **5.** ☐ Patient education   **6.** ☐ Case management   **7.** ☐ Other

18. FOREIGN EDUCATED NURSES

a. Did your facility hire more foreign-educated nurses (including contract or agency nurses) to help fill RN vacancies in 2022 vs. 2021?

More ☐   Less ☐   Same ☐   Did not hire foreign nurses ☐

b. From which countries/continents are you recruiting foreign-educated nurses? (check all that apply)

Africa ☐   South Korea ☐   Canada ☐   Philippines ☐   China ☐   India ☐   Other ☐

19. WORKFORCE

a. Does your hospital use artificial intelligence (AI) or machine learning in the following? (Check all that apply)

1. ☐ Predicting staffing needs

2. ☐ Predicting patient demand

3. ☐ Staff scheduling

4. ☐ Automating routine tasks

5. ☐ Optimizing administrative and clinical workflows

6. ☐ None of the above

b. How is your hospital incorporating workforce as part of the strategic planning process? (Check all that apply)

1. ☐ Conduct needs assessment

2. ☐ Leadership succession planning

3. ☐ Talent development plan

4. ☐ Recruitment & retention planning

5. ☐ Partnerships with elementary/HS to develop interest in health care careers

6. ☐ Training program partnership with community colleges, vocational training programs

7. ☐ None of the above

F. ADDRESSING PATIENT SOCIAL NEEDS AND COMMUNITY SOCIAL DETERMINANTS OF HEALTH

1. Which social needs of patients/social determinants of health in communities does your hospital or health system have programs or strategies to address? (Check all that apply)

   a. ☐ Housing (instability, quality, financing)
   b. ☐ Food insecurity or hunger
   c. ☐ Utility needs
   d. ☐ Interpersonal violence
   e. ☐ Transportation
   f. ☐ Employment and income
   g. ☐ Education
   h. ☐ Social isolation (lack of family and social support)
   i. ☐ Health behaviors
   j. ☐ Other, please describe: _____

2. Does your hospital or health system screen patients for social needs?

   ☐ Yes, for all patients   ☐ Yes, for some patients   ☐ No (skip to question 3)

   2a. If yes, please indicate which social needs are assessed. (Check all that apply)

   1. ☐ Housing (instability, quality, financing)
   2. ☐ Food insecurity or hunger
   3. ☐ Utility needs
   4. ☐ Interpersonal violence
   5. ☐ Transportation
   6. ☐ Employment and income
   7. ☐ Education
   8. ☐ Social isolation (lack of family and social support)
   9. ☐ Health behaviors
   10. ☐ Other, please describe: _____

   2b. If yes, does your hospital or health system record the social needs screening results in your electronic health record?   Yes ☐   No ☐

3. Does your hospital or health system utilize outcome measures (for example, cost of care or readmission rates) to assess the effectiveness of the interventions to address patients' social needs?   Yes ☐   No ☐

4. Has your hospital or health system been able to gather data indicating that activities used to address the social determinants of health and patient social needs have resulted in any of the following? (Check all that apply)

   a. ☐ Better health outcomes for patients
   b. ☐ Decreased utilization of hospital or health system services
   c. ☐ Decreased health care costs
   d. ☐ Improved community health status
   e. ☐ None of the above

F. ADDRESSING PATIENT SOCIAL NEEDS AND COMMUNITY SOCIAL DETERMINANTS OF HEALTH (continued)

5. Who in your hospital or health care system is accountable for meeting health equity goals? (Check all that apply)

    a. ☐ CEO
    b. ☐ Designated Senior Executive (Chief Diversity Office, VP for DEI, etc.)
    c. ☐ Middle Management
    d. ☐ Committee or Task Force
    e. ☐ Division/Department Leaders
    f. ☐ Employee Resource Group
    g. ☐ None of the above

6. Who in your hospital or health care system is accountable for implementing strategies for health equity goals? (Check all that apply)

    a. ☐ CEO
    b. ☐ Designated Senior Executive (Chief Diversity Office, VP for DEI, etc.)
    c. ☐ Middle Management
    d. ☐ Committee or Task Force
    e. ☐ Division/Department Leaders
    f. ☐ Employee Resource Group
    g. ☐ None of the above

7. Does your hospital or health care system use DEI disaggregated data to inform decisions on the following? (Check all that apply)

    a. ☐ Patient outcomes
    b. ☐ Procurement
    c. ☐ Supply chain
    d. ☐ Training
    e. ☐ Professional Development
    f. ☐ None of the above

8. Does your hospital or health care system have a health equity strategic plan for the following? (Check all that apply)

    a. ☐ Equitable and inclusive organizational policies
    b. ☐ Systematic and shared accountability for health equity
    c. ☐ Diverse representation in hospital and health care system leadership
    d. ☐ Diverse representation in hospital and health care system governance
    e. ☐ Community engagement
    f. ☐ Collection and use of segmented data to drive action
    g. ☐ Culturally appropriate patient care
    h. ☐ None of the above

AHA Hospital Statistics © 2024 Health Forum LLC, an affiliate of the American Hospital Association

F. ADDRESSING PATIENT SOCIAL NEEDS AND COMMUNITY SOCIAL DETERMINANTS OF HEALTH (continued)

9. Please indicate the extent of your hospital's current partnerships with external partners for population and/or community health initiatives. Which types of organizations do you currently partner with in each of the following activities? (Check all that apply)

	(1) Not Involved	(2) Work together to meet patient social needs (e.g., referral arrangement or case management)	(3) Participates in our Community Health Needs Assessment process	(4) Work together to implement community-level initiatives to address social determinants of health
a. Health care providers outside your system	☐	☐	☐	☐
b. Health insurance providers outside of your system	☐	☐	☐	☐
c. Local or state public health departments/organizations	☐	☐	☐	☐
d. Other local or state government agencies or social service organizations	☐	☐	☐	☐
e. Faith-based organizations	☐	☐	☐	☐
f. Local organizations addressing food insecurity	☐	☐	☐	☐
g. Local organizations addressing transportation needs	☐	☐	☐	☐
h. Local organizations addressing housing insecurity	☐	☐	☐	☐
i. Local organizations providing legal assistance for individuals	☐	☐	☐	☐
j. Other community non-profit organizations	☐	☐	☐	☐
k. K-12 schools	☐	☐	☐	☐
l. Colleges or universities	☐	☐	☐	☐
m. Local businesses or chambers of commerce	☐	☐	☐	☐
n. Law enforcement/safety forces	☐	☐	☐	☐
o. Area Behavioral Health Service Providers	☐	☐	☐	☐
p. Area Agencies on Aging (AAA)	☐	☐	☐	☐

G. SUPPLEMENTAL INFORMATION

1. Does the hospital participate in a group purchasing arrangement? YES ☐ NO ☐
If yes, please provide the name, city, and state of your primary group purchasing organization.

Name: _____ City: _____ State: _____

2. Does the hospital purchase medical/surgical supplies directly through a distributor? YES ☐ NO ☐
If yes, please provide the name of your primary distributor.

Name: _____

3. If your hospital hired RNs during the reporting period, how many were new graduates from nursing schools? _____

4. Does your hospital have an established patient and family advisory council that meets regularly to actively engage the perspectives of patients and families? Yes ☐ No ☐

5. Utilization of telehealth/virtual care
The definitions used herein represent one approach to understanding telehealth/virtual care. The AHA is aware that different organizations use different definitions for these terms and that Medicare defines them in a more narrow way than they are used in the field. The definitions we chose are meant to balance the statutory and regulatory use of the terms with the way they are understood by providers on the ground.

a. Number of video visits: Synchronous visits between patient and provider that are not co-located, through the use of two-way, interactive, real-time audio and video communication. _____

b. Number of audio visits: Synchronous visits between a patient and a provider that are not co-located, through the use of two-way, interactive, real-time audio-only communication. _____

c. Number of patients being monitored through remote patient monitoring (RPM): Asynchronous or synchronous interactions between and patient and a provider that are not co-located involving the collection, transmission, evaluation, and communication of physiological data. _____

d. Number of patients receiving other virtual services: All other synchronous or asynchronous interactions between a provider and patient or provider and provider delivered remotely including messages, eConsults, and virtual check-ins. _____

6. Does your hospital have a partnership with a Community Mental Health Center or a Certified Community Behavioral Health Center?

a. Community Mental Health Center Yes ☐ No ☐

b. Certified Community Behavioral Health Center Yes ☐ No ☐

7. Which of the following best describes your organization's decarbonization efforts?

a. ☐ We have set a decarbonization percentage reduction goal

      1. % reduction goal _____
      2. Target year to meet goal _____
      3. Baseline year _____

b. ☐ We have set a "net-zero emissions" goal
      1. Target year to meet goal _____
      2. Baseline year _____

c. ☐ We have set both a decarbonization percentage reduction and a "net-zero emissions goal"

      % Reduction Goal
      1. % reduction goal _____
      2. Target year to meet goal _____
      3. Baseline year _____
      "Net-Zero Emissions" Goal
      4. Target year to meet goal _____
      5. Baseline year _____

d. ☐ We have not set any decarbonization targets/goals but plan to within the year

e. ☐ We have not set any decarbonization targets/goals and uncertain if any plans to within the year

G. SUPPLEMENTAL INFORMATION (continued)

f.   Please free to expand on your response:

_____

_____

_____

8. The federal government has recently released ambitious goals for federal facilities. They include achieving a carbon-pollution free electricity sector by 2035 and net-zero emissions economy-wide by no later than 2050 with a 65% reduction in Scope 1 and 2 GHG emissions from federal operation by 2050 (from 2008 levels). Irrespective of the exact targets and years, would your organization, in principle, be willing to support similar types of goals for the health sector?

Yes ☐   No ☐   Unsure ☐

Please feel free to expand on your response: _____

_____

_____

9. Do you believe the decarbonization goals for the health sector should be similar, more ambitious, or less ambitious than the targets set by the federal government?

Similar ☐   More ambitious ☐   Less ambitious ☐   Unsure ☐

Please feel free to expand on your response: _____

_____

_____

10. Does your organization have an executive leader responsible for environmental sustainability, including climate change mitigation?

Yes ☐   No ☐

Please feel free to expand on your response: _____

_____

_____

_____

G. SUPPLEMENTAL INFORMATION (continued)

Use this space for comments or to elaborate on any information supplied on this survey. Refer to the response by page, section and item name.

_____

_____

_____

_____

_____

_____

_____

_____

_____

As declared previously, hospital specific revenue data are treated as confidential. AHA's policy is not to release these data without written permission from your institution. The AHA will however, share these data with your respective state hospital association and if requested with your appropriate metropolitan/regional association.

On occasion, the AHA is asked to provide these data to external organizations, both public and private, for their use in analyzing crucial health care policy or research issues. The AHA is requesting your permission to allow us to release your confidential data to those requests that we consider legitimate and worthwhile. In every instance of disclosure, the receiving organization will be prohibited from releasing hospital specific information.

Please indicate below whether or not you agree to these types of disclosure:

[　] I hereby grant AHA permission to release my hospital's revenue data to external users that the AHA determines have a legitimate and worthwhile need to gain access to these data subject to the user's agreement with the AHA not to release hospital specific information.

_____

Chief Executive Officer　　　　　　　　Date

[　] I do not grant AHA permission to release my confidential data.

_____

Chief Executive Officer　　　　　　　　Date

With the exception of restrictions protecting certain confidential information, the results of this survey may be publically released.

Thank you for your cooperation in completing this survey. If there are any questions about your responses to this survey, who should be contacted?

		( )
Name (please print)	Title	(Area Code) Telephone Number

___/___/___		( )
Date of Completion	Chief Executive Officer	Hospital's Main Fax Number

Contact Email address: _____

NOTE: PLEASE PHOTOCOPY THE INFORMATION FOR YOUR HOSPITAL FILE BEFORE RETURNING THE ORIGINAL FORM TO THE AMERICAN HOSPITAL ASSOCIATION. ALSO, PLEASE FORWARD A PHOTOCOPY OF THE COMPLETED QUESTIONNAIRE TO YOUR STATE HOSPITAL ASSOCIATION.

THANK YOU

SECTION A
REPORTING PERIOD
Instructions

INSTRUCTIONS AND DEFINITIONS FOR THE 2022 ANNUAL SURVEY OF HOSPITALS.
For purposes of this survey, a hospital is defined as the organization or corporate entity licensed or registered as a hospital by a state to provide diagnostic and therapeutic patient services for a variety of medical conditions, both surgical and nonsurgical.

1. **Reporting period used (beginning and ending date**): Record the beginning and ending dates of the reporting period in an eight-digit number: for example, January 1, 2022 should be shown as 01/01/2022. Number of days should equal the time span between the two dates that the hospital was open. If you are reporting for less than 365 days, utilization and finances should be presented for days reported only.
2. **Were you in operation 12 full months at the end of your reporting period?** If you are reporting for less than 365 days, utilization and finances should be presented for days reported only.
3. **Number of days open during reporting period:** Number of days should equal the time span between the two dates that the hospital was open.

SECTION B
ORGANIZATIONAL STRUCTURE
Instructions and Definitions

1. **CONTROL**
   Check the box to the left of the type of organization that is responsible for establishing policy for overall operation of the hospital.
   Government, nonfederal.
   State. Controlled by an agency of state government.
   County. Controlled by an agency of county government.
   City. Controlled by an agency of municipal government.
   City-County. Controlled jointly by agencies of municipal and county governments.
   Hospital district or authority. Controlled by a political subdivision of a state, county, or city created solely for the purpose of establishing and maintaining medical care or health-related care institutions.
   Nongovernment, not for profit. Controlled by not-for-profit organizations, including religious organizations (Catholic hospitals, for example), community hospitals, cooperative hospitals, hospitals operated by fraternal societies, and so forth.
   Investor owned, for profit. Controlled on a for profit basis by an individual, partnership, or a profit making corporation.
   Government, federal. Controlled by an agency or department of the federal government.

2. **SERVICE**
   Indicate the ONE category that best describes the type of service that your hospital provides to the majority of patients.
   General medical and surgical. Provides diagnostic and therapeutic services to patients for a variety of medical conditions, both surgical and nonsurgical.
   Hospital unit of an institution. Provides diagnostic and therapeutic services to patients in an institution.
   Hospital unit within a facility for persons with intellectual disabilities. Provides diagnostic and therapeutic services to persons with intellectual disabilities.
   Surgical. An acute care specialty hospital where 2/3 or more of its inpatient claims are for surgical/diagnosis related groups.
   Psychiatric. Provides diagnostic and therapeutic services to patients with mental or emotional disorders.
   Tuberculosis and other respiratory diseases. Provides medical care and rehabilitative services to patients for whom the primary diagnosis is tuberculosis or other respiratory diseases.
   Cancer. Provides medical care to patients for whom the primary diagnosis is cancer.
   Heart. Provides diagnosis and treatment of heart disease.
   Obstetrics and gynecology. Provides medical and surgical treatment to pregnant women and to mothers following delivery. Also provides diagnostic and therapeutic services to women with diseases or disorders of the reproductive organs.
   Eye, ear, nose, and throat. Provides diagnosis and treatment of diseases and injuries of the eyes, ears, nose, and throat.
   Rehabilitation. Provides a comprehensive array of restoration services for people with disabilities and all support services necessary to help them attain their maximum functional capacity.
   Orthopedic. Provides corrective treatment of deformities, diseases, and ailments of the locomotive apparatus, especially affecting the limbs, bones, muscles, and joints.
   Chronic disease. Provides medical and skilled nursing services to patients with long-term illnesses who are not in an acute phase, but who require an intensity of services not available in nursing homes.
   Intellectual disabilities. Provides health-related care on a regular basis to patients with developmental or intellectual disabilities who cannot be treated in a skilled nursing unit.
   Acute long-term care hospital. Provides high acuity interdisciplinary services to medically complex patients that require more intensive recuperation and care than can be provided in a typical nursing facility.
   Substance use disorder. Provides diagnostic and therapeutic services to patients with a medical illness characterized by clinically significant impairments in health, social function, and voluntary control over use of substances such as alcohol, prescription and non-prescription drugs. Substance use disorders range in severity, duration and complexity from mild to severe.

3. **OTHER**
   a. **Children admissions.** A hospital whose primary focus is the health and treatment of children and adolescents.
   b. **Subsidiary.** A company that is wholly controlled by another or one that is more than 50% owned by another organization.
   c. **Contract managed.** General day-to-day management of an entire organization by another organization under a formal contract. Managing organization reports directly to the board of trustees or owners of the managed organization; managed organization retains total legal responsibility and ownership of the facility's assets and liabilities.
   d. **Physician group.** Cooperative practice of medicine by a group of physicians, each of whom as a rule specializes in some particular field.
   f. **Co-located hospitals.** Co-location refers to two or more entities, with separate CMS Certification Numbers occupying the same building, or conjoined buildings.

244 AHA Hospital Statistics © 2024 Health Forum LLC, an affiliate of the American Hospital Association

SECTION C
FACILITIES AND SERVICES
Definitions

Owned/provided by the hospital or its subsidiary. All patient revenues, expenses and utilization related to the provision of the service are reflected in the hospital's statistics reported elsewhere in this survey.

Provided by my health system (in my local community). Another health care provider in the same system as your hospital provides the service and patient revenue, expenses, and utilization related to the provision of the service are recorded at the point where the service was provided and would not be reflected in your hospital's statistics reported elsewhere in this survey. (A system is a corporate body that owns, leases, religiously sponsors and/or manages health providers)

Provided through a partnership or joint venture with another provider that is not in my system. All patient revenues and utilization related to the provision of the service are recorded at the site where the service was provided and would not be reflected in your hospital statistics reported elsewhere in this survey. (A joint venture is a contractual arrangement between two or more parties forming an unincorporated business. The participants in the arrangement remain independent and separate outside of the venture's purpose.)

1. **General medical-surgical care.** Provides acute care to patients in medical and surgical units on the basis of physicians' orders and approved nursing care plans.
2. **Pediatric medical-surgical care.** Provides acute care to pediatric patients on the basis of physicians' orders and approved nursing care plans.
3. **Obstetrics.** For service owned or provided by the hospital, level should be designated: (1) unit provides services for uncomplicated maternity and newborn cases; (2) unit provides services for uncomplicated cases, the majority of complicated problems, and special neonatal services; and (3) unit provides services for all serious illnesses and abnormalities and is supervised by a full-time maternal/fetal specialist.
4. **Medical-surgical intensive care.** Provides patient care of a more intensive nature than the usual medical and surgical care, on the basis of physicians' orders and approved nursing care plans. These units are staffed with specially trained nursing personnel and contain monitoring and specialized support equipment for patients who because of shock, trauma or other life-threatening conditions require intensified comprehensive observation and care. Includes mixed intensive care units.
5. **Cardiac intensive care.** Provides patient care of a more specialized nature than the usual medical and surgical care, on the basis of physicians' orders and approved nursing care plans. The unit is staffed with specially trained nursing personnel and contains monitoring and specialized support or treatment equipment for patients who, because of heart seizure, open-heart surgery, or other life-threatening conditions, require intensified, comprehensive observation and care. May include myocardial infarction, pulmonary care, and heart transplant units.
6. **Neonatal intensive care.** A unit that must be separate from the newborn nursery providing intensive care to all sick infants including those with the very lowest birth weights (less than 1500 grams). NICU has potential for providing mechanical ventilation, neonatal surgery, and special care for the sickest infants born in the hospital or transferred from another institution. A full-time neonatologist serves as director of the NICU.
7. **Neonatal intermediate care.** A unit that must be separate from the normal newborn nursery and that provides intermediate and/or recovery care and some specialized services, including immediate resuscitation, intravenous therapy, and capacity for prolonged oxygen therapy and monitoring.
8. **Pediatric intensive care.** Provides care to pediatric patients that is of a more intensive nature than that usually provided to pediatric patients. The unit is staffed with specially trained personnel and contains monitoring and specialized support equipment for treatment of patients who, because of shock, trauma, or other life-threatening conditions, require intensified, comprehensive observation and care.
9. **Burn care.** Provides care to severely burned patients. Severely burned patients are those with any of the following: (1) second-degree burns of more than 25% total body surface area for adults or 20% total body surface area for children: (2) third-degree burns of more than 10% total body surface area; (3) any severe burns of the hands, face, eyes, ears, or feet; or (4) all inhalation injuries, electrical burns, complicated burn injuries involving fractures and other major traumas, and all other poor risk factors.
10. **Other special care.** Provides care to patients requiring care more intensive than that provided in the acute area, yet not sufficiently intensive to require admission to an intensive care unit. Patients admitted to this area are usually transferred here from an intensive care unit once their condition has improved. These units are sometimes referred to as definitive observation, step-down or progressive care units.
11. **Other intensive care.** A specially staffed, specialty equipped, separate section of a hospital dedicated to the observation, care, and treatment of patients with life-threatening illnesses, injuries, or complications from which recovery is possible. It provides special expertise and facilities for the support of vital function and utilizes the skill of medical nursing and other staff experienced in the management of these problems.
12. **Physical rehabilitation.** Provides care encompassing a comprehensive array of restoration services for people with disabilities and all support services necessary to help patients attain their maximum functional capacity.
13. **Substance use disorder care.** Provides diagnostic and therapeutic services to patients with a medical illness characterized by clinically significant impairments in health, social function, and voluntary control over use of substances such as alcohol, prescription and non-prescription drugs Substance use disorders range in severity, duration and complexity from mild to severe. Includes care for inpatient/residential treatment for patients whose course of treatment involves more intensive care than provided in an outpatient setting or where patient requires supervised withdrawal.
14. **Psychiatric care.** Provides acute or long-term care to patients with mental or emotional disorders, including patients admitted for diagnosis and those admitted for treatment of psychiatric disorders, on the basis of physicians' orders and approved nursing care plans. Long-term care may include intensive supervision to persons with chronic/severe mental illness.
15. **Skilled nursing care.** Provides non-acute medical and skilled nursing care services, therapy, and social services under the supervision of a licensed registered nurse on a 24-hour basis.
16. **Intermediate nursing care.** Provides health-related services (skilled nursing care and social services) to residents with a variety of physical conditions or functional disabilities. These residents do not require the care provided by a hospital or skilled nursing facility, but do need supervision and support services.
17. **Acute long-term care.** Provides specialized acute hospital care to medically complex patients who are critically ill, have multisystem complications and/or failure, and require hospitalization averaging 25 days, in a facility offering specialized treatment programs and therapeutic intervention on a 24-hour/7 days a week basis.
18. **Other long-term care.** Provision of long-term care other than skilled nursing care or intermediate care for those who do not require daily medical or nursing services, but may requires some assistance in the activities of daily living. This can include residential care, elderly care, or care facilities for those with developmental or intellectual disabilities
19. **Biocontainment patient care unit.** A permanent unit that provides the first line of treatment for people affected by bio-terrorism or highly hazardous communicable diseases. The unit is equipped to safely care for anyone exposed to a highly contagious and dangerous disease. Please do not report temporary COVID-19 units on this line.
20. **Other care.** (specify) Any type of care other than those listed above.
    The sum of the beds reported in Section C 1-20 should equal what you have reported in Section E(1b) for beds set up and staffed.
21. **Adult day care program.** Program providing supervision, medical and psychological care, and social activities for older adults who live at home or in another family setting, but cannot be alone or prefer to be with others during the day. May include intake assessment, health monitoring, occupational therapy, personal care, noon meal, and transportation services.

AHA Hospital Statistics © 2024 Health Forum LLC, an affiliate of the American Hospital Association **245**

22. **Airborne infection isolation room.** A single-occupancy room for patient care where environmental factors are controlled in an effort to minimize the transmission of those infectious agents, usually spread person to person by droplet nuclei associated with coughing and inhalation. Such rooms typically have specific ventilation requirements for controlled ventilation, air pressure and filtration.
23. **Alzheimer center.** Facility that offers care to persons with Alzheimer's disease and their families through an integrated program of clinical services, research, and education.
24. **Ambulance services.** Provision of ambulance service to the ill and injured who require medical attention on a scheduled and unscheduled basis.
25. **Air ambulance services.** Aircraft and especially a helicopter equipped for transporting the injured or sick. Most air ambulances carry critically ill or injured patients, whose condition could rapidly change for the worse.
26. **Ambulatory surgery center.** Facility that provides care to patients requiring surgery that are admitted and discharged on the same day. Ambulatory surgery centers are distinct from same day surgical units within the hospital outpatient departments for purposes of Medicare payment.
27. **Arthritis treatment center.** Specifically equipped and staffed center for the diagnosis and treatment of arthritis and other joint disorders.
28. **Auxiliary.** A volunteer community organization formed to assist the hospital in carrying out its purpose and to serve as a link between the institution and the community.
29. **Bariatric/weight control services.** The medical practice of weight reduction.
30. **Birthing room/LDR room/LDRP room.** A single-room type of maternity care with a more homelike setting for families than the traditional three-room unit (labor/delivery/recovery) with a separate postpartum area. A birthing room combines labor and delivery in one room. An LDR room accommodates three stages in the birthing process--labor, delivery, and recovery. An LDRP room accommodates all four stages of the birth process--labor, delivery, recovery, and postpartum.
31. **Blood donor center.** A facility that performs, or is responsible for the collection, processing, testing or distribution of blood and components.
32. **Breast cancer screening/mammograms.** Mammography screening - The use of breast x-ray to detect unsuspected breast cancer in asymptomatic women. Diagnostic mammography - The x-ray imaging of breast tissue in symptomatic women who are considered to have a substantial likelihood of having breast cancer already.
33. **Cardiology and cardiac surgery services.** Services which include the diagnosis and treatment of diseases and disorders involving the heart and circulatory system.
    a. -b. **Cardiology services.** An organized clinical service offering diagnostic and interventional procedures to manage the full range of heart conditions.
    c. -d. **Diagnostic catheterization.** (Also called coronary angiography or coronary arteriography) is used to assist in diagnosing complex heart conditions. Cardiac angiography involves the insertion of a tiny catheter into the artery in the groin then carefully threading the catheter up into the aorta where the coronary arteries originate. Once the catheter is in place, a dye is injected which allows the cardiologist to see the size, shape, and distribution of the coronary arteries. These images are used to diagnose heart disease and to determine, among other things, whether or not surgery is indicated.
    e. -f. **Interventional cardiac catheterization.** Nonsurgical procedure that utilizes the same basic principles as diagnostic catheterization and then uses advanced techniques to improve the heart's function. It can be a less invasive alternative to heart surgery.
    g. -h. **Cardiac surgery.** Includes minimally invasive procedures that include surgery done with only a small incision or no incision at all, such as through a laparoscope or an endoscope and more invasive major surgical procedures that include open chest and open heart surgery.
    i. -j. **Cardiac electrophysiology.** Evaluation and management of patients with complex rhythm or conduction abnormalities, including diagnostic testing, treatment of arrhythmias by catheter ablation or drug therapy, and pacemaker/defibrillator implantation and follow-up.
    k. **Cardiac rehabilitation.** A medically supervised program to help heart patients recover quickly and improve their overall physical and mental functioning. The goal is to reduce risk of another cardiac event or to keep an already present heart condition from getting worse. Cardiac rehabilitation programs include: counseling to patients, an exercise program, helping patients modify risk factors such as smoking and high blood pressure, providing vocational guidance to enable the patient to return to work, supplying information on physical limitations and lending emotional support.
34. **Case management.** A system of assessment, treatment planning, referral and follow-up that ensures the provision of comprehensive and continuous services and the coordination of payment and reimbursement for care.
35. **Chaplaincy/pastoral care services.** A service ministering religious activities and providing pastoral counseling to patients, their families, and staff of a health care organization.
36. **Chemotherapy.** An organized program for the treatment of cancer by the use of drugs or chemicals.
37. **Children's wellness program.** A program that encourages improved health status and a healthful lifestyle of children through health education, exercise, nutrition and health promotion.
38. **Chiropractic services.** An organized clinical service including spinal manipulation or adjustment and related diagnostic and therapeutic services.
39. **Community outreach.** A program that systematically interacts with the community to identify those in need of services, alerting persons and their families to the availability of services, locating needed services, and enabling persons to enter the service delivery system.
40. **Complementary and alternative medicine services.** Organized hospital services or formal arrangements to providers that provide care or treatment not based solely on traditional western allopathic medical teachings as instructed in most U.S. medical schools. Includes any of the following: acupuncture, chiropractic, homeopathy, osteopathy, diet and lifestyle changes, herbal medicine, massage therapy, etc.
41. **Computer assisted orthopedic surgery (CAOS).** Orthopedic surgery using computer technology, enabling three-dimensional graphic models to visualize a patient's anatomy.
42. **Crisis prevention.** Services provided in order to promote physical and mental wellbeing and the early identification of disease and ill health prior to the onset and recognition of symptoms so as to permit early treatment.
43. **Dental services.** An organized dental service or dentists on staff, not necessarily involving special facilities, providing dental or oral services to inpatients or outpatients.
44. **Diabetes prevention program.** Program to prevent or delay the onset of type 2 diabetes by offering evidence-based lifestyle changes based on research studies, which showed modest behavior changes helped individuals with prediabetes reduce their risk of developing type 2 diabetes.
45. **Emergency services.** Health services that are provided after the onset of a medical condition that manifests itself by symptoms of sufficient severity, including severe pain, that the absence of immediate medical attention could reasonably be expected by a prudent layperson, who possesses an average knowledge of health and medicine, to result in placing the patient's health in serious jeopardy.
    a. **On-campus emergency department.** Hospital facilities for the provision of unscheduled outpatient services to patients whose conditions require immediate care.
    b. **Off-campus emergency department.** A facility owned and operated by the hospital but physically separate from the hospital for the provision of unscheduled outpatient services to patients whose conditions require immediate care. A freestanding ED is not physically connected to a hospital but has all the necessary emergency staffing and equipment on site.
    c. **Pediatric emergency department.** A recognized hospital emergency department capable of identifying those pediatric patients who are critically ill or injured, stabilizing pediatric patients, including the management of airway, breathing and circulation and providing an appropriate transfer to a definitive care facility.

246 AHA Hospital Statistics © 2024 Health Forum LLC, an affiliate of the American Hospital Association

d–e. Trauma Center. A facility to provide emergency and specialized intensive care to critically ill and injured patients. For the facility to be provided by the hospital, it must be located in your hospital. In addition, the utilization, expense, and revenue from the provision of trauma services must be reported in Section E of the survey. For the service owned or provided by the hospital, please specify the trauma center level. "Level 1 A regional resource trauma center, which is capable of providing total care for every aspect of injury and plays a leadership role in trauma research and education. Level 2: A community trauma center, which is capable of providing trauma care to all but the most severely injured patients who require highly specialized care. Level 3: A rural trauma hospital, which is capable of providing care to a large number of injury victims and can resuscitate and stabilize more severely injured patients so that they can be transported to level 1 or 2 facilities.

46. **Enabling services.** A program that is designed to help the patient access health care services by offering any of the following: transportation services and/or referrals to local social services agencies.

47. **Endoscopic services.**
    a. **Optical colonoscopy.** An examination of the interior of the colon using a long, flexible, lighted tube with a small built-in camera.
    b. **Endoscopic ultrasound.** Specially designed endoscope that incorporates an ultrasound transducer used to obtain detailed images of organs in the chest and abdomen. The endoscope can be passed through the mouth or the anus. When combined with needle biopsy the procedure can assist in diagnosis of disease and staging of cancer.
    c. **Ablation of Barrett's esophagus.** Premalignant condition that can lead to adenocarcinoma of the esophagus. The nonsurgical ablation of premalignant tissue in Barrett's esophagus by the application of thermal energy or light through an endoscope passed from the mouth into the esophagus.
    d. **Esophageal impedance study.** A test in which a catheter is placed through the nose into the esophagus to measure whether gas or liquids are passing from the stomach into the esophagus and causing symptoms.
    e. **Endoscopic retrograde cholangiopancreatography (ERCP).** A procedure in which a catheter is introduced through an endoscope into the bile ducts and pancreatic ducts. Injection of contrast material permits detailed x-ray of these structures. The procedure is used diagnostically as well as therapeutically to relieve obstruction or remove stones.

48. **Enrollment (insurance) assistance services.** A program that provides enrollment assistance for patients who are potentially eligible for public health insurance programs such as Medicaid, State Children's Health Insurance, or local/state indigent care programs. The specific services offered could include explanation of benefits, assist applicants in completing the application and locating all relevant documents, conduct eligibility interviews, and/or forward applications and documentation to state/local social service or health agency.

49. **Employment support services.** Services designed to support individuals with significant disabilities to seek and maintain employment.

50. **Extracorporeal shock wave lithotripter (ESWL).** A medical device used for treating stones in the kidney or urethra. The device disintegrates kidney stones noninvasively through the transmission of acoustic shock waves directed at the stones.

51. **Fertility clinic.** A specialized program set in an infertility center that provides counseling and education as well as advanced reproductive techniques such as: injectable therapy, reproductive surgeries, treatment for endometriosis, male factor infertility, tubal reversals, in vitro fertilization (IVF), donor eggs, and other such services to help patients achieve successful pregnancies.

52. **Fitness center.** Provides exercise, testing, or evaluation programs and fitness activities to the community and hospital employees.

53. **Freestanding outpatient care center.** A facility owned and operated by the hospital that is physically separate from the hospital and provides various medical treatments and diagnostic services on an outpatient basis only. Laboratory and radiology services are usually available.

54. **Geriatric services.** The branch of medicine dealing with the physiology of aging and the diagnosis and treatment of disease affecting the aged. Services could include: adult day care; Alzheimer's diagnostic-assessment services; comprehensive geriatric assessment; emergency response system; geriatric acute care unit; and/or geriatric clinics.

55. **Health fair.** Community health education events that focus on the prevention of disease and promotion of health through such activities as audiovisual exhibits and free diagnostic services.

56. **Community health education.** Education that provides health information to individuals and populations as well as support for personal, family and community health decisions with the objective of improving health status.

57. **Genetic testing/counseling.** A service equipped with adequate laboratory facilities and directed by a qualified physician to advise patients on potential genetic diagnosis of vulnerabilities to inherited diseases. A genetic test is the analysis of human DNA, RNA, chromosomes, proteins, and certain metabolites in order to detect heritable disease-related genotypes, mutations, phenotypes, or karyotypes for clinical purposes. Genetic tests can have diverse purposes, including the diagnosis of genetic diseases in newborns, children, and adults; the identification of future health risks; the prediction of drug responses; and the assessment of risks to future children.

58. **Health screening.** A preliminary procedure such as a test or examination to detect the most characteristic sign or signs of a disorder that may require further investigation.

59. **Health research.** Organized hospital research program in any of the following areas: basic research, clinical research, community health research, and/or research on innovative health care delivery.

60. **Hemodialysis.** Provision of equipment and personnel for the treatment of renal insufficiency on an inpatient or outpatient basis.

61. **HIV/AIDS services.** Diagnosis, treatment, continuing care planning, and counseling services for HIV/AIDS patients and their families. Could include: HIV/AIDS unit, special unit or designated team, general inpatient care, or specialized outpatient program.

62. **Home health services.** Service providing nursing, therapy, and health-related homemaker or social services in the patient's home.

63. **Hospice.** A program providing palliative care, chiefly medical relief of pain and supportive services, addressing the emotional, social, financial, and legal needs of terminally ill patients and their families. Care can be provided in a variety of settings, both inpatient and at home.

64. **Hospital-based outpatient care center-services.** Organized hospital health care services offered by appointment on an ambulatory basis. Services may include outpatient surgery, examination, diagnosis, and treatment of a variety of medical conditions on a nonemergency basis, and laboratory and other diagnostic testing as ordered by staff or outside physician referral.

65. **Housing Services**
    a. **Assisted living.** A special combination of housing, supportive services, personalized assistance and health care designed to respond to the individual needs of those who need help in activities of daily living and instrumental activities of daily living. Supportive services are available, 24 hours a day, to meet scheduled and unscheduled needs, in a way that promotes maximum independence and dignity for each resident and encourages the involvement of a resident's family, neighbor and friends.
    b. **Retirement housing.** A facility that provides social activities to senior citizens, usually retired persons, who do not require health care but some short-term skilled nursing care may be provided. A retirement center may furnish housing and may also have acute hospital and long-term care facilities, or it may arrange for acute and long-term care through affiliated institutions.
    c. **Supportive housing services.** A hospital program that provides decent, safe, affordable, community-based housing with flexible support services designed to help the individual or family stay housed and live a more productive life in the community.

66. **Immunization program.** Program that plans, coordinates and conducts immunization services in the community.

67. **Indigent care clinic.** Health care services for uninsured and underinsured persons where care is free of charge or charged on a sliding scale. This would include "free clinics" staffed by volunteer practitioners, but could also be staffed by employees with the sponsoring health care organization subsidizing the cost of service.

68. **Linguistic/translation services.** Services provided by the hospital designed to make health care more accessible to non-English speaking patients and their physicians.

AHA Hospital Statistics © 2024 Health Forum LLC, an affiliate of the American Hospital Association **247**

69. **Meal delivery services.** A hospital sponsored program which delivers meals to people, usually the elderly, who are unable to prepare their own meals. Low cost, nutritional meals are delivered to individuals' homes on a regular basis.
70. **Mobile health services.** Vans and other vehicles used for delivery of primary care services.
71. **Neurological services.** Services provided by the hospital dealing with the operative and nonoperative management of disorders of the central, peripheral, and autonomic nervous systems.
72. **Nutrition programs.** Services within a health care facility which are designed to provide inexpensive, nutritionally sound meals to patients.
73. **Occupational health services.** Includes services designed to protect the safety of employees from hazards in the work environment.
74. **Oncology services.** Inpatient and outpatient services for patients with cancer, including comprehensive care, support and guidance in addition to patient education and prevention, chemotherapy, counseling and other treatment methods.
75. **Orthopedic services.** Services provided for the prevention or correction of injuries or disorders of the skeletal system and associated muscles, joints and ligaments.
76. **Outpatient surgery.** Scheduled surgical services provided to patients who do not remain in the hospital overnight. The surgery may be performed in operating suites also used for inpatient surgery, specially designated surgical suites for outpatient surgery, or procedure rooms within an outpatient care facility.
77. **Pain management program.** A recognized clinical service or program providing specialized medical care, drugs or therapies for the management of acute or chronic pain and other distressing symptoms, administered by specially trained physicians and other clinicians, to patients suffering from acute illnesses of diverse causes.
78. **Palliative care program.** An organized program providing specialized medical care, drugs or therapies for the management of acute or chronic pain and/or the control of symptoms administered by specially trained physicians and other clinicians; and supportive care services, such as counseling on advanced directives, spiritual care, and social services, to patients with advanced diseases and their families.
79. **Palliative care inpatient unit.** An inpatient palliative care ward is a physically discreet, inpatient nursing unit where the focus is palliative care. The patient care focus is on symptom relief for complex patients who may be continuing to undergo primary treatment. Care is delivered by palliative medicine specialists.
80. **Patient controlled analgesia (PCA).** Intravenously administered pain medicine under the patient's control. The patient has a button on the end of a cord than can be pushed at will, whenever more pain medicine is desired. This button will only deliver more pain medicine at predetermined intervals, as programmed by the doctor's order.
81. **Patient education center.** Written goals and objectives for the patient and/or family related to therapeutic regimens, medical procedures, and self-care.
82. **Patient representative services.** Organized hospital services providing personnel through whom patients and staff can seek solutions to institutional problems affecting the delivery of high quality care and services.
83. **Physical rehabilitation services.** Program providing medical, health-related, therapy, social, and/or vocational services to help people with disabilities attain or retain their maximum functional capacity.
    a. **Assistive technology center.** A program providing access to specialized hardware and software with adaptations allowing individuals greater independence with mobility, dexterity, or increased communication options.
    b. **Electrodiagnostic services.** Diagnostic testing services for nerve and muscle function such as nerve conduction studies and needle electromyography.
    c. **Physical rehabilitation outpatient services.** Outpatient program providing medical, health-related, therapy, social, and/or vocational services to help people with disabilities attain or retain their maximum functional capacity.
    d. **Prosthetic and orthotic services.** Services providing comprehensive prosthetic and orthotic evaluation, fitting, and training.
    e. **Robot-assisted walking therapy.** A form of physical therapy that uses a robotic device to assist patients who are relearning how to walk.
    f. **Simulated rehabilitation environment.** Rehabilitation focused on retraining functional skills in a contextually appropriate environment (simulated home and community settings) or in a traditional setting (gymnasium) using motor learning principles.
84. **Primary care department.** A unit or clinic within the hospital that provides primary care services (e.g., general pediatric care, general internal medicine, family practice, gynecology) through hospital-salaried medical and/or nursing staff, focusing on evaluating and diagnosing medical problems and providing medical treatment on an outpatient basis.
85. **Psychiatric services.** Services provided by the hospital that offer immediate initial evaluation and treatment to patients with mental or emotional disorders.
    a. **Psychiatric consultation-liaison services.** Provides organized psychiatric consultation/liaison services to nonpsychiatric hospital staff and/or departments on psychological aspects of medical care that may be generic or specific to individual patients. Consultation-liaison psychiatrists work to help people suffering from a combination of mental and physical illness by consulting with them and liaising with other members of their care team.
    b. **Psychiatric pediatric services.** The branch of medicine focused on the diagnosis, treatment and prevention of mental, emotional and behavioral disorders in pediatric patients. Please report the number of staffed beds. The beds reported here should be included in the staffed bed count for 14 psychiatric care.
    c. **Psychiatric geriatric services.** Provides care to elderly patients with mental or emotional disorders, including those admitted for diagnosis and those admitted for treatment. Please report the number of staffed beds. The beds reported here should be included in the staffed bed count for 14 psychiatric care.
    d. **Psychiatric education services.** Provides psychiatric educational services to community agencies and workers such as schools, police, courts, public health nurses, welfare agencies, clergy, and so forth. The purpose is to expand the mental health knowledge and competence of personnel not working in the mental health field and to promote good mental health through improved understanding, attitudes, and behavioral patterns.
    e. **Psychiatric emergency services.** Services of facilities available on a 24-hour basis to provide immediate unscheduled outpatient care, diagnosis, evaluation, crisis intervention, and assistance to persons suffering acute emotional or mental distress.
    f. **Psychiatric outpatient services.** Provides medical care, including diagnosis and treatment, of psychiatric outpatients.
    g. **Psychiatric intensive outpatient services.** A prescribed course of treatment in which the patient receives outpatient care no less than three times a week (which might include more than one service/day)
    h. **Social and community psychiatric services.** Social psychiatry deals with social factors associated with psychiatric morbidity, social effects of mental illness, psycho-social disorders and social approaches to psychiatric care. Community psychiatry focuses on detection, prevention, early treatment and rehabilitation of emotional and behavioral disorders as they develop in a community.
    i. **Forensic psychiatric services.** A medical subspecialty that includes research and clinical practice in many areas in which psychiatric is applied to legal issues.
    j. **Prenatal and postpartum psychiatric services.** Psychiatric care during and post-pregnancy. Includes perinatal depression and postpartum depression.
    k. l. **Psychiatric partial hospitalization program – adult/pediatric.** Organized hospital services providing intensive day/evening outpatient services of three hours or more duration, distinguished from other outpatient visits of one hour.
    m. n. **Psychiatric residential treatment – adult/pediatric.** Overnight psychiatric care in conjunction with an intensive treatment program in a setting other than a hospital.

o. **Suicide prevention services.** A collection of efforts to reduce the risk of suicide. These efforts may occur at the individual, relationship, community and society levels.

86. **Radiology, diagnostic.** The branch of radiology that deals with the utilization of all modalities of radiant energy in medical diagnoses and therapeutic procedures using radiologic guidance. This includes, but is not restricted to, imaging techniques and methodologies utilizing radiation emitted by x-ray tubes, radionuclides, and ultrasonographic devices and the radiofrequency electromagnetic radiation emitted by atoms.

   a. **CT Scanner.** Computed tomographic scanner for head or whole body scans.

   5. **Diagnostic radioisotope facility.** The use of radioactive isotopes (Radiopharmaceuticals) as tracers or indicators to detect an abnormal condition or disease.

   6. **Electron beam computed tomography (EBCT).** A high tech computed tomography scan used to detect coronary artery disease by measuring coronary calcifications. This imaging procedure uses electron beams which are magnetically steered to produce a visual of the coronary artery and the images are produced faster than conventional CT scans.

   d. **Full-field digital mammography (FFDM).** Combines the x-ray generators and tubes used in analog screen-film mammography (SFM) with a detector plate that converts the x-rays into a digital signal.

   e. **Magnetic resonance imaging (MRI).** The use of a uniform magnetic field and radio frequencies to study tissue and structure of the body. This procedure enables the visualization of biochemical activity of the cell in vivo without the use of ionizing radiation, radioisotopic substances or high-frequency sound.

   f. **Intraoperative magnetic resonance imaging.** An integrated surgery system which provides an MRI system in an operating room. The system allows for immediate evaluation of the degree to tumor resection while the patient is undergoing a surgical resection. Intraoperative MRI exists when a MRI (low-field or high-field) is placed in the operating theater and is used during surgical resection without moving the patient from the operating room to the diagnostic imaging suite.

   g. **Magnetoencephalography (MEG).** A noninvasive neurophysiological measurement tool used to study magnetic fields generated by neuronal activity of the brain. MEG provides direct information about the dynamics of evoked and spontaneous neural activity and its location in the brain. The primary uses of MEG include assisting surgeons in localizing the source of epilepsy, sensory mapping, and the study of brain function. When it is combined with structural imaging, it is known as *magnetic source imaging* (MSI).

   h. **Multi-slice spiral computed tomography (<64+slice CT).** A specialized computed tomography procedure that provides three-dimensional processing and allows narrower and multiple slices with increased spatial resolution and faster scanning times as compared to a regular computed tomography scan.

   i. **Multi-slice spiral computed tomography (64+ slice CT).** Involves the acquisition of volumetric tomographic x-ray absorption data expressed in Hounsfield units using multiple rows of detectors. 64+ systems reconstruct the equivalent of 64 or more slices to cover the imaged volume.

   j. **Positron emission tomography (PET).** A nuclear medicine imaging technology which uses radioactive (positron emitting) isotopes created in a cyclotron or generator and computers to produce composite pictures of the brain and heart at work. PET scanning produces sectional images depicting metabolic activity or blood flow rather than anatomy.

   k. **Positron emission tomography/CT (PET/CT).** Provides metabolic functional information for the monitoring of chemotherapy, radiotherapy and surgical planning.

   l. **Single photon emission computerized tomography (SPECT).** A nuclear medicine imaging technology that combines existing technology of gamma camera imaging with computed tomographic imaging technology to provide a clearer and more precise image.

   m.**Ultrasound.** The use of acoustic waves above the range of 20,000 cycles per second to visualize internal body structures.

87. **Radiology, therapeutic.** The branch of medicine concerned with radioactive substances and using various techniques of visualization, with the diagnosis and treatment of disease using any of the various sources of radiant energy. Services could include: megavoltage radiation therapy; radioactive implants; stereotactic radiosurgery; therapeutic radioisotope facility; X-ray radiation therapy.

   a. **Image-guided radiation therapy (IGRT).** Automated system for image-guided radiation therapy that enables clinicians to obtain high-resolution x-ray images to pinpoint tumor sites, adjust patient positioning when necessary, and complete a treatment, all within the standard treatment time slot, allowing for more effective cancer treatments.

   b. **Intensity-Modulated Radiation Therapy (IMRT).** A type of three-dimensional radiation therapy which improves treatment delivery by targeting a tumor in a way that is likely to decrease damage to normal tissues and allows for varying intensities.

   c. **Proton beam therapy.** A form of radiation therapy which administers proton beams. While producing the same biologic effects as x-ray beams, the energy distribution of protons differs from conventional x-ray beams: proton beams can be more precisely focused in tissue volumes in a three-dimensional pattern, resulting in less surrounding tissue damage than conventional radiation therapy, permitting administration of higher doses.

   d. **Shaped beam radiation system.** A precise, noninvasive treatment that involves targeted beams of radiation that mirror the exact size and shape of a tumor at a specific area to shrink or destroy cancerous cells. This procedure delivers a therapeutic dose of radiation that conforms precisely to the shape of the tumor, thus minimizing the risk to nearby tissues.

   e. **Stereotactic radiosurgery.** A radiotherapy modality that delivers a high dosage of radiation to a discrete treatment area in as few as one treatment session. Includes Gamma Knife, Cyberknife, etc.

   f. **Basic interventional radiology.** Therapies include embolization, angioplasty, stent placement, thrombus management, drainage and ablation among others. Facilities providing interventional radiology should have a radiologist with additional certification and training in diagnostic radiology, interventional radiology, or radiation oncology.

88. **Robotic surgery.** The use of mechanical guidance devices to remotely manipulate surgical instrumentation.

89. **Rural health clinic.** A clinic located in a rural, medically under-served area in the United States that has a separate reimbursement structure from the standard medical office under the Medicare and Medicaid programs.

90. **Sleep center.** Specially equipped and staffed center for the diagnosis and treatment of sleep disorders.

91. **Social work services.** Could include: organized services that are properly directed and sufficiently staffed by qualified individuals who provide assistance and counseling to patients and their families in dealing with social, emotional, and environmental problems associated with illness or disability, often in the context of financial or discharge planning coordination.

92. **Sports medicine.** Provision of diagnostic screening, assessment, clinical and rehabilitation services for the prevention and treatment of sports-related injuries.

93. **Substance use disorder services.**

   a. **Substance use disorder – pediatric services.** Provides diagnostic and therapeutic services to pediatric patients with alcoholism or other drug dependencies. Includes care for inpatient/residential treatment for patients whose course of treatment involves more intensive care that provided in an outpatient setting or where patients require supervised withdrawal. Please report staffed beds. The beds reported here should be included in the staffed bed count for 13 substance use disorder care.

   b. **Substance use disorder outpatient.** Organized hospital services that provide medical care and/or rehabilitative treatment services to outpatients for whom the primary diagnosis is alcoholism or other chemical dependency.

   c. **Substance use disorder partial hospitalization services.** Organized hospital services providing intensive day/evening outpatient services of three hour or more duration, distinguished from other outpatient visits of one hour

   d. **Medication assisted treatment for Opioid Use Disorder.** Medication assisted treatment (MAT) is the use of medications, in combination with counseling and behavioral therapies, to provide a "whole-patient" approach to the treatment of substance use disorders. Medications used in MAT are approved by the Food and Drug Administration (FDA) and MAT programs are clinically driven and tailed to meet each patient's needs.

AHA Hospital Statistics © 2024 Health Forum LLC, an affiliate of the American Hospital Association **249**

e. **Medication assisted treatment for other substance use disorders.** Medication assisted treatment (MAT) is the use of medications, in combination with counseling and behavioral therapies, to provide a "whole-patient" approach to the treatment of substance use disorders. Medications used in MAT are approved by the Food and Drug Administration (FDA) and MAT programs are clinically driven and tailed to meet each patient's needs.

94. **Support groups.** A hospital sponsored program that allows a group of individuals with common experiences or issues who meet periodically to share experiences, problems, and solutions in order to support each other.

95. **Swing bed services.** A hospital bed that can be used to provide either acute or long-term care depending on community or patient needs. To be eligible a hospital must have a Medicare provider agreement in place, have fewer than 100 beds, be located in a rural area, not have a 24-hour nursing service waiver in effect, have not been terminated from the program in the prior two years, and meet various service conditions.

96. **Teen outreach services.** A program focusing on the teenager which encourages an improved health status and a healthful lifestyle including physical, emotional, mental, social, spiritual and economic health through education, exercise, nutrition and health promotion.

97. **Tobacco treatment/cessation program.** Organized hospital services with the purpose of ending tobacco-use habits of patients addicted to tobacco/nicotine.

98. **Telehealth.** A broad variety of technologies and tactics to deliver virtual medical, public health, health education delivery and support services using telecommunications technologies. Telehealth is used more commonly as it describes the wide range of diagnosis and management, education, and other related fields of health care. This includes, but are not limited to: dentistry, counseling, physical and occupational therapy, home health, chronic disease monitoring and management, disaster management and consumer and professional education.

    b. **eICU.** An electronic intensive care unit (eICU), also referred to as a tele-ICU, is a form of telemedicine that uses state of the art technology to provide an additional layer of critical care service. The goal of an eICU is to optimize clinical experience and facilitate 24-hour a day care by ICU caregivers.

    c. **Stroke care.** Stroke telemedicine is a consultative modality that facilitates the care of patients with acute stroke by specialists at stroke centers.

    d. **Psychiatric and addiction treatment.** Telepsychiatry can involve a range of services including psychiatric evaluations, therapy, patient education, and medication management.

    e. **Remote patient monitoring.** The use of digital technologies to collect medical and other forms of health data from individuals in one location and electronically transmit the information securely to health care providers in a different location for assessment and recommendation.

99. **Transplant services.** The branch of medicine that transfers an organ or tissue from one person to another or from one body part to another, to replace a diseased structure or to restore function or to change appearance. Services could include: Bone marrow, heart, lung, kidney, intestine, or tissue transplant. <u>Please include heart/lung or other multi-transplant surgeries in 'other'.</u>

100. **Transportation to health facilities. (non-emergency)** A long-term care support service designed to assist the mobility of the elderly. Some programs offer improved financial access by offering reduced rates and barrier-free buses or vans with ramps and lifts to assist the elderly or people with disabilities; others offer subsidies for public transport systems or operate mini-bus services exclusively for use by senior citizens.

101. **Urgent care center.** A facility that provides care and treatment for problems that are not life threatening but require attention over the short term.

102. **Violence Prevention**

    a. **Workplace.** A violence prevention program with goals and objectives for preventing workplace violence against staff and patients.

    b. **Community**. An organized program that attempts to make a positive impact on the type(s) of violence a community is experiencing. For example, it can assist victims of violent crimes, e.g., rape, or incidents, e.g., bullying, to hospital or to community services to prevent further victimization or retaliation. A program that targets the underlying circumstances that contribute to violence such as poor housing, insufficient job training, and/or substance abuse through means such direct involvement and support, education, mentoring, anger management, crisis intervention and training programs would also qualify.

103. **Virtual colonoscopy.** Noninvasive screening procedure used to visualize, analyze and detect cancerous or potentially cancerous polyps in the colon.

104. **Volunteer services department.** An organized hospital department responsible for coordinating the services of volunteers working within the institution.

105. **Women's health center/services.** An area set aside for coordinated education and treatment services specifically for and promoted to women as provided by this special unit. Services may or may not include obstetrics but include a range of services other than OB.

106. **Wound management services**. Services for patients with chronic wounds and nonhealing wounds often resulting from diabetes, poor circulation, improper seating and immunocompromising conditions. The goals are to progress chronic wounds through stages of healing, reduce and eliminate infections, increase physical function to minimize complications from current wounds and prevent future chronic wounds. Wound management services are provided on an inpatient or outpatient basis, depending on the intensity of service needed.

107. **a-b. Consultation-liaison** psychiatrists, medical physicians, or advance practice providers (APPs) work to help people suffering from a combination of mental and physical illness by consulting with them and liaising with other members of their care team.

108a-b. **Physician arrangements.** An integrated healthcare delivery program implementing physician compensation and incentive systems for managed care services. Please report the number of physicians and ownership percentage for each arrangement.

    1. **Independent practice association (IPA).** A legal entity that holds managed care contracts. The IPA then contracts with physicians, usually in solo practice, to provide care either on a fee-for-service or capitated basis. The purpose of an IPA is to assist solo physicians in obtaining managed care contracts.

    2. **Group practice without walls.** Hospital sponsors the formation of, or provides capital to physicians to establish, a "quasi" group to share administrative expenses while remaining independent practitioners.

    3. **Open physician-hospital organization (PHO).** A joint venture between the hospital and all members of the medical staff who wish to participate. The PHO can act as a unified agent in managed care contracting, own a managed care plan, own and operate ambulatory care centers or ancillary services projects, or provide administrative services to physician members.

    4. **Closed physician-hospital organization (PHO).** A PHO that restricts physician membership to those practitioners who meet criteria for cost effectiveness and/or high quality.

    5. **Management services organization (MSO).** A corporation, owned by the hospital or a physician/hospital joint venture, that provides management services to one or more medical group practices. The MSO purchases the tangible assets of the practices and leases them back as part of a full-service management agreement, under which the MSO employs all non-physician staff and provides all supplies/administrative systems for a fee.

    6. **Integrated salary model.** Physicians are salaried by the hospital or another entity of a health system to provide medical services for primary care and specialty care.

    7. **Equity model.** Allows established practitioners to become shareholders in a professional corporation in exchange for tangible and intangible assets of their existing practices.

    8. **Foundation.** A corporation, organized either as a hospital affiliate or subsidiary, which purchases both the tangible and intangible assets of one or more medical group practices. Physicians remain in a separate corporate entity but sign a professional services agreement with the foundation.

109. Of all physician arrangements listed in question 108a. (1-9), indicate the total number of physicians (count each physician only once) that are engaged in an arrangement with your hospital that allows for joint contracting with payers or shared responsibility for financial risk or clinical performance between the hospital and physician (arrangement may be any type of ownership). *Joint contracting* does not include contracting between physicians participating in an independent practice.

110a-d. **Joint venture.** A contractual arrangement between two or more parties forming an unincorporated business. The participants in the arrangement remain independent and separate outside of the venture's purpose.

114. **Ventilators.** Report both transport and regular ventilators. Count non-invasive ventilators that can be converted to invasive ventilators. For ventilators that can be used for both adult and pediatric patients, please report these as adult ventilators; do not report on both lines (i.e., pediatric ventilators can only be used for pediatric patients. The exception is pediatric hospitals – ventilators that can be used for both adult and pediatric patients should be reported on the pediatric lines for these hospitals.)

SECTION D
INSURANCE AND ALTERNATIVE PAYMENT MODELS
Definitions

4. Insurance Products

   a. **Medicare Advantage.** Health Insurance program within Part C of Medicare. Medicare Advantage plans provide a managed health care plan (typically a health maintenance organization (HMO) but also often a preferred provider organization (PPO) or another type of managed care arrangement) that is paid based on a monthly capitated fee. This Part of Medicare provides beneficiaries an alternative to "Original Medicare" Parts A and B Medicare, which provides insurance for the same medical services but pays providers a fee for service (FFS) directly rather than through managed care plans.

   b. **Medicaid Managed Care.** Services in through an arrangement between a state Medicaid agency and managed care organizations (MCOs) that accept a set payment – "capitation" – for these services.

   c. **Health Insurance Marketplace.** Also called health exchanges, are organizations set up to facilitate the purchase of health insurance in each state in accordance with Patient Protection and Affordable Care Act. Marketplaces provide a set of government-regulated and standardized health care plans from which individuals may purchase health insurance policies eligible for federal subsidies.

   d. **Other Individual Market.** Health insurance coverage offered to individuals other than in connection with a group health plan.

   e. **Small Group.** A group health plan that covers employees of an employer that has less than 50 employees.

   f. **Large Group.** A group health plan that covers employees of an employer that has 51 or more employees.

8. Self-administered health plan. A health plan in which the employer assumes the financial risk for providing health care benefits to its employees. The employer may or may not also be responsible for claims processing and the provider network.

9. Capitation. An at-risk payment arrangement in which an organization receives a fixed prearranged payment and in turn guarantees to deliver or arrange all medically necessary care required by enrollees in the capitated plan. The fixed amount is specified within contractual agreements between the payer and the involved organization. The fixed payment amount is based on an actuarial assessment of the services required by enrollees and the costs of providing these services, recognizing enrollees' adjustment factors such as age, sex, and family size.

10-11. Bundling. Bundling is a payment mechanism whereby a provider entity receives a single payment for services provided across one or parts of the care continuum. For example, an entity might receive a single payment for the hospital and physician services provided as part of an inpatient stay or might receive a single payment for the post-acute care services involved in a single episode of care. The entity then has responsibility for compensating each of the individual providers involved in the episode of care.

12. Shared risk payments. A payment arrangement in which a hospital and a managed care organization share the risk of adverse claims experience. Methods for sharing risk could include: capitation with partial refunds or supplements if billed hospital charges or costs differ from capitated payments, and service or discharge-based payments with withholds and bonus payouts that depend on expenditure targets

15. Accountable Care Organization (ACO) Contract. An ACO contract has two essential elements: (1) accountability for the total costs of care for the population of patients attributed to the primary care physicians in the organization; (2) financial incentives that link the magnitude of bonus payments to performance on quality measures (which could include technical quality, patient experience and/or health outcome measures) This will generally involve a contract where the payer establishes a target budget for one or more years for the total costs of care for the agreed-upon patient population, the payer tracks actual spending and performance on quality; and the provider receives bonus payments that could include a share of savings that are (or are not) contingent on meeting quality targets, with (or without) additional bonuses related to performance on those quality measures.

15c. Traditional Medicare ACO Programs

   MSSP. Medicare Shared Savings Program. For fee-for-service beneficiaries. The Shared Savings Program has different tracks that allow ACOs to select an arrangement that makes the most sense for their organization.

   NextGen. The Next Generation ACO Model is an initiative for ACOs that are experienced in coordinating care for populations of patients. It allows these provider groups to assume higher levels of financial risk and reward.

   Comprehensive ESRD Care. The model is designed to identify, test, and evaluate new ways to improve care for Medicare beneficiaries with End-Stage Renal Disease (ESRD.)

18. Patient-Centered Medical Home. The medical home concept refers to the provision of comprehensive primary care services that facilitates communication and shared decision-making between the patient, his/her primary care providers, other providers, and the patient's family.

SECTION E
TOTAL FACILITY BEDS, UTILIZATION, FINANCES, AND STAFFING
Instructions and Definitions

For the purposes of this survey, a nursing home type unit/facility provides **long-term care for the elderly or other patients requiring chronic care** in a non-acute setting in any of the following categories: *Skilled nursing care *Intermediate care *Other long-term care (see page 30) The nursing home type unit/facility is to be owned and operated by the hospital. Only one legal entity may be vested with title to the physical property or operate under the authority of a duly executed lease of the physical property.

a. **Total licensed beds.** Report the total number of beds authorized by the state licensing (certifying) agency.

b. **Beds set up and staffed.** Report the number of beds regularly available (those set up and staffed for use) at the end of the reporting period. Report only operating beds, not constructed bed capacity. Include all bed facilities that are set up and staffed for use by inpatients that have no other bed facilities, such as pediatric bassinets, isolation units and quiet rooms. Exclude newborn bassinets and bed facilities for patients receiving special procedures for a portion of their stay and who have other bed facilities assigned to or reserved for them. Exclude, for example, labor room, post anesthesia, or postoperative recovery room beds, psychiatric holding beds, observation beds, and beds that are used only as holding facilities for patients prior to their transfer to another hospital.

c. **Bassinets set up and staffed.** Report the number of normal newborn bassinets. Do not include neonatal intensive care or intermediate care bassinets. These should be reported on page 3, C6 and C7 and included in E1b. Beds set up and staffed.

d. **Births.** Total births should exclude fetal deaths.

e. **Admissions.** Include the number of adult and pediatric admissions (exclude births). This figure should include all patients admitted during the reporting period, including neonatal and swing admissions.

f. **Inpatient days.** Report the number of adult and pediatric days of care rendered during the entire reporting period. Do not include days of care rendered for normal infants born in the hospital, but do include those for their mothers. Include days of care for infants born in the hospital and transferred into a neonatal care unit. Also include swing bed inpatient days. An inpatient day of care (also commonly referred to as a <u>patient day</u> or a <u>census day</u>, or by some federal hospitals as an <u>occupied bed day</u>) is a period of service between the census-taking hours on two successive calendar days, the day of discharge being counted only when the patient was admitted the same day.

g. **Emergency department visits.** Should reflect the number of visits to the emergency unit. Emergency outpatients can be admitted to the inpatient areas of the hospital, but they are still counted as emergency visits and subsequently as inpatient admissions.

h. **Total outpatient visits.** A visit by a patient who is not lodged in the hospital while receiving medical, dental, or other services. Each appearance of an outpatient in each unit constitutes one visit regardless of the number of diagnostic and/or therapeutic treatments that the patient receives. Total outpatient visits should include all clinic visits, referred visits, observation services, outpatient surgeries (also reported on line E1k), home health service visits, telehealth visits and emergency department visits (also reported on line E1g).

    Clinic visits should reflect total number of visits to each specialized medical unit that is responsible for the diagnosis and treatment of patients on an outpatient, nonemergency basis. (e.g., alcoholism, dental, gynecology.) Visits to the satellite clinics and primary group practices should be included if revenue is received by the hospital.

    Referred visits should reflect total number of outpatient ancillary visits to each specialty unit of the hospital established for providing technical aid used in the diagnosis and treatment of patients. Examples of such units are diagnostic radiology, EKG, and pharmacy.

    Observation services are those services furnished on a hospital's premises, including use of a bed and periodic monitoring by a hospital's nursing or other staff, which are reasonable and necessary to evaluate an outpatient's condition or determine the need for a possible admission to the hospital as an inpatient. Observation services usually do not exceed 24 hours; however, there is no hourly limit on the extent to which they may be used.

    Home health service visits are visits by home health personnel to a patient's residence.

    Telehealth visits are synchronous visits between a patient and provider that are not co-located through the use of two-way, interactive, real-time audio and/or video communication.

i. **Inpatient surgical operations.** Count each patient undergoing surgery as one surgical operation regardless of the number of surgical procedures that were performed while the patient was in the operating or procedure room.

j. **Operating room.** A unit/room of a hospital or other health care facility in which surgical procedures requiring anesthesia are performed.

k. **Outpatient surgical operations.** For outpatient surgical operations, please record operations performed on patients who do not remain in the hospital overnight. Include all operations whether performed in the inpatient operating rooms or in procedure rooms located in an outpatient facility. Include an endoscopy only when used as an operative tool and not when used for diagnosis alone. Count each patient undergoing surgery as one surgical operation regardless of the number of surgical procedures that were performed while the patient was in the operating or procedure room.

2a2. Managed Care Medicare Discharges. A discharge day where a Medicare Managed Care Plan is the source of payment.

2b2. Managed Care Medicare Inpatient Days. An inpatient day where a Medicare Managed Care Plan is the source of payment.

2c2. Managed Care Medicaid Discharges. A discharge day where a Medicaid Managed Care Plan is the source of payment.

2d2. Managed Care Medicaid Inpatient Days. An inpatient day where a Medicaid Managed Care Plan is the source of payment.

3a. Net patient revenue. Reported at the estimated net realizable amounts from patients, third-party payers, and others for services rendered, including estimated retroactive adjustments under reimbursement agreements with third-party payers. Retroactive adjustments are accrued on an estimated basis in the period the related services are rendered and adjusted in future periods, as final settlements are determined.

3b. Tax appropriations. A predetermined amount set aside by the government from its taxing authority to support the operation of the hospital.

3c. Other operating revenue. Revenue that arises from the normal day-to-day operations from services other than health care provided to patients. Includes sales and services to nonpatients, and revenue from miscellaneous sources (rental of hospital space, sale of cafeteria meals, gift shop sales). Also include operating gains in this category.

3d. Nonoperating revenue. Includes investment income, extraordinary gains and other nonoperating gains.

3e. Total revenue. Add net patient revenue, tax appropriations, other operating revenue and nonoperating revenue.

3f. Payroll expenses. Include payroll for all personnel including medical and dental residents/interns and trainees.

3g. Employee benefits. Includes social security, group insurance, retirement benefits, workman's compensation, unemployment insurance, etc.

3h. Depreciation expense (for reporting period only). Report only the depreciation expense applicable to the reporting period. The amount should also be included in accumulated depreciation. (E9b)

3i. Interest expense. Report interest expense for the reporting period only.

3j. Pharmacy expense. Includes the cost of drugs and pharmacy supplies requested to patient care departments and drugs charged to patients.

3k. Supply expense. The net cost of all tangible items that are expensed including freight, standard distribution cost, and sales and use tax minus rebates. This would exclude labor, labor-related expenses and services as well as some tangible items that are frequently provided as part of labor costs.

3l. All other expenses. Any total facility expenses not included in E3f-E3k.

3m. Total expenses. Add 3f-3l. Include all payroll and nonpayroll expenses as well as any nonoperating losses (including extraordinary losses.)
    Treat bad debt as a deduction from gross patient revenue and not as an expense.

4a. Total gross inpatient revenue. The hospital's full-established rates (charges) for all services rendered to inpatients.

4b. Total gross outpatient revenue. The hospital's full-established rates (charges) for all services rendered to outpatients.

4c. Total gross patient revenue. Add total gross inpatient revenue and total gross outpatient revenue.

5. Uncompensated care. Care for which no payment is expected or no charge is made. It is the sum of bad debt and charity care absorbed by a hospital or other health care organization in providing medical care for patients who are uninsured or are unable to pay.

5a. Bad debt. The provision for actual or expected uncollectables resulting from the extension of credit. Report as a deduction from gross revenue. <u>For Question 6 (Revenue by payer), if you cannot break out your bad debt by payer, deduct the amount from self-pay.</u>

5b. Financial Assistance (Includes charity care). Financial assistance and charity care refer to health services provided free of charge or at reduced rates to individuals who meet certain financial criteria. <u>For purposes of this survey, charity care is measured on the basis of revenue forgone, at full-established rates.</u>

5d. Medicaid Provider Tax, Fee or Assessment. Dollars paid as a result of a state law that authorizes collecting revenue from specified categories of providers. Federal matching funds may be received for the revenue collected from providers and some or all of the revenues may be returned directly or indirectly back to providers in the form of a Medicaid payment.

6. REVENUE BY PAYER

6a1. Medicare. Should agree with the Medicare utilization reported in questions E2a1-E2b2.

6a1a. Fee for service patient revenue. Include traditional Medicare fee-for-service.

6a1c. Total. Medicare revenue (add Medicare fee for service patient revenue and Medicare managed care revenue).

6a2. Medicaid. Should agree with Medicaid utilization reported in questions E2c1-E2d2.

6a2a. Fee for service patient revenue. Do not include Medicaid disproportionate share payments (DSH) or other Medicaid supplemental payments.

6a2c. Medicaid Graduate Medical Education (GME) payments. Payments for the cost of approved graduate medical education (GME) programs. <u>Report in 'net' column only.</u>

6a2d. Medicaid disproportionate share payment (DSH). DSH minus associated provider taxes or assessments. <u>Report in 'net' column only.</u>

6a2e. Medicaid supplemental payments. Supplemental payments the Medicaid program pays the hospital that are NOT Medicaid DSH, minus associated provider taxes or assessments. <u>Report in 'net' column only.</u>

6a2f. Other Medicaid. Any Medicaid payments such as delivery system reform incentive program (DSRIP) payments that are not included in lines 6a2a-e. <u>Report in 'net' column only.</u>

6e. Medicaid Intergovernmental Transfers (IGT) or certified public expenditure program. Exchange of public funds between different levels of government (e.g., county, city, or another state agency) to the state Medicaid agency.

7. COVID RELIEF FUNDS. Include all funds received from federal and state government for COVID relief, such as CARES Act Provider Relief Fund payments. Do not include any funds that constitute a loan and may be on the balance sheet as a liability.

8. FINANCIAL PERFORMANCE – MARGIN

8a. Total Margin. Total income over total revenue. Nonoperating income is included in revenue in the total margin.

8b. Operating Margin. Measure of profit per dollar of revenue calculated by dividing net operating income by operating revenues.

8c. EBITDA Margin. Earnings before interest, tax depreciation and amortization (EBITDA) divided by total revenue.

8d. Medicare margin. (Medicare revenue-Medicare expenses)/Medicare revenue.

<u>Medicare revenue</u> = Patient revenue received from the Medicare program including traditional Medicare, Medicare Advantage, and any ACO, Bundled Payment, or other pilot program (net of disallowances)

<u>Medicare expenses</u> = Cost of patient care for Medicare beneficiaries in traditional Medicare, Medicare Advantage and any ACO, bundled payment, or other pilot program. If actual costs cannot be obtained, use cost-to-charge ratios to estimate based on Medicare charges.

8e. Medicaid margin. (Medicaid revenue-Medicaid expenses)/Medicaid revenue.

<u>Medicaid revenue</u> = Patient revenue received from the Medicaid program including traditional Medicaid, Medicaid Managed Care, and any ACO, Bundled Payment, or other pilot program (net of disallowances)

<u>Medicaid expenses</u> = Cost of patient care for Medicaid beneficiaries in traditional Medicaid, Medicaid Managed Care and any ACO, bundled payment, or other pilot program. If actual costs cannot be obtained, use cost-to-charge ratios to estimate based on Medicaid charges.

9. Fixed Assets. Represent land and physical properties that are consumed or used in the creation of economic activity by the health care entity. The historical or acquisition costs are used in recording fixed assets. Net plant, property, and equipment represent the original costs of these items less accumulated depreciation and amortization.

9d. Gross Square Footage. Include all inpatient, outpatient, office, and support space used for or in support of your health care activities. Exclude exterior, roof, and garage space in the figure.

10. Capital Expenses. Expenses used to acquire assets, including buildings, remodeling projects, equipment, or property.

11. Information Technology and Cybersecurity.

b. Number of Internal IT staff (in FTEs). Number of full-time equivalent (FTE) staff employed in the IT department/organization and on the payroll.

c. Cybersecurity. Measures taken to protect against the criminal or unauthorized use of electronic data.

d. Number of internal staff devoted to cybersecurity (in FTEs). FTEs on the organization's payroll devoted to cybersecurity.

e. Number of outsourced staff devoted to cybersecurity (in FTEs). i.e., contracted staff FTEs devoted to cybersecurity.

STAFFING

12. Full-Time Equivalent (FTE) is the total number of hours worked (excluding all non-worked hours such as PTO, etc.) by all employees over the full 12-month reporting period, divided by the normal number of hours worked by a full-time employee for that same time period. For example, if your hospital considers a normal workweek for a full-time employee to be 40 hours, a total of 2,080 would be worked over a full year (52 weeks). If the total number of hours worked by all employees on the payroll is 208,000, then the number of full-time equivalents (FTE) is 100 (employees). The FTE calculation for a specific occupational category such as registered nurses is exactly the same. The calculation for each occupational category should be based on the number of hours worked by staff employed in that specific category.

a.-b. Physicians and dentists. Include only those physicians and dentists engaged in clinical practice and on the payroll. Those who hold administrative positions should be reported in all other personnel. (12n)

e. Other trainees. A trainee is a person who has not completed the necessary requirements for certification or met the qualifications required for full salary under a related occupational category. Exclude medical and dental residents/interns who should be reported on line 12c-d.

f. Registered nurses. Nurses who have graduated from approved schools of nursing and who are currently registered by the state. They are responsible for the nature and quality of all nursing care that patients receive. Do not include any registered nurses more appropriately reported in other occupational categories, such as facility administrators, and therefore listed under all other personnel. (12n)

g. Licensed practical (vocational) nurses. Nurses who have graduated from an approved school of practical (vocational) nursing who work under the supervision of registered nurses and/or physicians.

h. Nursing assistive personnel. Certified nursing assistant or equivalent unlicensed staff who assist registered nurses in providing patient care related services as assigned by and under the supervision of a registered nurse.

i. Radiology technicians. Technical positions in imaging fields, including, but not limited to, radiology, sonography, nuclear medicine, radiation therapy, CT, MRI.

j. **Laboratory technicians.** Professional and technical positions in all areas of the laboratory, including, but not limited to, histology, phlebotomy, microbiology, pathology, chemistry, etc.

k. **Pharmacists, licensed.** Persons licensed within the state who are concerned with the preparation and distribution of medicinal products.

l. **Pharmacy technicians.** Persons who assist the pharmacist with selected activities, including medication profile reviews for drug incompatibilities, typing labels and prescription packaging, handling of purchase records and inventory control.

m. **Respiratory Therapists.** An allied health professional who specializes in scientific knowledge and theory of clinical problems of respiratory care. Duties include the collection and evaluation of patient data to determine an appropriate care plan, selection and assembly of equipment, conduction of therapeutic procedures, and modification of prescribed plans to achieve one or more specific objectives.

n. **All other personnel.** This should include all other personnel not already accounted for in other categories.

o. **Total facility personnel.** Add 12a-12n. Includes the total facility personnel - hospital plus nursing home type unit/facility personnel (for those hospitals that own and operate a nursing home type unit/facility.)

p. q. **Nursing home type unit/facility personnel.** These lines should be filled out only by hospitals that own and operate a nursing home type unit/facility, where only one legal entity is vested with title to the physical property or operates under the authority of a duly executed lease of the physical property. If nursing home type unit/facility personnel are reported on the total facility personnel lines (12a-12n) but cannot be broken out, please leave blank.

r. **Direct patient care RN.** Registered nurses providing care directly to patients. Direct patient care responsibilities are patient-centered nursing activities carried out in the presence of the patient (such as admission, transfer/discharge, patient teaching, patient communication, treatments, counseling, and administration of medication.)

14. **Privileged Physicians.** Report the total number of physicians (by type) on the medical staff with privileges except those with courtesy, honorary and provisional privileges. Do not include residents or interns. Physicians that provide only non-clinical services (administrative services, medical director services, etc.) should be excluded.

Employed by your hospital. Physicians that are either direct hospital employees or employees of a hospital subsidiary corporation.

Individual contract. An independent physician under a formal contract to provide services at your hospital including at outpatient facilities, clinics and offices

Group contract. A physician that is part of a group (group practice, faculty practice plan or medical foundation) under a formal contract to provide services at your hospital including at inpatient and outpatient facilities, clinics and offices.

Not employed or under contract. Other physicians with privileges that have no employment or contractual relationship with the hospital to provide services.

The sum of the physicians reported in 16a-16g should equal the total number of privileged physicians in the hospital.

a. **Primary care.** A physician that provides primary care services including general practice, general internal medicine, family practice, general pediatrics and geriatrics.

b. **Obstetrics/gynecology.** A physician who provides medical and surgical treatment to pregnant women and to mothers following delivery. Also provides diagnostic and therapeutic services to women with diseases or disorders of the reproductive organs.

c. **Emergency medicine.** Physicians who provide care in the emergency department.

d. **Hospitalist.** Physicians whose primary professional focus is the care of hospitalized medical patients (through clinical, education, administrative and research activity).

e. **Intensivist.** A physician with special training to work with critically ill patients. Intensivists generally provided medical-surgical, cardiac, neonatal, pediatric and other types of intensive care.

f. **Radiologist/pathologist/anesthesiologist. Radiologist.** A physician who has specialized training in imaging, including but not limited to radiology, sonography, nuclear medicine, radiation therapy, CT, MRI. **Pathologist.** A physician who examines samples of body tissues for diagnostic purposes. **Anesthesiologist.** A physician who specializes in administering medications or other agents that prevent or relieve pain, especially during surgery.

g. **Other specialist.** Other physicians not included in the above categories that specialize in a specific type of medical care.

17. **Advanced Practice Registered Nurses/Physician Assistants.** Registered nurses with advanced didactic and clinical education, knowledge, skills, and scope of practice. **Physician assistant.** A healthcare professional licensed to practice medicine with supervision of a licensed physician. Includes: **Nurse practitioner.** A registered nurse with at least a master's degree in nursing and advanced education in primary care, capable of independent practice in a variety of settings. **Certified Registered Nurse anesthetist.** An advanced practice registered nurse who is certified to administer anesthesia to patients typically during surgical, diagnostic, or obstetric procedures. **Clinical nurse specialist (CNS).** A registered nurse who, through a formal graduate degree (masters or doctorate) CNS education program, has expertise in a specialty area of nursing practice. CNSs are clinical experts in the diagnosis and treatment of illness, and the delivery of evidence-based nursing interventions.

17c. **Primary care.** Medical services including general practice, general internal medicine, family practice, general pediatrics.

Emergency department care. The provision of unscheduled outpatient services to patients whose conditions require immediate care in the emergency department setting.

Other specialty care. A clinic that provides specialized medical care beyond the scope of primary care.

Patient education. Goals and objectives for the patient and/or family related to therapeutic regimens, medical procedures and self-care.

Case management. A system of assessment, treatment planning, referral and follow-up that ensures the provision of comprehensive and continuous services and the coordination of payment and reimbursement for care.

Other. Any type of care other than those listed above.

18. **Foreign-educated nurses.** Individuals who are foreign born and received basic nursing education in a foreign country. In general many of these nurses come to the US on employment-based visas which allow them to obtain a green card.

SECTION G. SUPPLEMENTAL INFORMATION
DEFINITIONS

1. **Group Purchasing Organization.** An organization whose primary function is to negotiate contracts for the purpose of purchasing for members of the group or has a central supply site for its members.

2. **Distributor.** An entity that typically does not manufacture most of its own products but purchases and re-sells these products. Such a business usually maintains an inventory of products for sales to hospitals and physician offices and others.

4. **Patient and family advisory council.** Advisory council dedicated to the improvement of quality in patient and family care. The advisory council is comprised of past/present patients, family members, and hospital staff.

5. **Utilization of telehealth/virtual care.** The definitions used herein represent one approach to understanding telehealth/virtual care. The AHA is aware that different organizations use different definitions for these terms and that Medicare defines them in a more narrow way than they are being used in the field. The definitions we chose are meant to balance the statutory and regulatory use of the terms with the way they are understood by providers on the ground. Please report only hospital-based services on these lines. Please do not report system-level numbers.

a. **Video visits.** Synchronous visits between patient and provider that are not co-located, through the use of two-way, interactive, real-time audio and video communication.

---

254 AHA Hospital Statistics © 2024 Health Forum LLC, an affiliate of the American Hospital Association

b. **Audio visits.** Synchronous visits between a patient and a provider that are not co-located, through the use of two-way, int audio-only communication.

c. **Remote patient monitoring.** Asynchronous or synchronous interactions between patient and provider that are not co-loca collection, transmission, evaluation, and communication of physiological data.

d. **Other virtual services.** All other synchronous or asynchronous interactions between a provider and patient, or provider ar delivered remotely including messages, eConsults, and virtual check-ins.

6. **6a.Certified Community Behavioral Health Clinics (CCBHCs).** These entities, a new provider type in Medicaid, are designec comprehensive range of mental health and substance use disorder services to vulnerable individuals. In return, CCBHCs receiv Medicaid reimbursement rate based on their anticipated costs of expanding services to meet the needs of these complex popul are non-profit organizations or units of a local government behavioral health authority. They must directly provide (or contract w organizations to provide) nine types of services, with an emphasis on the provision of 24-hour crisis care, evidence-based pract coordination with local primary care and hospital partners, and integration with physical health care.

6b.Community Mental Health Centers: According to the American Psychological Association, a community mental health cer facilities that are community-based and provide mental health services, sometimes as an alternative to the care that mental hos provide. SAMHSA reported that, as of 2019, approximately 2,700 community mental health centers were in operation. They are sources such as county and state funding programs, federal funding through programs such as Medicaid and Medicare, private cash payments. The centers treat both children and adults, including individuals who are chronically mentally ill or have been di inpatient mental health facility.

7. **Decarbonization.** Decarbonization is the key term used to describe phasing out carbon dioxide equivalent emissions, both ope embodied carbon. In the strictest sense, decarbonization means removing carbon from the process chain as well as carbon rele producing building materials.

Net-Zero Emissions. Net-zero is a balance between all emissions produced and the emissions removed from the atmosphere. building that generates as much energy as it uses.